Respiratory Infections

Editor

MICHAEL J. LOEFFELHOLZ

CLINICS IN LABORATORY MEDICINE

www.labmed.theclinics.com

June 2014 • Volume 34 • Number 2

ELSEVIER

1600 John F. Kennedy Boulevard • Suite 1800 • Philadelphia, Pennsylvania, 19103-2899

http://www.theclinics.com

CLINICS IN LABORATORY MEDICINE Volume 34, Number 2
June 2014 ISSN 0272-2712, ISBN-13: 978-0-323-29924-4

Editor: Joanne Husovski
Developmental Editor: Yonah Korngold

Reprints. For copies of 100 or more, of articles in this publication, please contact the Commercial Reprints Department, Elsevier Inc., 360 Park Avenue South, New York, New York 10010-1710. Tel. 212-633-3874, Fax: 212-633-3820, E-mail: reprints@elsevier.com.

Clinics in Laboratory Medicine (ISSN 0272-2712) is published quarterly by Elsevier Inc., 360 Park Avenue South, New York, NY 10010-1710. Months of issue are March, June, September, and December. Business and Editorial offices: 1600 John F. Kennedy Blvd., Suite 1800, Philadelphia, PA 19103-2899. Periodicals postage paid at NewYork, NY and additional mailing offices. Subscription prices are $250.00 per year (US individuals), $419.00 per year (US institutions), $135.00 per year (US students), $305.00 per year (Canadian individuals), $510.00 per year (Canadian institutions), $185.00 per year (Canadian students), $390.00 per year (foreign individuals), $510.00 per year (foreign institutions), $185.00 (foreign students). Foreign air speed delivery is included in all Clinics subscription prices. All prices are subject to change without notice. POSTMASTER: Send address changes to *Clinics in Laboratory Medicine*, Elsevier Health Sciences Division, Subscription Customer Service, 3251 Riverport Lane, Maryland Heights, MO 63043. **Customer Service: 1-800-654-2452 (US). From outside of the US and Canada, call 1-314-447-8871. Fax: 1-314-447-8029. E-mail: journalscustomerservice-usa@elsevier.com (for print support) or journalsonlinesupport-usa@elsevier. com (for online support).**

Clinics in Laboratory Medicine is covered in *EMBASE/Exerpta Medica*, *MEDLINE/PubMed (Index Medicus)*, *Cinahl*, *Current Contents/Clinical Medicine*, *BIOSIS* and *ISI/BIOMED*.

Contributors

EDITOR

MICHAEL J. LOEFFELHOLZ, PhD
Professor, Department of Pathology, University of Texas Medical Branch, Galveston, Texas

AUTHORS

BARBARA D. ALEXANDER, MD, MHS
Division of Infectious Diseases, Department of Medicine, Duke University Medical Center; Clinical Microbiology Laboratory, Department of Pathology, Duke University Medical Center, Durham, North Carolina

ROBERT BELKNAP, MD
Assistant Professor of Medicine, Denver Public Health and University of Colorado School of Medicine, Denver, Colorado

MARC ROGER COUTURIER, PhD, D(ABMM)
ARUP Laboratories, Institute for Clinical and Experimental Pathology; Department of Pathology, University of Utah School of Medicine, Salt Lake City, Utah

CHARLES L. DALEY, MD
Chief, Division of Mycobacterial and Respiratory Infections; Professor of Medicine, National Jewish Health and University of Colorado School of Medicine, Denver, Colorado

GERALD A. DENYS, PhD, D(ABMM)
Visiting Professor of Pathology and Laboratory Medicine and Medical Microbiologist, Division of Clinical Microbiology, Department of Pathology and Laboratory Medicine, Indiana University School of Medicine, Indianapolis, Indiana

EDWARD P. DESMOND, PhD
Chief of Mycobacteriology and Mycology Section, Microbial Diseases Laboratory, California Department of Public Health, Richmond, California

JAMES J. DUNN, PhD, DABMM
Department of Pathology and Laboratory Medicine, Cook Children's Medical Center, Fort Worth, Texas

PETER H. GILLIGAN, PhD, DABMM, FAAM
Professor, Pathology-Laboratory Medicine and Microbiology-Immunology, Director, Clinical Microbiology-Immunology Laboratories, UNC Health Care, UNC Hospitals, UNC School Medicine, Chapel Hill, North Carolina

ERIN H. GRAF, PhD
Department of Pathology, University of Utah School of Medicine, Salt Lake City, Utah

ALLEN T. GRIFFIN, MD
Department of Pathology, University of Utah School of Medicine, Salt Lake City, Utah

KEVIN C. HAZEN, PhD, D(ABMM), FAAM, FIDSA
Director of Clinical Microbiology, Professor of Pathology, Duke University Health System, Durham, North Carolina

FRÉDÉRIC LAMOTH, MD
Division of Infectious Diseases, Department of Medicine, Duke University Medical Center; Clinical Microbiology Laboratory, Department of Pathology, Duke University Medical Center, Durham, North Carolina; Infectious Diseases Service and Institute of Microbiology, Lausanne University Hospital, Lausanne, Switzerland

MARIE L. LANDRY, MD
Professor, Departments of Laboratory Medicine and Internal Medicine, Yale University School of Medicine, New Haven, Connecticut

JENNIFER LAPLANTE, BS
Research Scientist, Laboratory of Viral Diseases, Wadsworth Center, New York State Department of Health, Albany, New York

AMY L. LEBER, PhD, D(ABMM)
Assistant Professor of Pediatrics and Pathology, Department of Laboratory Medicine, Nationwide Children's Hospital, The Ohio State University College of Medicine, Columbus, Ohio

SHOU-YEAN GRACE LIN, MS
Research Scientist, Microbial Diseases Laboratory, California Department of Public Health, Richmond, California

MELISSA B. MILLER, PhD, DABMM
Associate Professor, Department of Pathology and Laboratory Medicine, University of North Carolina School of Medicine, Chapel Hill, North Carolina

DAVID R. PEAPER, MD, PhD
Assistant Professor of Laboratory Medicine, Department of Laboratory Medicine, Yale University School of Medicine, New Haven; Section of Pathology and Laboratory Medicine, VA Connecticut Healthcare System, West Haven, Connecticut

RYAN F. RELICH, PhD, MLS(ASCP)^{CM}
Visiting Assistant Professor of Pathology and Laboratory Medicine and Medical Microbiologist, Division of Clinical Microbiology, Department of Pathology and Laboratory Medicine, Indiana University School of Medicine, Indianapolis, Indiana

MAX SALFINGER, MD
Laboratory Director, Mycobacteriology and Pharmacokinetics, Department of Medicine, National Jewish Health, Denver, Colorado

AKOS SOMOSKOVI, MD, PhD, DSc
Chief, Mycobacteriology Laboratory, Institute of Medical Microbiology, Swiss National Reference Center for Mycobacteria, University of Zurich, Zurich, Switzerland

KIRSTEN St. GEORGE, MAppSc, PhD
Chief, Laboratory of Viral Diseases, Wadsworth Center, New York State Department of Health, Albany, New York

Contents

> Survival has improved in patients with cystic fibrosis (CF), in part because of aggressive antimicrobial management. Two multidrug-resistant environmental bacteria, the *Burkholderia cepacia* group and nontuberculous mycobacteria, have emerged. Improving genomic and proteomic technologies are allowing better identification of bacteria and fungi found in the CF lung and detection of viral agents that may be associated with pulmonary exacerbations. Anaerobic bacteria and *Streptococcus angionsus* group organisms may play a role in chronic CF lung infections. The diversity of organisms declines perhaps as a result of aggressive antimicrobial therapy, and an apex predator, *Pseudomonas aeruginosa*, may emerge in many patients with CF.

> Urinary antigen testing has grown in popularity for several significant respiratory infections, particularly *Legionella pneumophila*, *Streptococcus pneumoniae*, and *Histoplasma capsulatum*. By capitalizing on the concentration of shed antigen from a variety of pathogens in the kidneys for excretion in the urine, urinary antigen testing can be used to obtain rapid test results related to respiratory infection, independent of an invasive collection such as a bronchoalveolar lavage. This article describes the 3 aforementioned organisms, their role in respiratory disease, and the current status of urinary antigen testing in their respective diagnosis.

> Pertussis is increasing due to multiple factors including increasing awareness by clinicians, decreased effectiveness of vaccines, and improved testing. While *Bordetella pertussis* is the causative agent of pertussis other *Bordetella* species such as *B. parapertussis*, and *B. holmesii*, have been associated with pertussis-like illness. Laboratory diagnosis is made using various tests with molecular methods supplanting culture due to increased sensitivity. Serology is useful but standardized methods that are needed. The targets used for molecular detection are varied and have differing sensitivities and specificities. Laboratorians must consider if differentiation of various *Bordetella* species is necessary when choosing an amplified testing approach.

other microbiological and radiologic tools in preemptive antifungal strategies.

Robert Belknap and Charles L. Daley

Diagnosis of latent tuberculosis infection (LTBI) should be targeted toward individuals and groups with high risk of progression to active tuberculosis (TB). Low-risk populations should not be screened. Interferon-gamma release assays (IGRAs) perform as well or better than the tuberculin skin test in most targeted populations. IGRAs are preferred for bacille Calmette-Guérin (BCG)-vaccinated populations. A positive IGRA in a person at low risk for TB exposure should be confirmed with a repeat test or another method before recommending LTBI treatment. The choice of which IGRA to use is generally based on the costs and feasibility of performing the test.

Kevin C. Hazen

Fungal infection of the respiratory tract can take several forms, the most common of which is pneumonia. Fungal infection can occur in the immunocompetent typically as a result of inhalation of a large inoculum of fungal elements. However, the number of etiologic agents attacking immunocompetent individuals and causing significant infection is limited. Molecular assays are a potential additional and sensitive weapon that can be added to the diagnostic arsenal used by physicians to determine whether a fungus is definitively, probably, or possibly causing infection in a patient.

David R. Peaper and Marie L. Landry

Much effort has been expended developing testing modalities for influenza viruses that are capable of providing rapid results to clinicians. Antigen-detection techniques, historically the only methods able to deliver results quickly, are still widely used despite concerns about sensitivity. Recently, nucleic acid amplification tests (NAATs), which can achieve rapid turnaround times and high sensitivity, have become available. In addition, NAATs can detect other respiratory pathogens. Although there are many theoretical advantages to rapid influenza testing, the clinical impact of testing in various patient populations must be considered against the cost and the analytical performance of the tests.

Jennifer Laplante and Kirsten St. George

Influenza continues to be a significant health care issue. Although vaccination is the major line of defense, antiviral drugs play an important role in prophylaxis and disease management. Approved drugs for influenza are currently limited to those that target the viral matrix protein or neuraminidase enzyme. Resistance-associated sequence changes in the genes encoding these proteins have been extensively studied. Available methods for genotypic and phenotypic antiviral susceptibility testing have expanded and are being further developed and improved. The sporadic emergence of drug-resistant variants and the global spread of resistant strains have demonstrated the ongoing need for vigilant testing and surveillance.

Non-influenza respiratory virus infections are common worldwide and contribute to morbidity and mortality in all age groups. The recently identified Middle East respiratory syndrome coronavirus has been associated with rapidly progressive pneumonia and high mortality rate. Adenovirus 14 has been increasingly recognized in severe acute respiratory illness in both military and civilian individuals. Rhinovirus C and human bocavirus type 1 have been commonly detected in infants and young children with respiratory tract infection and studies have shown a positive correlation between respiratory illness and high viral loads, mono-infection, viremia, and/or serologically-confirmed primary infection.

CLINICS IN LABORATORY MEDICINE

RELATED INTEREST

Clinics in Chest Medicine March 2013 (Vol. 34, No. 1)
Pleural Disease
Jonathan Puchalski, *Editor*
Available at: http://www.chestmed.theclinics.com/

NOW AVAILABLE FOR YOUR iPhone and iPad

CLINICS IN LABORATORY MEDICINE

Preface

Respiratory Infections

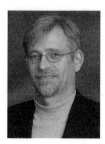

Michael J. Loeffelholz, PhD
Editor

Infections of the respiratory tract include both acute and chronic processes, ranging from the common cold to tuberculosis. Acute respiratory infections are responsible for an estimated 4 million deaths annually worldwide and are the leading cause of death in children younger than 5 years. Over 1 million people in the United States are hospitalized each year with pneumonia. *Mycobacterium tuberculosis* infects one-third of the world's population. There are more than 1 million tuberculosis-related deaths worldwide each year. Emerging resistance to multiple available antimicrobial agents has hampered the ability to treat tuberculosis and hospital-acquired respiratory infections. Laboratory diagnosis is an important part of the management and treatment of patients with respiratory infections.

In addition to appraising current microbiology and epidemiology, this issue provides a comprehensive review of the most current and relevant issues in the laboratory diagnosis of respiratory infections, including pertussis, tuberculosis, and influenza, as well as the detection of nontuberculous mycobacteria, fungi, emerging respiratory viruses, and agents affecting cystic fibrosis patients. Antigen tests, interferon gamma release assays, and molecular methods used to diagnose various respiratory infections are reviewed. Finally, the challenge of emerging resistance to antimicrobial and antiviral agents and its detection in the laboratory is reviewed.

I'd like to thank Alexander McAdam, MD, PhD for enlightening discussion and his contributions to the development of the article content. I'd also like to thank the Elsevier staff, particularly, Yonah Korngold and Joanne Husovski.

Michael J. Loeffelholz, PhD
Professor
Department of Pathology
University of Texas Medical Branch
Galveston, Texas 77555-0740, USA

E-mail address:
mjloeffe@UTMB.EDU

Clin Lab Med 34 (2014) xi
http://dx.doi.org/10.1016/j.cll.2014.03.002
0272-2712/14/$ – see front matter © 2014 Elsevier Inc. All rights reserved.

ns in Patients with
ibrosis

Microbiology Update

hD, DABMM

fibrosis • Diagnostic microbiology • Update

e most important genetic disease in Caucasians. Patients with this dis-
ely primarily as a result of chronic lung infection. *Staphylococcus aureus*
omonas aeruginosa continue to be the key pulmonary pathogens.

oved in patients with CF in part because of aggressive antimicrobial
unintended consequence of this therapy has been the emergence of
nt environmental bacteria: the *Burkholderia cepacia* group and nontu-
cteria.

cepacia, a species within the *Burkholderia cepacia* complex, is associ-
tality and is a contraindication for lung transplantation. The key nontu-
cterial pathogen, *Mycobacterium abscessus*, is not so virulent and is
intation contraindication. Both present an infection control challenge,
be spread from person to person.

c and proteomic technologies are allowing better identification of bac-
ad in the CF lung and to detect viral agents that may be associated with
oations. Chronic rhinovirus infections are of particular interest.

s have identified 2 groups of bacteria that may play a role in chronic CF
aerobic bacteria and *Streptococcus angionsus* group organisms. Mi-
lso show that as the diversity of organisms decline, perhaps as a result
microbial therapy, an apex predator, etc., *Pseudomonas aeruginosa*,
ny patients with CF.

DEMIOLOGY, AND CLINICAL PRESENTATION

is the most common autosomal-recessive genetic disease that
anic Caucasians populations, although other racial groups may
well.[1] Affected individuals have mutation in the CF transmembrane

ce gene (CFTR), a membrane protein involved in sodium and chloride trans-
thelial cells.[2] The resulting dysregulation in electrolyte transport leads to
n airway surface liquid on bronchial epithelial cell surfaces. As a result, pa-
CF have thick, dry, tenacious mucus, which impairs mucociliary clearance
tes, especially bacteria and fungal conidia, from the airways. This environ-
al for the growth of a limited number of organisms, primarily those that thrive
nvironments such as water. This thickened mucus provides an ideal niche for
shment of chronic infection. It is this chronic infection that results in the pre-
ath that in seen in CF.[3]

n 1800 CFTR mutations have been associated with CF.[4] The most common
F508del, which is found in ~85% of people in the United States; approx-
% are homozygous for this mutated gene.[4] Further carrier rate for mutated
es is estimated to range from 1/25 for non-Hispanic Caucasians to 1/61
Americans to 1/94 for Asian Americans.[1] CF is seen most frequently in North
lorthern Europe, Australia, New Zealand, Brazil, and Argentina. It is esti-
1 in 3500 live births result in clinical disease.[4]

y life expectancy in US patients with CF is approximately 38 years, signifi-
than that of the general population.[4] Cardiopulmonary failure secondary to
g disease is responsible for 85% of premature deaths in CF. The airways of
th CF become infected in infancy. This situation begins periods of chronic
d lung inflammation with accompanying cough, which is a lifelong reality in
th CF. A hallmark of chronic infection and airway inflammation is periods of
exacerbations. Pulmonary exacerbations are characterized by worsening
, including increased cough and sputum production, hemoptysis, shortness
increased respiratory rate, loss of appetite, weight loss, increased neutro-
s, and declining pulmonary function.[5] The events that trigger these pulmo-
rbations are not clearly understood, although viral infections and perhaps
n the microbiome may be important.[6,7] Exacerbations are characterized
cruitment of neutrophils, cytokine release, and high level of neutrophil-
astases in the bronchi and bronchioles, causing significant lung disease.[8]
ial therapy has been shown to be effective in treating exacerbations symp-
.[9] However, over time, lung function deteriorates and becomes so low, that
ger compatible with life (**Fig. 1**). Only lung transplantation can successfully
s disease course.[8]

FEV₁ Normal/Mild (greater than or equal to 70% predicted)
FEV₁ Moderate (40% to 69% predicted)
FEV₁ Severe (less than 40% predicted)

**IAGNOSTIC CONSIDERATIONS, AND SUSCEPTIBILITY TESTING OF
NIC INFECTION**

cades, our understanding of the complex nature of chronic lung in-
y expanded. Over the past 3 decades, there has been more than a
ectancy in the population with CF.[4] Three factors have been central
nt:

antimicrobial therapy and treatment strategies, with early eradica-
ionas aeruginosa being a key strategy
airway clearance techniques
n infection control techniques to prevent the spread of organisms
i patients with CF, especially Burkholderia cenocepacia[2,9]

broader-spectrum antimicrobials, we are seeing a plethora of
sistant bacteria and fungi in the CF airways. Our understanding
e organisms in chronic infection and inflammation is poorly delin-
the past decades, new technologies (**Fig. 2**) have been developed
understanding. These technologies include nucleic acid amplifica-
AATs) for direct organism detection, including multiplex NAAT for
DNA sequence analysis for organism identification; molecularly
iic techniques, including pulsed field gel electrophoresis (PFGE),
ce type, whole genome sequencing; and matrix-assisted laser
on–time of flight mass spectroscopy (MALDI-TOF MS).
t exciting development in the application of new technologies is the
ncing technique to study the CF microbiome.[5,10–13] These studies
ir new understanding of the disease process, with accompanying
t strategies.

AUREUS

obial era, few children with CF survived past the age of 2 years. The
rily from failure to thrive, coupled with bacterial pneumonia. The or-
e lungs at autopsy in these children was almost always *Staphylo-*
With the advent of antistaphylococcal antimicrobial therapy,
v S aureus decreased substantially, but it continues to be the pre-
ogen from birth to adolescence, with 80% of children infected in
ce and early adolescence.[4] Improvements in antistaphylococcal
v the use of oral agents such as oral cephalosporins and
nethoxazole (TMP-SMX), are likely to have contributed to the
ctancy seen in patients with CF.[3,15] However this effective antista-
y is not without its costs.
ial resistance issues have arisen, which must be considered in the
i CF. First, the use of oral TMP-SMX has been associated with the
colony variants (SCV) of S aureus.[16–18] The resistance mechanism

potential of commonly recovered organisms from chronic CF airway infections or exacerbations

monas aeruginosa

ococcus aureus

icillin resistant

l colony variant

lderia multivorans

lderia cenocepacia

lderia dolosa

illus spp

orium spp

acterium abscessus

za virus

tory syncytial virus

kely

philus influenzae

acterium avium complex

bic bacteria especially Prevotella spp

coccus anginosus group

tory viruses other than influenza virus and respiratory syncytial virus

ia spp

aea spp

members of the Burkholderia cepacia complex

us spp

ooron spp

ophomonas maltophilia

obacter spp

ia spp

lderia gladioli

coccus pneumoniae

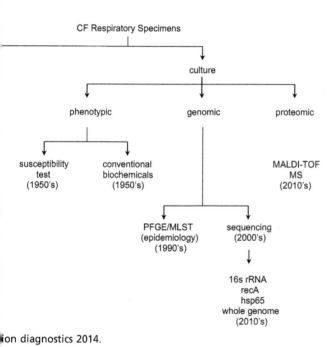

CF Respiratory Specimens

culture

phenotypic   genomic   proteomic

susceptibility test (1950's)   conventional biochemicals (1950's)   MALDI-TOF MS (2010's)

PFGE/MLST (epidemiology) (1990's)   sequencing (2000's)

16s rRNA
recA
hsp65
whole genome
(2010's)

ion diagnostics 2014.

higher mortality than those patients with CF without this organ-
SA isolates can be divided into 2 molecular types based on staph-
mal cassette (SCC) *mecA* type and whether they have the gene
e leukocidin (*pvl*). Approximately 70% are SCC*mecA* type II *pvl*
re SCC*mecA* type IV *pvl* positive; the other 13% are SCC*mecA*
[20] SCC*mecA* type IV, *pvl* positive MRSA isolates are also referred
quired (CA)-MRSA strains. Initial studies of respiratory infections
used by CA-MRSA suggested that this organism caused severe,

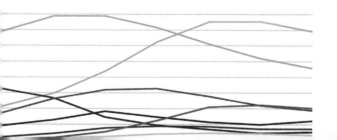

pneumonia, with significant morbidity and mortality in excess of 50% in
s.[22] We were concerned that this organism would be a problem in patients
well. In a survey performed between 2005 and 2007, we found that approx-
of patients with CF in our institution had CA-MRSA recovered from their
specimen and that approximately 1% of patients in our center were chron-
ted. Further, no episodes of necrotizing pneumonia were seen in our pop-
atients with CF during that period.[23]
d antimicrobial resistance issue we have observed is vancomycin-
te S aureus (VISA). The mechanism of resistance is believed to be a thick-
vall, which prevents vancomycin from reaching the site of peptidoglycan
[24] We have screened S aureus isolates for the VISA phenotype (a vancomy-
m inhibitory concentration [MIC] of 4–8 μg/mL) for the past 5 years by the
comycin E-test or the Vitek 2 susceptibility testing (Biomerieux, Durham,
ave tested in excess of 1500 isolates from more than 700 patients with
M and Gilligan P, 2013, unpublished data). We have found VISA in only 1 pa-
atient had been chronically infected with MRSA for more than 10 years and
ed repeated courses of vancomycin. Over time, her pulmonary function
Vith the emergence of VISA, she was treated with multiple courses of line-
eftaroline. Neither was successful in eradicating the organism. Because of
ung function, she received a double lung transplant. On her most recent
opy culture 9 months after transplant, she had positive S aureus infection
e organism was both vancomycin and oxacillin susceptible, but the VISA
not been recovered from multiple bronchoscopy specimens obtained dur-
ttransplant period (Miller M and Gilligan P, 2013, unpublished data).
ory detection and identification of S aureus from patients with CF is straight-
ecause these patients often are infected with other organisms, especially
eruginosa, selective media for the recovery should be used.[25] Two media,
alts agar (**Fig. 4**) and chromogenic S aureus agar, are effective in the recov-
/ and wild-type strains.[16,26] SCV S aureus have typical morphology on
alts agar, whereas on chromogenic media, these organisms may grow

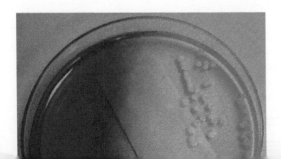

ot give typical phenotypic reactions.[16,26] Organism identification is
ch catalase and latex agglutination or coagulase testing being highly
-TOF MS works well for identification of S aureus from patients with
ility to speciate SCV has not been reported.[28] Susceptibility testing
except for the detection of VISA strains. For those isolates, the most
s an MIC-based method. Because E-test MICs tend to run higher
ional agar or broth dilution methods, all S aureus isolates with a
f 4 μg/mL or greater should be confirmed by a conventional MIC

ERUGINOSA

n chronic lung disease is an unusual morphotype of P aeruginosa,
oid. The organism is typically obtained from the patient's environ-
ient-to-patient spread of virulent clones does occur.[30] The patho-
nosa is dependent on the transition of the organism from a motile,
d organism to a nonmotile, comparatively avirulent, mucoid organ-
apted to living in the CF airways. The transition is believed to be
is that inactivate the mucA gene, which regulates alginate produc-
ucing organisms grow in a biofilm within the mucous layer in bron-
ng. These organisms may be observed as microcolonies when the
served microscopically.[31] On agar plates, these organisms appear
(Fig. 5). In the lung, these organisms are resistant to mechanical
ytosis, and antimicrobial therapy.[3,31] Although they are compara-
y induce a chronic inflammatory response, which is believed to
he lung damage that results in the patient's demise.[31] This disease
e over a period of years to decades.
tes, 60% to 75% of adults are infected with this organism.[4] The
n remain free of chronic infection with P aeruginosa, the longer
is. A highly aggressively antimicrobial therapeutic approach, first
tients with CF, for eradicating early infection with P aeruginosa
o lengthen the time that patients with CF remain P aeruginosa
anish patients with CF have perhaps the longest life expectancy
ons in the world, at 42 years.[9]

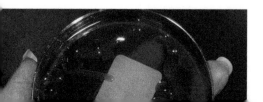

y diagnosis of infections with this organism is easily accomplished. It is
vered on both nonselective agar (chocolate) or selective agar (MacCon-
ve agar specific for P aeruginosa is not required. In addition, identification
complished. The organism is oxidase positive, mucoid, and produces
erdin) or blue-green (pyocyanin) pigments. These characteristics identify
% of CF isolates.[25] MALDI-TOF MS has been shown to accurately identify
d and nonmucoid strains of P aeruginosa.[28,32]

ility testing of P aeruginosa from patients with CF can be challenging. Anti-
usceptibility results using automated susceptibility systems correlate
reference methods and are not recommended. Rather, disk diffusion or
recommended.[33] Paradoxically, it is unlikely that conventional susceptibil-
ccurately predicts in vivo response.[34] The reasons for this situation are
t can be explained in part by comparing susceptibility of P aeruginosa
robials when the organism is grown in a conventional manner or planktoni-
a biofilm mode of growth. When P aeruginosa is grown as a biofilm, it is 8
more resistant to all classes of β-lactams than when it is grown planktoni-
. difference can be explained in part by reduced growth rates of mucoid
d by the possibility that these antimicrobials cannot penetrate to the cell
alginate layer. There is little difference between the MICs for aminoglcyo-
oroquinolones grown under these 2 conditions.[35] Further complicating
n of these results is a growing body of literature that suggests that P aer-
y grow under anaerobic conditions behind mucous plugs or in the thick-
s of the airway.[36] Tobramycin is not active under anaerobic conditions,
poor transport into bacteria. Aerosolized tobramycin therapy, a key strat-
eradication of P aeruginosa,[9,31] may act only against organisms in the
are growing in the superficial layer of mucus. Chronic P aeruginosa infec-
established only when the organism is growing as a biofilm in the anoxic
e mucous layer. Further complexity in susceptibility testing is caused by
ead use of aerosolized antimicrobials, tobramycin, colistin, and aztreo-
to prevent the establishment of chronic P aeruginosa or to suppress the
aeruginosa in those patients chronically infected.[37] Because antimicrobial
ty is based on achievable serum drug concentrations, susceptibility testing
curately predict resistance in patients receiving aerosolized antimicrobials,
airway levels at least 10 to 25 times greater than serum levels.

2 additional problems that confront laboratorians when determining anti-
usceptibility of P aeruginosa. Technically, susceptibility testing of mucoid P
is poorly reproducible and operator dependent.[38] In the late stages of
eruginosa infection, after many rounds of intravenous and aerosolized anti-
erapy, the organism may become resistant to all classes of antimicrobial.[34]
e strategies was to perform multicombinational bactericidal testing
n this method, 2-drug, 3-drug, and 4-drug combinations at serum achiev-
ntrations are placed in a microtiter well, inoculated with a bacteria, incu-
night and then subcultured to determine which combinations were

BURKHOLDERIA CEPACIA COMPLEX AND RELATED ORGANISMS

In the early 1980s, a significant new pathogen, then called *Pseudomonas cepacia*, was recognized in lung infections in patients with CF cared for at 3 different major CF centers.[41–43] In approximately 20% of patients with CF, the organism caused a fatal illness called the cepacia syndrome. In this syndrome, the patients had respiratory infections, with hallmarks of rapid decline in pulmonary function and frequent bacteremia, a highly unusual finding in patients with CF.[41,42] Subsequently, *P cepacia* was reclassified as belonging to the genus *Burkholderia*.[44] Vandamme and colleagues[45] showed that the organisms identified as *Burkholderia cepacia* represented multiple species of bacteria, which they called genomovars. The *B cepacia* complex is now recognized to consistent of 18 different species.[46,47] The species within this complex that is believed to be primarily responsible for the cepacia syndrome is *B cenocepacia*, although both *B multivorans* and *B dolosa* have also been associated with it.[46] *B cenocepacia* or *B multivorans* are recovered from 80% of the *B cepacia* complex infections seen in patients with CF.[46] The molecular epidemiology of *B cenocepacia* is reasonably well understood. Three different *B cenocepacia* clones, designated ET12,[42] PHDC,[43] and Midwest,[44] were associated with the initial description of *B cepacia* as a pathogen in patients with CF.[46] All 3 of these clones can be spread from person to person, although many patients have unique clones, which they likely acquired from their environment.[48] It has been shown that the ET-12 strain has been spread from Toronto to Europe and that it is the predominant strain in Canada.[46,49] The organism has an unusual appendage called a cable pilin, which is believed to be responsible for its high transmissibility.[50]

Because *B cepacia* and *B multivorans* were associated with accelerated lung function decline and high mortality and were often panresistant to antimicrobials, lung transplantation was believed to be a life-saving therapy in those patients. Early molecular epidemiology studies using PFGE showed that patients infected with *B cepacia* complex after transplant had the same highly antimicrobial-resistant strain of *B cepacia* complex before transplant.[51] It was subsequently observed that patients with CF chronically infected with *B cenocepacia* who received lung transplant had a higher mortality at years 1, 3, and 5 years after transplant than those who were infected with other bacteria.[52,53] Early in the posttransplant period, some patients infected with *B cenocepacia* had a sepsis with positive blood cultures. Some of the transplants were further complicated by wound dehiscence. Posttransplant patients with *B cenocepacia* sepsis had a grim prognosis, with few survivors. Bronchiolitis obliterans was an additional problem seen in this patient population.[52] Other studies also showed increased risk of death after transplant in patients with CF infected before transplant with *B cenocepacia*.[53,54] As result, most centers no longer transplant patients with CF who are infected with *B cenocepacia*.

One of the difficulties in recovering *B cepacia* from respiratory specimens of patients with CF is that the organism grows slowly compared with mucoid *P aeruginosa*. Consequently, the growth of *B cepacia* may be obscured on most media. Three different groups developed isolation media for the recovery of *B cepacia* complex organism. *B cepacia* selective agar (BCSA)[55] was superior for *B cepacia* recovery compared with *P cepacia* agar[56] and oxidation-fermentation polymyxin-bacitracin-lactose agar.[57] All 3 media contain polymixin as a selective agent. Not only were *B cepacia* complex organisms isolated on these media from CF respiratory specimens but also a large group of environmental glucose nonfermenters, which were similar to *B cepacia*, were also recovered. These organisms were often phenotypically difficult to separate from *B cepacia* using commercially available kits, resulting in misidentification of non-*B cepacia* isolates as *B cepacia* complex ones.[58,59] Alternatively, some isolates were relatively inert biochemically, making them difficult to identify using commercially available phenotypic methods.[58,59]

Misidentification of non-*B cepacia* organisms as *B cepacia* has grim consequences for the patient with CF. In addition to no longer being candidates for lung transplantation in most centers, the patients are completely segregated from other children and adults with CF. They are likely to have a different clinic day, must always be on isolation when hospitalized, meaning no trips to the playroom to interact with other children, may no longer attend any CF sponsored social function or meetings, or participate in camps with other patients with CF.[60] The result is social isolation for these individuals and potential exclusion from a life-saving therapy. These draconian measures have been successful in blunting the spread of this organism among patients with CF.[60] Perhaps just as importantly, misidentifying *B cepacia* complex organism as some other species or genera results in failure to isolate patients with a potentially deadly organism, which can be spread to both patients with CF and those who do not have CF.[49,61]

Burkholderia gladioli was the first organism recovered on *B cepacia*–selective media and recognized to be misidentified as *B cepacia* using phenotypic means.[59,62] By the early part of this century, it was recognized that 16s ribosomal RNA (rRNA) sequencing was superior to phenotypic methods for differentiating *B cepacia* complex organisms from other genera growing on *B cepacia*–selective media such as *B gladioli*.[63] Our experience with 16s rRNA sequencing over the past 6 years is shown in **Table 1**. With the exception of the unusual *P aeruginosa* phenotypes identified by sequencing, the rest of the organisms identified were recovered on BCSA, the *B cepacia* selective medium that we use. Many more non-*B cepacia* complex organisms requiring identification grow on BCSA. Almost all the organisms listed in **Table 1** are recovered primarily from patients with CF. Most of them, including *Ralstonia*, *Chyseobacterium*, *Inquilinus*, and *Pandoraea*, are infrequently recovered and are believed to be of limited clinical importance. One group is reported in our laboratory as gram-negative rods,

Table 1
Organisms identified by 16S rRNA sequencing from patients with CF at UNC Hospitals from Jan 2008 to Nov 2013

Achromobacter	67
Burkholderia cepacia complex[a]	64
Burkholderia gladioli	63
Chryseobacterium	38
Gram-negative rods not *Burkholderia cepacia* complex, *Ralstonia* or *Pandoraea*[b]	35
Ralstonia spp	32
Pandoraea	12
Pseudomonas aeruginosa	10
Pseudomonas not *aeruginosa*	10
Acinetobacter spp	4
Inquilinus	2

[a] Isolates speciated by recA sequencing at *Burkholderia cepacia* Reference Laboratory and Repository, University of Michigan.
[b] Includes isolates of *Bordetella bronchiseptica*, *Comamonas*, *Herbaspirillium*, *Elizabethkingia*, and *Cupriavidus*.

not *Burkholderia*, *Ralstonia*, or *Pandoraea*. Included in this group are *Bordetella* spp, including *Bordetella broncoseptica*, *Comamonas*, *Herbaspirillium*, *Elizabethkingia*, and *Cupriavidus*. These organisms have not been associated with pulmonary exacerbation in patients with CF.

Although there are few published data suggesting a role for *B gladioli* in patients with CF,[64] the exception seems to be in lung transplant recipients, who have decreased survival compared with those transplant recipients who do not have *Burkholderia*.[53]

Both *Stenotrophomonas* and *Achromobacter* spp are recovered with frequency in patients with CF, especially older patients who have received many rounds of antipseudomonal antimicrobials. These species are the subject of the next section of this article.

One of the problems with 16s rRNA sequence identification is that it cannot accurately differentiate the members of the *B cepacia* complex. Because there seem to be differences in virulence among the different species within the complex, accurate speciation is important.[46] Three species are recognized as being pathogenic in patients with CF and being able to be spread from person to person: *B cenocepacia*, *B multivorans*, and *B dolosa*.[46] Other species seen with some degree of frequency in our patient population include *B vietnamiensis* and *B cepacia*. In our experience, the other 13 species within the complex are rarely if ever isolated. Accurate speciation of isolates of the *B cepacia* complex can be accomplished by sequencing of the *recA* gene.[65]

The requirement to use 2 sequencing steps to accurately identify isolates belonging to the *B cepacia* complex is time consuming and expensive, requiring days to obtain an accurate answer. As a result, alternative identification methods have been sought. The most promising of these is MALDI-TOF MS. We[66] and others[28,65,67] have shown that MALDI-TOF accurately identifies organisms to the *B cepacia* complex and can differentiate them readily from other genera of organisms that grow on BCSA, most importantly *B gladioli*. Preliminary studies suggest that the Bruker system more accurately identifies *B cenocepacia* isolates than the Vitek system.[65,67] Both systems accurately speciate *B multivorans* and *B vietnamiensis*. The Bruker system misidentifies *B contaminans* primarily as *B cepacia* but may also misidentify it as *B cenocepacia* or *B multivorans*. With database improvements, it is likely that the 2 major CF pathogens, *B cenocepacia* and *B multivorans*, will be accurately identified by both systems.

B cepacia complex is one of the most antimicrobial-resistant group of organisms. These organisms are intrinsically resistant to both colistin and aminoglycosides.[68] Clinical and Laboratory Standards Institute susceptibility breakpoints exist for ceftazidime, ticarcillin-clavulanic acid, TMP-SMX, meropenem. minocycline, and fluoroquinolones.[69] Although a large percentage of isolates may be initially susceptible to these agents, resistance develops over time, and many strains become resistant to all these antimicrobial agents.[68] Further complicating treatment is the lack of evidence that any specific antimicrobial treatment regimen is effective in treating *B cepacia* complex pulmonary exacerbations.[70]

STENOTROPHOMONAS AND ACHROMOBACTER

Both *Stenotrophomonas* and *Achromobacter* are glucose nonfermenting rods, which are found more frequently in patients with CF than are *B cepacia* complex organisms. *Stenotrophomonas* is found in approximately 10% to 20% of patients with CF, whereas *Achromobacter* is found in between 5% and 10%.[4] The incidence of these organisms increases with age and likely reflects patients who have had multiple rounds of antipseudomonal antimicrobial therapy.

The clinical significance of both of these organisms has been debated. One study suggested that patients who had precipitating antibodies to *Achromobacter* antigens have a more rapid decline in lung function.[71] Other studies do not support the notion that *Achromobacter* is pathogenic.[72,73] The story is similar with *Stenotrophmonas*. Patients may be more likely to have poor pulmonary function and may require lung transplantation. What is not clear is whether this organism represents a marker of severe lung disease or is the cause of this disease.[74,75]

Three different approaches have been used to identify these 2 organism: conventional phenotypic methods, 16s rRNA sequencing, and MALDI-TOF MS. Phenotypic methods work reasonably well for these organisms, although we have greater confidence in the use of the VITEK 2 for *Stenotrophomonas maltophilia* compared with *Achromobacter* spp.[76] MADLI-TOF MS accurately identifies both species.[66,67]

Both organisms are resistant to aminoglycosides and may develop resistance to colistin.[77] In addition, *Stenotrophomonas* produces a metallo-β-lactamase, which confers resistance to carbapenems.[78] The organism may be initially susceptible to levofloxacin and TMP-SMX but can develop resistance over time.[78] The initial susceptibility of *Achromobacter* is similar to that of *B cepacia* complex, with susceptibility to ceftazidime, meropenem, fluoroquinolones, and TMP-SMX being common.[79] However, drug resistance can develop over time and panresistant organisms can be seen.[80]

MYCOBACTERIUM

Over the past 25 years, mycobacteria are being recognized as an increasingly important agent of chronic lung infection in patients with CF.[81] Although we have been culturing patients with CF for *Mycobacterium* for more than 25 years in our institution, we have never recovered *Mycobacterium tuberculosis* from them.[82] The mycobacterial species most frequently associated with these infections are the nontuberculous mycobacteria, *M avium* complex and *M abscessus* complex.[82,83] There is an increasing body of evidence that both *M avium* complex and *M abscessus* complex can cause chronic infection in patients with CF and may be responsible for decline in pulmonary function, although it is not as dramatic as *B cepacia* or *P aeruginosa*.[81,84,85] In addition, the patient population infected with *M avium* complex seems to be older and does not have as severe disease as those infected with the *M abscessus* group, who seem to be younger and to have more severe lung disease.[85] Recent studies using whole genome sequencing have suggested that the *M abscessus* group show the potential for spread from person to person in CF centers, making it another target for infection prevention.[86]

Attempting to recover nontuberculous mycobacteria from a CF respiratory specimen is challenging for the laboratory. Approximately 50% to 70% of specimens contain *P aeruginosa*, which is resistant to 0.25% N-acetyl cysteine-1% sodium hydroxide decontamination, the standard method used in the culture respiratory specimens for mycobacteria. Contamination rates between 35% and 70% may be seen using this decontamination method in CF respiratory specimens. When a second step is added, 2.5% oxalic acid, the contamination rate is reduced to 3% to 5%, although low numbers of *M avium* complex may not be recovered.[87,88] Chlorohexidine alone has been shown to be an effective means of decontaminating CF respiratory specimens for the recovery of nontuberculous mycobacteria.[89]

A useful observation concerning the recovery of *M abscessus* group organisms is the observation that this group of organisms can be recovered on medium that is routinely used for bacterial isolation, specifically BCSA. *M abscessus* group clinical isolates were recovered on BCSA from 65% to 75% of infected individuals, whereas the organism was recovered from 85% using mycobacterial-specific culture methods. Twenty-five percent of patients with CF with *M abscessus* complex had it first recovered on routine culture. In addition, incubation of BCSA plates for 14 days greatly enhanced recovery compared with 5-day incubation.[90] As a result, we routinely examine BCSA plates for the presence of rapidly growing *Mycobacterium*.

Phenotypic identification of nontuberculous mycobacteria is challenging and not particularly accurate. As a result, we have used 16S rRNA sequence analysis for identification of these organisms. A 16S rRNA sequence works well for identification of *M avium* complex, but *M abscessus* complex isolates cannot be distinguished from *M chelonae*.[91] As a result, a second target is needed. Both *rpoB* and *hsp65* have been used for this purpose, with both being useful for differentiating *M abscessus* complex from *M chelonae*.[91] Whole genome sequencing has shown that in 1 center, *M abscessus* subspecies *massilense* was predominant and there was evidence of person-to-person spread.[86] Whole genome sequencing of *M abscessus* complex isolates from more than 100 patients with CF in our center showed *M abscessus* subspecies *abscessus* to be predominant (Grogono, Floto, Gilligan unpublished).

Antimicrobial resistance is a major problem in nontuberculous mycobacteria treatment. Anti–*M tuberculosis* therapy is ineffective against these organisms. Further complicating treatment is the lack of randomized, controlled trials of antimicrobial treatment against this group of organisms.[92] Susceptibility testing using broth dilution is helpful in guiding antimicrobial choice, because susceptibility is not predictable.[81] Broth MIC susceptibility tests of macrolides against the *M abscessus* group should be incubated for 14 days to detect inducible macrolide resistance. Clarithromycin seems to be a more potent inducer of this resistance than azithromycin, making azithromycin central to the treatment of *M abscessus* infections.[93]

A potential life-saving therapy for patients with CF infected with severe *M abscessus* is lung transplantation. However, based on anecdotal experience and case reports, *M abscessus* complex infection has been a contraindication for this life-saving procedure.[81] This strategy seems logical, given some of the similarities between *B cepacia* and *M abscessus*. Both organisms are environment organisms, which are highly drug resistant, making them difficult to treat, able to be spread from person to person, and associated with wound dehiscence after transplant. A recent single-center study with 13 patients with CF with *M abscessus* receiving double lung transplant showed the same survival rate as the control population, suggesting that this organism is not a contraindication to lung transplantation.[94]

FUNGI

Fungi have long been recognized as having a role in CF lung disease. In particular, 2 fungi, *Aspergillus fumigatus* and *Scedosporium apiospermum*, have been shown to be long-term colonizers in patients with CF.[95] Both organisms are most frequently associated with allergic bronchopulmonary disease, characterized by subacute clinical disease with eosinophilia, increased IgE levels, skin test reactivity in the case of *Aspergillus*, presence of serum IgE specific for the *Aspergillus* when it is the cause, and chest imaging changes that are not attributable to bacterial agents.[95] In addition, post–lung transplant infections are well described for both organisms, although colonization with these organisms is not a contraindication for lung transplantation.[96,97] *Candida* spp are found in as many as 70% of patients with CF, especially when selective media are used. Because patients with CF receive antibacterials from an early age, the presence of these organisms colonizing the airways is not surprising. The clinical significance of *Candida* in patients with CF is not clearly understood, but most clinicians discount these organisms as not significant.[98]

NAAT allows the detection of *Pneumocystis jirovecii* in the airway of patients with CF. In a prospective study, 12.5% of adults with CF were found to have *Pneumocystis jirovecii* in sputum. Lung function in these patients was better than in those without *Pneumocystis jirovecii.* These patients were more likely to have mild disease and be free of *P aeruginosa.*[99]

A fungal agent that has recently emerged in patients with CF is *Trichosporon*. With the increasing use of antifungal agents to treat disease associated with *Aspergillus* and *Scedosporium*, *Trichosporon,* which is resistant to the antifungals amphotericin and the echinocandins, may find a niche in the CF airway.[100] Fungemia caused by *Trichosporon* has been reported in 2 patients with CF, 1 of whom was a double lung transplant recipient.[101,102] Without using a selective fungal medium, we found it in 0.2% of our patients with CF,[103] and these patients tend to have more rapid decline in lung function. Whether this situation is directly attributable to *Trichosporon* infections is unknown.

Isolation of *Aspergillus, Scedosporium*, and *Trichosporon* can all be accomplished with media used for bacterial isolation. Because of its highly selective nature, BCSA is particularly useful for the isolation of fungi. Conventional techniques are sufficient for identification of these organisms. Susceptibility testing is not recommended.

RESPIRATORY VIRUSES

For many years, viral agents have been considered to play a prime role in the initial steps of establishing chronic lung infections.[15] However, almost all the data to support this theory were based on serologic data, with few culture data to support the theory, in part because of frequent contamination of viral respiratory culture, especially in patients infected with *P aeruginosa.*[15] With the advent of NAAT testing for viruses, a clearer picture of the role of viruses will likely emerge. It is now well recognized that acute exacerbations are associated with both influenza and respiratory syncytial virus.[104–106] One of the most interesting observations was the high rate of detection of rhinovirus, approximately 30% when a multiplex polymerase chain reaction was used.[107,108] Rhinovirus tends to persist in the CF airway, and viral loads increase during pulmonary exacerbations.[108] Using a CF airway epithelial model, it has been shown that rhinovirus superinfection of *P aeruginosa*–infected cells causes a release of planktonic bacteria. This release of planktonic bacteria during viral infection may be an important trigger of CF pulmonary exacerbations.[6]

Diagnosis of CF respiratory viral infections has been revolutionized by the use of NAAT. NAAT diagnostics approved by the US Food and Drug Administration are available for influenza A/B only, the combination of influenza A/B and respiratory syncytial virus (RSV), and multiplex NAAT for adenovirus, coronavirus, influenza viruses A/B, metapneumovirus, parainfluenza virus 1-4, RSV, and rhinovirus.[109–111] Because there have been no evaluations comparing these different methods specifically in patients with CF, the reliability of these methods is unknown in this patient population. Given the unusual nature of the matrix in which the virus may be found, specific evaluation of NAAT performance in these specimens would be useful. A meta-analysis[112] for influenza antigen detection assays suggested that these methods lack sensitivity in patients with low viral loads. Because they have not been evaluated in patients with CF, they cannot be recommended for that patient population.

MICROBIOME CONSIDERATIONS

Microbiome analysis is changing our way of thinking about chronic infections. In patients with CF, we have learned that other organisms beyond those that we have already discussed may play an important role in CF lung disease. Organisms typically believed as belonging to the normal microflora of the oropharynx, *Prevotella, Veillonella*, and the *Streptococcus anginosus* group, are all found in respiratory tract of patients with CF.[5,13] It is speculated that these organisms might upregulate or downregulate virulence genes in pathogens such as *P aeruginosa* to obtain essential nutrients through the activity of these pathogens.[12] Another observation that has arisen as a result of microbiome studies is that microbial communities are remarkably stable, even in the face of repeated rounds of antimicrobial therapy.[11,13] In addition, as chronic *P aeruginosa* infection is established, the diversity of the microbial community declines.[10] Is this a result of *P aeruginosa* being the apex predator in the CF airway microbiome eliminating competitors and adapting itself by downregulating virulence genes to allow long-term survival of its human host? Over the next decade, we should get closer to this answer.

REFERENCES

1. ACOG Committee Opinion No. 486: update on carrier screening for cystic fibrosis. Obstet Gynecol 2011;117:1028–31.
2. Goss CH, Ratjen F. Update in cystic fibrosis 2012. Am J Respir Crit Care Med 2013;187:915–9.
3. Donaldson SH, Wolgang MC, Gilligan PG, et al. Cystic fibrosis. In: Mandell GL, Bennett JE, Dolin R, editors. Principles and practices of infectious diseases. 7th edition. New York: Churchill Livingstone; 2006. p. 947–55.
4. Cystic Fibrosis Foundation. Cystic Fibrosis Foundation patient registry 2012 annual data report. 2013.
5. Goss CH, Burns JL. Exacerbations in cystic fibrosis. 1: epidemiology and pathogenesis. Thorax 2007;62:360–7.
6. Sibley CD, Grinwis ME, Field TR, et al. Culture enriched molecular profiling of the cystic fibrosis airway microbiome. PLoS One 2011;6:e22702.
7. Chattoraj SS, Ganesan S, Jones AM, et al. Rhinovirus infection liberates planktonic bacteria from biofilm and increases chemokine responses in cystic fibrosis airway epithelial cells. Thorax 2011;66:333–9.
8. Flume PA, Mogayzel PJ Jr, Robinson KA, et al. Cystic fibrosis pulmonary guidelines: treatment of pulmonary exacerbations. Am J Respir Crit Care Med 2009; 180:802–8.
9. Hansen CR, Pressler T, Hoiby N. Early aggressive eradication therapy for intermittent *Pseudomonas aeruginosa* airway colonization in cystic fibrosis patients: 15 years experience. J Cyst Fibros 2008;7:523–30.
10. Klepac-Ceraj V, Lemon KP, Martin TR, et al. Relationship between cystic fibrosis respiratory tract bacterial communities and age, genotype, antibiotics and *Pseudomonas aeruginosa*. Environ Microbiol 2010;12:1293–303.
11. Zhao J, Schloss PD, Kalikin LM, et al. Decade-long bacterial community dynamics in cystic fibrosis airways. Proc Natl Acad Sci U S A 2012;109:5809–14.
12. Sibley CD, Parkins MD, Rabin HR, et al. The relevance of the polymicrobial nature of airway infection in the acute and chronic management of patients with cystic fibrosis. Curr Opin Investig Drugs 2009;10:787–94.
13. Fodor AA, Klem ER, Gilpin DF, et al. The adult cystic fibrosis airway microbiota is stable over time and infection type, and highly resilient to antibiotic treatment of exacerbations. PLoS One 2012;7:e45001.
14. Anderson DH. Therapy and prognosis of fibrocystic disease of the pancreas. Pediatrics 1949;3:406–17.

15. Gilligan P, Kiska DL, Appleman MD. Cumitech 43: cystic fibrosis microbiology. Washington, DC: ASM Press; 2006.
16. Gilligan PH, Gage PA, Welch DF, et al. Prevalence of thymidine-dependent *Staphylococcus aureus* in patients with cystic fibrosis. J Clin Microbiol 1987;25:1258–61.
17. Proctor RA, von Eiff C, Kahl BC, et al. Small colony variants: a pathogenic form of bacteria that facilitates persistent and recurrent infections. Nat Rev Microbiol 2006;4:295–305.
18. Wolter DJ, Emerson JC, McNamara S, et al. *Staphylococcus aureus* small-colony variants are independently associated with worse lung disease in children with cystic fibrosis. Clin Infect Dis 2013;57:384–91.
19. Garcia LG, Lemaire S, Kahl BC, et al. Antibiotic activity against small-colony variants of *Staphylococcus aureus*: review of in vitro, animal and clinical data. J Antimicrob Chemother 2013;68:1455–64.
20. Champion EA, Miller MB, Popowitch EB, et al. Antimicrobial susceptibility and molecular typing of MRSA in cystic fibrosis. Pediatr Pulmonol 2014; 49:230–7.
21. Dasenbrook EC, Checkley W, Merlo CA, et al. Association between respiratory tract methicillin-resistant *Staphylococcus aureus* and survival in cystic fibrosis. JAMA 2010;303:2386–92.
22. David MZ, Daum RS. Community-associated methicillin-resistant *Staphylococcus aureus*: epidemiology and clinical consequences of an emerging epidemic. Clin Microbiol Rev 2010;23:616–87.
23. Goodrich JS, Sutton-Shields TN, Kerr A, et al. Prevalence of community-associated methicillin-resistant *Staphylococcus aureus* in patients with cystic fibrosis. J Clin Microbiol 2009;47:1231–3.
24. Cui L, Iwamoto A, Lian JQ, et al. Novel mechanism of antibiotic resistance originating in vancomycin-intermediate *Staphylococcus aureus*. Antimicrob Agents Chemother 2006;50:428–38.
25. Report of the UK Cystic Fibrosis Trust Microbiology Laboratory Standards Working Group: Laboratory standards for processing microbiological samples form people with cystic fibrosis. Cystic Fibrosis Trust 2010.
26. Kipp F, Kahl BC, Becker K, et al. Evaluation of two chromogenic agar media for recovery and identification of *Staphylococcus aureus* small-colony variants. J Clin Microbiol 2005;43:1956–9.
27. Kipp F, Becker K, Peters G, et al. Evaluation of different methods to detect methicillin resistance in small-colony variants of *Staphylococcus aureus*. J Clin Microbiol 2004;42:1277–9.
28. Desai AP, Stanley T, Atuan M, et al. Use of matrix assisted laser desorption ionisation-time of flight mass spectrometry in a paediatric clinical laboratory for identification of bacteria commonly isolated from cystic fibrosis patients. J Clin Pathol 2012;65:835–8.
29. Howden BP, Davies JK, Johnson PD, et al. Reduced vancomycin susceptibility in *Staphylococcus aureus*, including vancomycin-intermediate and heterogeneous vancomycin-intermediate strains: resistance mechanisms, laboratory detection, and clinical implications. Clin Microbiol Rev 2010;23:99–139.
30. Al-Aloul M, Crawley J, Winstanley C, et al. Increased morbidity associated with chronic infection by an epidemic *Pseudomonas aeruginosa* strain in CF patients. Thorax 2004;59:334–6.
31. Folkesson A, Jelsbak L, Yang L, et al. Adaptation of *Pseudomonas aeruginosa* to the cystic fibrosis airway: an evolutionary perspective. Nat Rev Microbiol 2012;10:841–51.

32. Marko DC, Saffert RT, Cunningham SA, et al. Evaluation of the Bruker Biotyper and Vitek MS matrix-assisted laser desorption ionization-time of flight mass spectrometry systems for identification of nonfermenting gram-negative bacilli isolated from cultures from cystic fibrosis patients. J Clin Microbiol 2012;50:2034–9.
33. Burns JL, Saiman L, Whittier S, et al. Comparison of two commercial systems (Vitek and MicroScan-WalkAway) for antimicrobial susceptibility testing of *Pseudomonas aeruginosa* isolates from cystic fibrosis patients. Diagn Microbiol Infect Dis 2001;39:257–60.
34. Gilligan PH. Is there value in susceptibility testing of *Pseudomonas aeruginosa* causing chronic infection in patients with cystic fibrosis? Expert Rev Anti Infect Ther 2006;4:711–5.
35. Moskowitz SM, Foster JM, Emerson J, et al. Clinically feasible biofilm susceptibility assay for isolates of *Pseudomonas aeruginosa* from patients with cystic fibrosis. J Clin Microbiol 2004;42:1915–22.
36. Su S, Hassett DJ. Anaerobic *Pseudomonas aeruginosa* and other obligately anaerobic bacterial biofilms growing in the thick airway mucus of chronically infected cystic fibrosis patients: an emerging paradigm or "old hat"? Expert Opin Ther Targets 2012;16:859–73.
37. Lo D, VanDevanter DR, Flume P, et al. Aerosolized antibiotic therapy for chronic cystic fibrosis airway infections: continuous or intermittent? Respir Med 2011;105(Suppl 2):S9–17.
38. Foweraker JE, Laughton CR, Brown DF, et al. Phenotypic variability of *Pseudomonas aeruginosa* in sputa from patients with acute infective exacerbation of cystic fibrosis and its impact on the validity of antimicrobial susceptibility testing. J Antimicrob Chemother 2005;55:921–7.
39. Aaron SD, Ferris W, Henry DA, et al. Multiple combination bactericidal antibiotic testing for patients with cystic fibrosis infected with *Burkholderia cepacia*. Am J Respir Crit Care Med 2000;161:1206–12.
40. Aaron SD, Vandemheen KL, Ferris W, et al. Combination antibiotic susceptibility testing to treat exacerbations of cystic fibrosis associated with multiresistant bacteria: a randomised, double-blind, controlled clinical trial. Lancet 2005;366:463–71.
41. Isles A, Maclusky I, Corey M, et al. *Pseudomonas cepacia* infection in cystic fibrosis: an emerging problem. J Pediatr 1984;104:206–10.
42. Tablan OC, Chorba TL, Schidlow DV, et al. *Pseudomonas cepacia* colonization in patients with cystic fibrosis: risk factors and clinical outcome. J Pediatr 1985;107:382–7.
43. Tablan OC, Martone WJ, Doershuk CF, et al. Colonization of the respiratory tract with *Pseudomonas cepacia* in cystic fibrosis. Risk factors and outcomes. Chest 1987;91:527–32.
44. Yabuuchi E, Kosako Y, Oyaizu H, et al. Proposal of *Burkholderia* gen. nov. and transfer of seven species of the genus *Pseudomonas* homology group II to the new genus, with the type species *Burkholderia cepacia* (Palleroni and Holmes 1981) comb. nov. Microbiol Immunol 1992;36:1251–75.
45. Vandamme P, Holmes B, Vancanneyt M, et al. Occurrence of multiple genomovars of *Burkholderia cepacia* in cystic fibrosis patients and proposal of *Burkholderia multivorans* sp. nov. Int J Syst Bacteriol 1997;47:1188–200.
46. Lipuma JJ. The changing microbial epidemiology in cystic fibrosis. Clin Microbiol Rev 2010;23:299–323.
47. Peeters C, Zlosnik JE, Spilker T, et al. *Burkholderia pseudomultivorans* sp. nov., a novel *Burkholderia cepacia* complex species from human respiratory samples and the rhizosphere. Syst Appl Microbiol 2013;36:483–9.

48. Heath DG, Hohneker K, Carriker C, et al. Six-year molecular analysis of *Burkholderia cepacia* complex isolates among cystic fibrosis patients at a referral center for lung transplantation. J Clin Microbiol 2002;40:1188–93.

49. Holmes A, Nolan R, Taylor R, et al. An epidemic of *Burkholderia cepacia* transmitted between patients with and without cystic fibrosis. J Infect Dis 1999;179: 1197–205.

50. Sun L, Jiang RZ, Steinbach S, et al. The emergence of a highly transmissible lineage of cbl+ *Pseudomonas* (*Burkholderia*) *cepacia* causing CF centre epidemics in North America and Britain. Nat Med 1995;1:661–6.

51. Steinbach S, Sun L, Jiang RZ, et al. Transmissibility of *Pseudomonas cepacia* infection in clinic patients and lung-transplant recipients with cystic fibrosis. N Engl J Med 1994;331:981–7.

52. Aris RM, Routh JC, LiPuma JJ, et al. Lung transplantation for cystic fibrosis patients with *Burkholderia cepacia* complex. Survival linked to genomovar type. Am J Respir Crit Care Med 2001;164:2102–6.

53. Murray S, Charbeneau J, Marshall BC, et al. Impact of *Burkholderia* infection on lung transplantation in cystic fibrosis. Am J Respir Crit Care Med 2008;178: 363–71.

54. Noone PG. Lung transplant and cystic fibrosis: what's new from the UK and France? Thorax 2008;63:668–70.

55. Henry D, Campbell M, McGimpsey C, et al. Comparison of isolation media for recovery of *Burkholderia cepacia* complex from respiratory secretions of patients with cystic fibrosis. J Clin Microbiol 1999;37:1004–7.

56. Gilligan PH, Gage PA, Bradshaw LM, et al. Isolation medium for the recovery of *Pseudomonas cepacia* from respiratory secretions of patients with cystic fibrosis. J Clin Microbiol 1985;22:5–8.

57. Welch DF, Muszynski MJ, Pai CH, et al. Selective and differential medium for recovery of *Pseudomonas cepacia* from the respiratory tracts of patients with cystic fibrosis. J Clin Microbiol 1987;25:1730–4.

58. Kiska DL, Kerr A, Jones MC, et al. Accuracy of four commercial systems for identification of *Burkholderia cepacia* and other gram-negative nonfermenting bacilli recovered from patients with cystic fibrosis. J Clin Microbiol 1996;34: 886–91.

59. Shelly DB, Spilker T, Gracely EJ, et al. Utility of commercial systems for identification of *Burkholderia cepacia* complex from cystic fibrosis sputum culture. J Clin Microbiol 2000;38:3112–5.

60. Saiman L, Siegel J. Infection control in cystic fibrosis. Clin Microbiol Rev 2004; 17:57–71.

61. Bressler AM, Kaye KS, LiPuma JJ, et al. Risk factors for *Burkholderia cepacia* complex bacteremia among intensive care unit patients without cystic fibrosis: a case-control study. Infect Control Hosp Epidemiol 2007;28:951–8.

62. Wilsher ML, Kolbe J, Morris AJ, et al. Nosocomial acquisition of *Burkholderia gladioli* in patients with cystic fibrosis. Am J Respir Crit Care Med 1997;155: 1436–40.

63. Ferroni A, Sermet-Gaudelus I, Abachin E, et al. Use of 16S rRNA gene sequencing for identification of nonfermenting gram-negative bacilli recovered from patients attending a single cystic fibrosis center. J Clin Microbiol 2002; 40:3793–7.

64. Kennedy MP, Coakley RD, Donaldson SH, et al. *Burkholderia gladioli*: five year experience in a cystic fibrosis and lung transplantation center. J Cyst Fibros 2007;6:267–73.

65. Fehlberg LC, Andrade LH, Assis DM, et al. Performance of MALDI-ToF MS for species identification of *Burkholderia cepacia* complex clinical isolates. Diagn Microbiol Infect Dis 2013;77:126–8.
66. Alby K, Gilligan PH, Miller MB. Comparison of matrix-assisted laser desorption ionization-time of flight (MALDI-TOF) mass spectrometry platforms for the identification of gram-negative rods from patients with cystic fibrosis. J Clin Microbiol 2013;51:3852–4.
67. Degand N, Carbonnelle E, Dauphin B, et al. Matrix-assisted laser desorption ionization-time of flight mass spectrometry for identification of nonfermenting gram-negative bacilli isolated from cystic fibrosis patients. J Clin Microbiol 2008;46:3361–7.
68. Leitao JH, Sousa SA, Cunha MV, et al. Variation of the antimicrobial susceptibility profiles of *Burkholderia cepacia* complex clonal isolates obtained from chronically infected cystic fibrosis patients: a five-year survey in the major Portuguese treatment center. Eur J Clin Microbiol Infect Dis 2008;27:1101–11.
69. Clinical and Laboratory Institute: Performance standards for antimicrobial susceptibility testing; 23rd Informational Supplement, M100–S23. Clinical and Laboratory Standards Institute 2013.
70. Horsley A, Jones AM. Antibiotic treatment for *Burkholderia cepacia* complex in people with cystic fibrosis experiencing a pulmonary exacerbation. Cochrane Database Syst Rev 2012;(10):CD009529.
71. Ronne Hansen C, Pressler T, Hoiby N, et al. Chronic infection with *Achromobacter xylosoxidans* in cystic fibrosis patients; a retrospective case control study. J Cyst Fibros 2006;5:245–51.
72. Raso T, Bianco O, Grosso B, et al. *Achromobacter xylosoxidans* respiratory tract infections in cystic fibrosis patients. APMIS 2008;116:837–41.
73. De Baets F, Schelstraete P, Van Daele S, et al. *Achromobacter xylosoxidans* in cystic fibrosis: prevalence and clinical relevance. J Cyst Fibros 2007;6:75–8.
74. Goss CH, Mayer-Hamblett N, Aitken ML, et al. Association between *Stenotrophomonas maltophilia* and lung function in cystic fibrosis. Thorax 2004;59:955–9.
75. Waters V, Atenafu EG, Lu A, et al. Chronic *Stenotrophomonas maltophilia* infection and mortality or lung transplantation in cystic fibrosis patients. J Cyst Fibros 2013;12:482–6.
76. Zbinden A, Bottger EC, Bosshard PP, et al. Evaluation of the colorimetric VITEK 2 card for identification of gram-negative nonfermentative rods: comparison to 16S rRNA gene sequencing. J Clin Microbiol 2007;45:2270–3.
77. Biswas S, Dubus JC, Reynaud-Gaubert M, et al. Evaluation of colistin susceptibility in multidrug-resistant clinical isolates from cystic fibrosis, France. Eur J Clin Microbiol Infect Dis 2013;32:1461–4.
78. Goncalves-Vidigal P, Grosse-Onnebrink J, Mellies U, et al. *Stenotrophomonas maltophilia* in cystic fibrosis: improved detection by the use of selective agar and evaluation of antimicrobial resistance. J Cyst Fibros 2011;10:422–7.
79. Wang M, Ridderberg W, Hansen CR, et al. Early treatment with inhaled antibiotics postpones next occurrence of *Achromobacter* in cystic fibrosis. J Cyst Fibros 2013;12:638–43.
80. Amoureux L, Bador J, Siebor E, et al. Epidemiology and resistance of *Achromobacter xylosoxidans* from cystic fibrosis patients in Dijon, Burgundy: First French data. J Cyst Fibros 2013;12:170–6.
81. Leung JM, Olivier KN. Nontuberculous mycobacteria: the changing epidemiology and treatment challenges in cystic fibrosis. Curr Opin Pulm Med 2013; 19:662–9.

82. Kilby JM, Gilligan PH, Yankaskas JR, et al. Nontuberculous mycobacteria in adult patients with cystic fibrosis. Chest 1992;102:70–5.
83. Olivier KN, Weber DJ, Lee JH, et al. Nontuberculous mycobacteria. II: nested-cohort study of impact on cystic fibrosis lung disease. Am J Respir Crit Care Med 2003;167:835–40.
84. Esther CR Jr, Esserman DA, Gilligan P, et al. Chronic *Mycobacterium abscessus* infection and lung function decline in cystic fibrosis. J Cyst Fibros 2010;9:117–23.
85. Catherinot E, Roux AL, Vibet MA, et al. *Mycobacterium avium* and *Mycobacterium abscessus* complex target distinct cystic fibrosis patient subpopulations. J Cyst Fibros 2013;12:74–80.
86. Bryant JM, Grogono DM, Greaves D, et al. Whole-genome sequencing to identify transmission of *Mycobacterium abscessus* between patients with cystic fibrosis: a retrospective cohort study. Lancet 2013;381:1551–60.
87. Whittier S, Hopfer RL, Knowles MR, et al. Improved recovery of mycobacteria from respiratory secretions of patients with cystic fibrosis. J Clin Microbiol 1993;31:861–4.
88. Bange FC, Kirschner P, Bottger EC. Recovery of mycobacteria from patients with cystic fibrosis. J Clin Microbiol 1999;37:3761–3.
89. Ferroni A, Vu-Thien H, Lanotte P, et al. Value of the chlorhexidine decontamination method for recovery of nontuberculous mycobacteria from sputum samples of patients with cystic fibrosis. J Clin Microbiol 2006;44:2237–9.
90. Esther CR Jr, Hoberman S, Fine J, et al. Detection of rapidly growing mycobacteria in routine cultures of samples from patients with cystic fibrosis. J Clin Microbiol 2011;49:1421–5.
91. Blauwendraat C, Dixon GL, Hartley JC, et al. The use of a two-gene sequencing approach to accurately distinguish between the species within the *Mycobacterium abscessus* complex and *Mycobacterium chelonae*. Eur J Clin Microbiol Infect Dis 2012;31:1847–53.
92. Waters V, Ratjen F. Antibiotic treatment for nontuberculous mycobacteria lung infection in people with cystic fibrosis. Cochrane Database Syst Rev 2012;(12):CD010004.
93. Choi GE, Shin SJ, Won CJ, et al. Macrolide treatment for *Mycobacterium abscessus* and *Mycobacterium massiliense* infection and inducible resistance. Am J Respir Crit Care Med 2012;186:917–25.
94. Lobo LJ, Chang LC, Esther CR Jr, et al. Lung transplant outcomes in cystic fibrosis patients with pre-operative *Mycobacterium abscessus* respiratory infections. Clin Transplant 2013;27:523–9.
95. Pihet M, Carrere J, Cimon B, et al. Occurrence and relevance of filamentous fungi in respiratory secretions of patients with cystic fibrosis–a review. Med Mycol 2009;47:387–97.
96. Bonvillain RW, Valentine VG, Lombard G, et al. Post-operative infections in cystic fibrosis and non-cystic fibrosis patients after lung transplantation. J Heart Lung Transplant 2007;26:890–7.
97. Morio F, Horeau-Langlard D, Gay-Andrieu F, et al. Disseminated *Scedosporium/Pseudallescheria* infection after double-lung transplantation in patients with cystic fibrosis. J Clin Microbiol 2010;48:1978–82.
98. Middleton PG, Chen SC, Meyer W. Fungal infections and treatment in cystic fibrosis. Curr Opin Pulm Med 2013;19:670–5.
99. Hernandez-Hernandez F, Frealle E, Caneiro P, et al. Prospective multicenter study of *Pneumocystis jirovecii* colonization among cystic fibrosis patients in France. J Clin Microbiol 2012;50:4107–10.

100. Miceli MH, Diaz JA, Lee SA. Emerging opportunistic yeast infections. Lancet Infect Dis 2011;11:142–51.
101. Hickey PW, Sutton DA, Fothergill AW, et al. *Trichosporon mycotoxinivorans*, a novel respiratory pathogen in patients with cystic fibrosis. J Clin Microbiol 2009;47:3091–7.
102. Hirschi S, Letscher-Bru V, Pottecher J, et al. Disseminated *Trichosporon mycotoxinivorans*, *Aspergillus fumigatus*, and *Scedosporium apiospermum* coinfection after lung and liver transplantation in a cystic fibrosis patient. J Clin Microbiol 2012;50:4168–70.
103. Paulson J, Kerr A, Gilligan P, et al. *Trichosporon* acquisition is linked to accelerated lung function decline in nontransplant cystic fibrosis patients. In: Am J Respir Crit Care Med. vol. 185. San Francisco (CA): American Thoracic Society International Meeting, poster discussion; 2012. p. A5274.
104. Burns JL, Emerson J, Kuypers J, et al. Respiratory viruses in children with cystic fibrosis: viral detection and clinical findings. Influenza Other Respir Viruses 2012;6:218–23.
105. Viviani L, Assael BM, Kerem E. Impact of the A (H1N1) pandemic influenza (season 2009-2010) on patients with cystic fibrosis. J Cyst Fibros 2011;10:370–6.
106. Etherington C, Naseer R, Conway SP, et al. The role of respiratory viruses in adult patients with cystic fibrosis receiving intravenous antibiotics for a pulmonary exacerbation. J Cyst Fibros 2014;13(1):49–55.
107. Esther CR Jr, Lin FC, Kerr A, et al. Respiratory viruses are associated with common respiratory pathogens in cystic fibrosis. Pediatr Pulmonol 2013. [Epub ahead of print].
108. Kieninger E, Singer F, Tapparel C, et al. High rhinovirus burden in lower airways of children with cystic fibrosis. Chest 2013;143:782–90.
109. Novak-Weekley SM, Marlowe EM, Poulter M, et al. Evaluation of the Cepheid Xpert Flu Assay for rapid identification and differentiation of influenza A, influenza A 2009 H1N1, and influenza B viruses. J Clin Microbiol 2013;50:1704–10.
110. Popowitch EB, O'Neill SS, Miller MB. Comparison of the Biofire FilmArray RP, Genmark eSensor RVP, Luminex xTAG RVPv1, and Luminex xTAG RVP fast multiplex assays for detection of respiratory viruses. J Clin Microbiol 2013;51: 1528–33.
111. Alby K, Popowitch EB, Miller MB. Comparative evaluation of the Nanosphere Verigene RV+ assay and the Simplexa Flu A/B & RSV kit for detection of influenza and respiratory syncytial viruses. J Clin Microbiol 2013;51:352–3.
112. Chartrand C, Leeflang MM, Minion J, et al. Accuracy of rapid influenza diagnostic tests: a meta-analysis. Ann Intern Med 2012;156:500–11.

Urine Antigen Tests for the Diagnosis of Respiratory Infections

Legionellosis, Histoplasmosis, Pneumococcal Pneumonia

Marc Roger Couturier, PhD, D(ABMM)[a,b,*], Erin H. Graf, PhD[b],
Allen T. Griffin, MD[b]

KEYWORDS

- Urine antigen tests • *Legionella* • *Histoplasma* • *Streptococcus pneumoniae*

KEY POINTS

- Because of their high specificity, urine antigen tests for *Legionella* and pneumococcus offer rapid pathogen identification for community-acquired pneumonia, allowing for targeted antimicrobial therapy.
- Although the urine antigen test provides many benefits over traditional methods, culture is still required for bacterial antimicrobial susceptibility profiles and epidemiologic data.
- Urinary antigen testing has revolutionized diagnostic testing particularly for disseminated histoplasmosis, largely supplanting serology.
- Recent commercial development of *Histoplasma* urine antigen reagents may allow institutions to perform testing in-house as an alternative to submitting specimens to reference laboratories.

INTRODUCTION

Diagnosing respiratory infections has historically relied on targeted culture of respiratory pathogens. Although this can provide adequate sensitivity for some organisms, not all causative organisms can be readily cultured from respiratory specimens. In addition, significant delays in turnaround time (TAT) are detrimental to patient care, particularly in the cases of pneumonia or severely immunocompromised hosts. As a

[a] ARUP Laboratories, Institute for Clinical and Experimental Pathology, 500 Chipeta Way, Salt Lake City, UT 84108, USA; [b] Department of Pathology, University of Utah School of Medicine, 15 North Medical Drive East, Suite #1100, Salt Lake City, UT, USA
* Corresponding author. ARUP Laboratories, Institute for Clinical and Experimental Pathology, 500 Chipeta Way, Salt Lake City, UT 84108.
E-mail address: marc.couturier@aruplab.com

Clin Lab Med 34 (2014) 219–236
http://dx.doi.org/10.1016/j.cll.2014.02.002
0272-2712/14/$ – see front matter © 2014 Elsevier Inc. All rights reserved.

result of these limitations, testing for pneumonia has evolved in recent decades to include so-called rapid culture-independent methods. However, not all modalities of culture-independent testing have measured up to clinical expectations. For instance, in the case of direct fluorescence antibody staining for *Legionella pneumophila*, the method has proved to be considerably less sensitive than conventionally used culture methods despite its shortened TAT.[1] In this case, the lack of result accuracy negates the rapidity of the result.

Urinary antigen testing has grown in popularity for several significant respiratory infections, particularly *Legionella pneumophila*, *Streptococcus pneumoniae*, and *Histoplasma capsulatum*. The broad concept of urinary antigen testing capitalizes on the concentration of shed antigen from a variety of pathogens in the kidneys for excretion in the urine. The antigens are then detected via an immunoassay such as an enzyme-linked immunosorbent assay (ELISA) or an immunochromatographic or lateral flow assay (LFA). Of importance is that the aforementioned pathogens are not present in the urine for culture, despite the target antigen being concentrated on this anatomic site. This situation allows for a noninvasive specimen collection to provide information on an infection occurring in a distal anatomic location. Urinary antigen testing can therefore be used to obtain rapid test results related to respiratory infection, independent of an invasive collection such as a bronchoalveolar lavage (BAL). This article describes the 3 aforementioned organisms, their role in respiratory disease, and the current status of urinary antigen testing in their respective diagnosis.

MICROBIOLOGY
Legionella

Legionella spp are fastidious, gram-negative bacilli that are ubiquitous in the aqueous environment, often parasitizing free-living amoebas.[2] The unusual nutritional requirements of this organism has led to a general difficulty in recovering the organism in many clinical cases of respiratory infections, with average cultures requiring 2 to 5 days for growth. While up to one-third of the validly named species have been isolated from humans, *L pneumophila* is conventionally considered the most clinically significant species, and within this species serogroup 1 is considered the most significant.[3]

Pneumococcus

S pneumoniae is a gram-positive coccus and a member of the viridans group of streptococcal bacteria. The pneumococcal genome is approximately 2 million base pairs, with more than 150 genes dedicated to virulence.[4] Pneumococci have to strike a balance between immune evasion and successful colonization of the human nasopharyngeal tract. To do this, they retain the ability to switch between thin, procolonization, polysaccharide capsules and more virulent, thicker capsules.[5,6] Prior colonization with certain bacteria or viral infection can also have dramatic effects on both propneumococcal and antipneumococcal colonization.[7,8]

Histoplasma

H capsulatum is a dimorphic mold of the Ascomycota phylum, Onygenales order. This organism exists in the body as a small, intracellular yeast (2–4 μm), exhibiting narrow-based budding, and in the environment as a mold with hyphae, tuberculate macroconidia, and smooth microconidia.[9] Environmentally, (+) and (−) forms of the perfect state (*Ajellomyces capsulatus*) combine sexually,[10] whereas replication in vivo transpires asexually by budding.

EPIDEMIOLOGY, DISEASE PRESENTATION, AND PATHOGENESIS
Legionella

Owing to the ubiquitous nature of *Legionella* in the environment, the epidemiology of disease is difficult to predict. In fact, *Legionella* can be found in almost any artificial water storage device. There are well-established environments that pose significantly higher risk for the organism being transmitted to humans, and these are more likely to cause community-associated outbreaks of disease. Of particular concern are devices found in institutional settings that use water in the cooling process for which aerosols are produced (eg, air-conditioners, evaporative coolers, cool-air humidifiers, warm-water spas, cooling towers, and plumbing/showers). In hospital settings, colonization of any number of these devices can be of significance, particularly in units housing severely immunocompromised patients.[3]

Legionella exist in the environment by parasitizing amoebas, and in the human host they also parasitize a conceptually analogous cell type, namely the macrophage.[2] *Legionella* interferes with phagocyte membrane trafficking, and can persist within a macrophage for an extended period of time in a protective vacuole where they replicate and subsequently infect other neighboring alveolar macrophages.[11] This subsequent proliferation leads to progressively amplified disease in the lung.

Legionella causes 2 distinct respiratory syndromes: Legionnaires disease (LD) and Pontiac fever (PF). LD is caused by *L pneumophila* and other *Legionella* spp. The disease is characterized as a mild to fatal (average 12% case-fatality rate) pneumonia. Symptoms include fever, nonproductive cough, myalgias, rigors, dyspnea, and diarrhea.[12] Features of LD are difficult to distinguish from those of other forms of community-acquired pneumonia (CAP) such as pneumococcal CAP, largely because of the nonspecific features of radiographic imaging, clinical presentation on admittance, and general laboratory tests. Specific risks for LD include advanced age, impaired airway function (cigarette smokers, emphysema, chronic obstructive pulmonary disease), use of nonchlorinated water supplies, cellular immune-system suppression, and chronic disease of major organ systems (heart, lung, or kidneys). Solid organ and bone marrow transplant recipients and patients receiving immune-suppressive therapy for autoimmune diseases (eg, systemic lupus erythematosus, Crohn disease, rheumatoid arthritis) that target tumor necrosis factor are also at risk.[3,13] The incubation period typically ranges from 4 to 7 days; however, the infection can incubate for up to 2 weeks after primary exposure, making epidemiologic investigations challenging.[14]

PF is an acute influenza-like illness that is self-limiting and nonfatal. The early presentation may appear similar to LD; however, patients do not progress to pneumonia.[15–17] Unlike LD, treatment of PF is not indicated and is not discussed here in any further detail.

Pneumococcus

Asymptomatic colonization of the nasopharyngeal tract by pneumococcus occurs early in infancy, with almost all children being colonized at least once by 1 year of age.[18,19] Carriage rates for children younger than 5 years vary by geographic region, but can be as high as 99% in some parts of the developing world.[20] Colonizing pneumococci are generally cleared within a month, but new serotypes can successfully colonize the same individual.[20,21] Adult colonization is less frequently detected (~10%).[22]

Disease is associated with recent colonization by a serotype not previously encountered.[19] Encapsulated pneumococci migrate from the nasopharynx to the lung and can enter the bloodstream by translocating across the lung interstitium,[4] although this process is not a requirement for invasive disease. Production of pneumococcal pneumolysin leads to massive inflammation and destruction of host lung tissue.

There are currently more than 90 recognized serotypes of *Pneumococcus*. Vaccine development has centered on serotypes that produce the most severe phenotypes. The pneumococcal polysaccharide vaccine was released in 1977 but was not sufficiently immunogenic in children younger than 2 years.[23] As a result, the pneumococcal conjugate vaccine (PCV) was developed and originally released in 2000 (PCV7), with an expanded serotype coverage version released in 2010 (PCV13). Vaccination programs have dramatically reduced the vaccine-serotype colonization rates, which have in turn reduced the rate of disease.[24,25] Nonvaccine serotypes have begun to replace colonization by vaccine serotypes,[22,26] although it remains to be determined if these serotypes cause less severe disease.

S pneumoniae is still the leading cause of CAP and meningitis worldwide,[27–30] although rates of both diseases have begun to decrease with conjugate vaccine introduction.[29,31] Pneumococcal infections can lead to a variety of additional presentations, the most common being otitis media.

Histoplasma

H capsulatum disease is most prevalent in the Ohio-Mississippi river valley, with highest rates of endemicity in Indiana, Arkansas, Kentucky, and Mississippi owing to the ideal soil, temperature, and moisture conditions in these regions. Areas laden with avian excrement are particularly favored by this organism. Having the distinction of being the most common endemic mycoses in the United States, histoplasmosis has a predilection for older men, particularly those with chronic lung disease.[32] As a continent, North America claims most infections attributable to this pathogen; however, genetic studies have revealed 8 clades within 3 varieties that are found across the world and are responsible for varying clinical manifestations by region.[33,34]

In North America, acute and chronic localized disease is noted in immunocompetent individuals, whereas disseminated variants are found in immunocompromised hosts. Acute localized illness, typically affecting healthy individuals exposed to an abundant inoculum, manifests as a mild to severe flu-like syndrome with or without pneumonia, whereas chronic localized illness, transpiring in those with existing lung disease, presents with pneumonic consolidation, cavitation, and cough resembling tuberculosis. Disseminated presentations have a proclivity for affecting the hematopoietic system, lung, liver, and gastrointestinal tract.[9] By contrast, African and South American varieties are marked by prominent cutaneous and osseous involvement resembling blastomycosis.[35,36] The ability of *H capsulatum* to bind CD11-CD18 cellular receptors, enter macrophages by expression of heat-shock protein 60, and circumvent acidification in phagosomes is its primary means of pathogenesis and evasion of the immune system.[9]

DIAGNOSIS

Clinical symptoms and radiologic evidence of pneumonia is often the first indication of LD, histoplasmosis, and pneumococcal pneumonia. For each of these specific infections, the gold-standard diagnostic laboratory test remains culture of the offending pathogen from an appropriate clinical specimen (typically sputum or BAL). For both LD and histoplasmosis, serologic testing has historically been used as an adjunctive diagnostic tool that can be particularly helpful in retrospective investigation of illness. Of importance, the immunoglobulin G (IgG) antibody response may take several weeks to become detectable, limiting its utility particularly in LD beyond outbreak investigations.[37] Molecular methodologies using nucleic acid amplification are limited primarily to reference laboratories as laboratory-developed tests, and as a result are not routinely used diagnostic tools despite their excellent analytical sensitivity and specificity. Comprehensive descriptions of these and other methods have been reviewed in detail.[13,38] Advantages and disadvantages of each method are compared in **Table 1**.

Legionella Urinary Antigen Testing

Urine antigen testing has become a routine test method for the diagnosis of LD. The current *Legionella* urine antigen assays cleared by the Food and Drug Administration (FDA) are shown in **Table 2**, and are the focus of this article. Attributes of urinary antigen testing that are advantageous for LD include the relatively short TAT (particularly for LFAs), ability for laboratories to perform the testing on-site (near point of care for some assays), and very high specificity (paramount test characteristic for a rare pathogen). Antigenuria can be detected in as little as 24 hours after onset of clinical symptoms, and the typical shedding period can persist for several days or weeks.[13] For this reason, the use of serial testing for "test of cure" is limited and should be discouraged in most clinical situations. In fact, one report demonstrated persistent antigenuria for 300 days.[39] Alternatively, for patients with high pretest probability of LD who have a negative test result shortly after symptom onset, repeat testing in 2 to 3 days is indicated. The clinical sensitivity of urinary antigen testing is also associated with the severity of disease, whereby hospitalized patients are more likely to test positive than those with mild illness.[40,41]

Legionella urine antigen assays use capture antibodies specific for *L pneumophila* serogroup 1, which is considered the leading cause of LD. As a result, these assays perform best in the setting of *L pneumophila* serogroup 1 infections, with a pooled clinical sensitivity and specificity of 74% and 99%, respectively, for LD.[42] These data are based on a comprehensive meta-analysis, and the sensitivity value is drastically lower than those claimed by each individual manufacturer (see **Table 2**).[42] Essentially, this pooled clinical test performance indicates that a positive *Legionella* antigen test can indicate LD, whereas a negative one cannot reliably exclude the diagnosis. Other serogroups of *L pneumophila* and non-*pneumophila Legionella* spp are poorly detected by these assays (sensitivity of 5%–40%), which likely results in underappreciation of the true clinical role of these organisms.[43]

ELISA

ELISA was once the most commonly used method for urine antigen detection, and was primarily performed in reference laboratories and large academic medical centers. According to the most recent (2013) College of American Pathologists survey results, LFAs are now the most frequently used methodology, accounting for more than 95% of respondent laboratories. The results from these surveys show equivalent performance for both ELISA and LFAs. LFAs are advantageous to perform because the results are available near point of care, but clinical studies are mixed in terms of performance when compared with ELISA. For instance, published studies have demonstrated comparable sensitivity for ELISA and LFAs (echoing CAP survey results), whereas more recent studies have shown significantly lower sensitivity for LFAs.[41,44]

LFA

All 3 FDA-cleared LFAs (Meridian, SAS, and Binax) show improved sensitivity when the test is incubated an additional 60 minutes longer than the manufacturer's recommendation (importantly, with no loss in specificity).[41,45,46] In addition, urine

Table 1
Comparison of detection methods for *Legionella*, *Pneumococcus*, and *Histoplasma*

Test	Time to Result	Advantages	Disadvantages
Blood culture[a]	3 d to 1 wk (for *Histoplasma*)	Likely to identify true pathogen if detected; isolate for susceptibility testing and further investigation (eg, serotyping, sequencing)	Bacteremia not always associated with pneumonia
Sputum stain and culture	Minutes (Gram stain/DFA) to 2 d	Potential quick result could lead to targeted therapy; isolate for susceptibility and further investigation	Difficult to obtain good-quality specimen; colonizing pneumococcus can be detected. *Histoplasma* requires unique stains
Other lower respiratory tract	1–2 d	Likely to identify true pathogen if detected; isolate for susceptibility and further investigation	Invasive procedure limits utility
Molecular assays	2–4 h	Quick result; high sensitivity; may be able to include susceptibility or other genetic markers (species or serotyping)	No isolate for further testing; not standardized; many different laboratory-developed tests; colonizing *Pneumococcus* can be detected
Serology	2 h to 2 d	Useful for epidemiologic investigation; prognostic indicator for *Histoplasma*; can differentiate serotypes of *Pneumococcus*	Not useful for acute diagnosis; no isolate for further testing; pneumococcal vaccination confounds results
UAT	15 min[b]	Quick[b]; high specificity allows for rapid modification of therapy based on positive result; FDA-approved tests available[b]	No isolate for further testing; *Histoplasma* UAT not widely available

Abbreviations: DFA, direct fluorescent antibody; FDA, Food and Drug Administration; UAT, urine antigen test.
[a] Blood culture is of limited utility for *Legionella* infections.
[b] These characteristics are specific to the *Legionella* and pneumococcal UATs.

Table 2
Legionella UATs currently cleared by the FDA with manufacturer's stated test characteristics

Manufacturer	Product Name	Method	Sensitivity[a]	Specificity[a]	Comparison Method
Binax	*Legionella* Urinary Antigen EIA	ELISA	87	86	Culture
Trinity Biotech	Bartels *Legionella* urinary antigen ELISA test	ELISA	94.7	91.1	Culture
Alere	BinaxNOW *Legionella pneumophila* urinary antigen test	LFA	97	98	Binax ELISA
Meridian Biosciences	TRU Legionella Assay	LFA	95.5	100	BinaxNOW
Sa Scientific	SAS Legionella Test	LFA	90.5	95	BinaxNOW

[a] The values are stated by the manufacturer based on clinical studies submitted to the FDA and represent agreement values for the comparison method stated.

concentration for LFAs is recommended to maximize sensitivity, but is not included in the package inserts.[40,47] Similarly, several reports suggest that concentration of urine before testing can significantly increase the sensitivity of ELISA tests.[47,48] However, The Bartels ELISA, if performed on nonconcentrated urine, is more sensitive than the Binax ELISA.[49,50]

Pneumococcal Urinary Antigen Test

The Alere BinaxNOW is the only FDA-approved pneumococcal urine antigen test (pUAT), and is available as an LFA with antibodies directed against the pneumococcal C-polysaccharide protein. The test was released in 2003 and is also approved by the FDA for detection in cerebrospinal fluid (not reviewed). The pUAT can be performed by the bedside with results available in 15 minutes. Manufacturer-defined sensitivities range from 86% to 90%, specificity from 71% to 94%, and positive and negative predictive values from 31% to 59% and 98%, respectively. It is reported to detect 100% of 23 of the most important serotypes. Cross-reactivity is only reported with *Streptococcus mitis*. Pneumococcal polysaccharide vaccination does not cause false-positive detection more than 48 hours after vaccination; however, the PCV was not evaluated by the manufacturer. As a result, testing is not recommended on individuals vaccinated against *Pneumococcus* in the last 5 days.

Effects of study design on the sensitivity of the pUAT

Several studies have been published evaluating the clinical accuracy of the BinaxNOW pUAT. A clear theme in many of these studies is that the choice of gold standard significantly affects pUAT performance (compared in **Table 3**).

Studies that definitively diagnosed pneumococcal infection via blood or pleural fluid culture showed the highest sensitivity, ranging from 77% to 87%,[51–59] overlapping with, but lower than values defined by the manufacturer. Studies comparing a probable diagnosis based on sputum Gram stain, sputum culture, or nasopharyngeal specimens had lower sensitivities ranging from 44% to 60%.[51,54,55,57–60] The difference in sensitivities could be due to the culture of colonizing *Pneumococcus* from respiratory samples, rather than detection of a true pathogen. However, because CAP is often unaccompanied by bacteremia, it is unclear as to what the appropriate gold-standard comparator should be.

Table 3
Published sensitivities and specificities for given pneumococcal urine antigen test studies

Authors,[Ref.] Year	Sensitivity (%)	Gold Standard for Sensitivity Evaluation	Specificity (%)	Negative Controls for Specificity Evaluation	Additional Findings
Marcos et al,[54] 2003	77 / 44	Blood, BAL or pleural fluid culture / Sputum culture	93	Non-pneumo CAP	Concentrating urine gives better sensitivity
Dominguez et al,[52] 2001	82	Blood culture	97	Non-pneumo CAP, non-pneumo bacteremia, UTI	
Smith et al,[56] 2009	87 / 72	Blood culture / *Blood culture (non-CAP bacteremia)*[a]	98	Non-pneumo bacteremia or UTI	
Briones et al,[51] 2006	81 / 59	Blood or pleural fluid culture / Sputum Gram stain and/or sputum culture	80	Non-pneumo CAP	
Gutierrez et al,[53] 2003	77 / 64	Blood culture / *Pleural fluid or sputum culture*	90	Non-pneumo CAP	
Murdoch et al,[55] 2001	80 / 52	Blood culture / Sputum culture	100	Non-CAP, illness not specified	False-positive vaccine recipients (>5 d postvaccination)
Stralin et al,[58] 2004	79 / 47 / 54	Blood culture / Sputum culture / Nasopharyngeal swab/aspirate	98	Skin infection, urinary tract infection, non-ID related surgery	Better sensitivity in severe CAP
Sorde et al,[57] 2011	78 / 57	Blood or pleural fluid culture / Sputum Gram stain and/or sputum culture	96	Non-pneumo CAP	
Boulware et al,[59] 2007	85 / 60	Blood culture / Sputum Gram stain and/or sputum culture	98	Non-pneumo CAP	HIV status does not affect pUAT result
Guchev et al,[60] 2005	52	Sputum culture	99/100	N/A	
Genne et al,[62] 2006	64	Blood or respiratory culture		Healthy controls/non-pneumo CAP	
Roson et al,[61] 2004	66	Blood or respiratory culture	100	Non-pneumo CAP	Better sensitivity in severe CAP

Gold standard represents the method used to diagnose pneumococcal CAP. Non-pneumo CAP or bacteremia refers to the isolation of a pathogen other than *Pneumococcus*. Methods in italics highlight studies that did not separate definitive (eg, blood culture) from presumptive (eg, respiratory culture) pneumococcal pneumonia.

Abbreviations: BAL, bronchoalveolar lavage; CAP, community-acquired pneumonia; HIV, human immunodeficiency virus; N/A, no data available; pUAT, pneumococcal urine antigen test; UTI, urinary tract infection.

[a] This study used patients with pneumococcal bacteremia without pneumonia as a gold standard.

Study design does not seem to affect specificity. Testing in individuals with CAP caused by an organism other than *Pneumococcus* had specificity similar to that in individuals with nonpneumococcal bacteremia, urinary tract infections, or other noninfectious conditions, and in healthy adults (range 80%–100%; see **Table 3**).

Initiation of antibiotics before specimen collection can also confound study results. Many of the prospective studies in **Table 3** were unable to detect a pathogen by classic microbiology methods, but a large proportion (~20%) of these patients had positive pUATs.[51,53,61,62] Antibiotic therapy may limit recovery of *Pneumococcus* from blood or respiratory sites while antigen is still detectable in urine. Indeed, pneumococcal antigens are still detectable in most infected patients as many as 7 days after the initiation of therapy.[63]

Similarly to LD, there is a strong correlation between severity of symptoms and sensitivity of the pUAT.[58,60,61] Limiting pUAT performance to these classes might be more cost-effective. In fact, the Infectious Disease Society of America (IDSA) and American Thoracic Society (ATS) recommend the pUAT only in cases of severe or critical CAP.[64]

Colonization and the pUAT

As discussed earlier, pneumococcal carriage varies by age group. Although the manufacturer does not recommend restricting the use of the BinaxNOW, the package insert does admit a lack of evaluation in children. At least 2 studies reported that a large percentage (22%–54%) of colonized children had positive pUATs whereas only a small percentage (4%–21%) of noncarriers had positive pUATs, although it is possible that sampling methods missed colonizing pneumococcus in some of these individuals.[65,66] Unfortunately, this is a high false-positive rate in the population most frequently affected by pneumococcal CAP.[29] More studies are needed in different geographic regions to fully evaluate the false-positive rate and guide recommendations for pUAT use.

Histoplasma Antigen Testing

As for LD and pneumococcal CAP, tests to detect antigenuria in the context of histoplasmosis are routinely ordered, although such assays are best utilized in disseminated infection. Two commercially available tests exist, one of which is approved by the FDA; a third can be obtained through a private diagnostic company (Miravista Diagnostics [MVD], Indianapolis, IN).

Miravista Diagnostics enzyme immunoassay

In 1986, MVD published results of an *H capsulatum* antigen capture sandwich immunoassay capable of use on urine or serum. Polyclonal rabbit anti-*Histoplasma* IgG was used as capture and detect antibodies, with detect antibodies conjugated to [125]I. Levels of *H capsulatum* antigen relative to a negative control, in turn, were then expressed semiquantitatively in radioimmunoassay (RIA) units. Despite low sensitivity in localized pulmonary disease, greater than 90% and 50% sensitivity, respectively, were demonstrated in disseminated disease with the urine and serum assays. Cross-reactions were documented to various endemic fungi.[67] Similar positive findings were found with this RIA in pediatric and HIV patients with dissemination.[68,69] A drawback, however, is the requirement for radioactive materials.

Second generation More palatable enzyme immunoassays (EIAs) were subsequently developed by MVD. Using microwells coated with polyclonal anti-*Histoplasma* IgG, urine specimens were incubated, washed, and later exposed to alkaline phosphatase or horseradish peroxidase (HRP) enzymes conjugated to similar detect antibodies. After repeat washing, 1 of 2 substrates was then added depending on the conjugated enzyme, and colorimetric enzymatic reactions were expressed as EIA units relative to a mean negative control. Results of both EIAs reached sensitivity comparable with that of the RIA in disseminated histoplasmosis (~90%). Specificities for all methods exceeded 92%, though superior with the RIA and HRP-EIA. All methods had poor sensitivity (18%–50%) in localized (predominantly pulmonary) disease.[70] Further investigation confirmed the high correlation between the HRP-EIA and RIA, making the HRP-EIA preferred.[71]

Additional modifications to the HRP-EIA on serum (heat-EDTA treatment)[72] and urine (ultrafiltration)[73] have been implemented to increase sensitivity. Furthermore, owing to false-positive results in serum specimens in patients treated with rabbit antithymocyte globulin, alterations of the detect antibody and the HRP enzyme were undertaken.[74] Thus, current techniques use a modified biotinylated rabbit detect antibody, a streptavidin-HRP enzyme, and a tetramethylbenzidine substrate. If antigen is present in a specimen, a semiquantitative, colorimetric value in EIA units relative to a control is provided.

Third generation Further enhancement applying graded, standard concentrations of *Histoplasma* antigen (ng/mL) to each run has negated the need to express a result in reference to a mean negative control.[75] This third-generation assay (MVista EIA) yields a best-fit curve from the included standards with optical density measurements on the x-axis and concentration (ng/mL) on the y-axis, making it possible to extrapolate optical density (absorbance) of a sample to quantitative vales from 0.4 to 19 ng/mL. A detectable antigen level greater than 19 ng/mL or less than 0.4 ng/mL is reported as positive, but cannot be quantified, although the clinical utility in particular of registering "detected" levels of less than 0.4 ng/mL has not been elucidated.[76] With these improvements, sensitivity for disseminated infection is 100% for urine and 92% for serum; specificity is 99%.[75] For optimum test performance, simultaneous urine and serum assays are advised.[76] As with previous versions, cross-reactions occur with *Blastomyces dermatitidis, Paracoccidioides brasiliensis, Penicillium marneffei,*[77] *Sporothrix* species, and, infrequently, *Aspergillus* and *Coccidioides* species.[76] While this assay has been used on additional body fluids,[78] it is particularly valuable in BAL specimens where sensitivity and specificity may exceed 90% in patients with localized cavitary disease or disseminated disease with lung involvement.[79] Furthermore, antigen dynamics parallel successful therapy and can be used to identify recurrence.[80,81]

Thus, through a series of refinements, MVD offers a sensitive and specific, quantitative *H capsulatum* antigen EIA that is most useful in disseminated disease. Furthermore, this assay makes it possible to monitor therapy and detect recurrence. Unfortunately, this test is not commercially available and can only be executed at MVD on physician request.

Immuno-Mycologics EIA
A commercially available, FDA-cleared EIA that uses (polyclonal) antibodies and reagents similar to those of the MVista EIA, namely the IMMY ALPHA Histoplasma EIA (Immuno-Mycologics, Norman, OK), has been developed for urine and found to have greater than 90% agreement with the MVista EIA. Values are reported in EIA units by using "standards" analogous to the MVista EIA; levels of 2 or more EIA units are considered positive. False-positive results occur with various dimorphic fungi.[82] This test has not been validated to confirm successful treatment or document relapse, and data on specific patient presentations (systemic vs localized disease) are not readily available. Although the high correlation initially reported with the MVista EIA[82] was not later corroborated by MVD,[83] these findings are debated.[84] Recently,

Immuno-Mycologics has also developed an EIA using analyte-specific reagents (ASR) and a monoclonal capture/detect antibody for *Histoplasma* urinary antigen. Using a threshold of 0.5 ng/mL to denote a positive result, the sensitivity of this assay is 64.5% with specificity of 99.8% when using the MVista EIA as the gold standard. Results correlate with the MVista EIA more than 90% of the time. Of note, nearly half of values not concordant with the MVista EIA were 0.4 ng/mL or less by the MVista EIA, a range of dubious clinical significance.[85] In a related analysis involving immunocompromised patients with dissemination, the ASR monoclonal assay was directly compared with the polyclonal IMMY ALPHA kit. Higher sensitivity (90.5%), specificity (96.3%), and correlation with the MVista assay were noted with the monoclonal ASR test when compared with the polyclonal IMMY ALPHA.[86]

TREATMENT
Empiric Therapy for LD/Pneumococcal Pneumonia

The CAP treatment guidelines issued by the IDSA and ATS recommend empiric therapy for outpatients.[64] Empiric therapy in most outpatients consists of a newer-generation macrolide. For patients with significant comorbidities, a respiratory quinolone and β-lactam in combination with a macrolide are recommended.[64] For inpatients without intensive care unit (ICU) admission, the same 2 options as indicated for outpatients with comorbidities is appropriate. For patients admitted to the ICU, a β-lactam plus either a respiratory quinolone or macrolide is recommended.[64] In light of the test performance described herein for both pneumococcal *Legionella* urinary antigen testing, a positive test result supports the use of pathogen-targeted therapy.

Targeted Therapy for LD/Pneumococcal Pneumonia

The intracellular nature of *Legionella* is particularly important in choosing appropriate pathogen-directed antimicrobial therapy, as directed therapy for *S pneumoniae* using β-lactams will not provide adequate therapy for LD.[64] The official CAP treatment guidelines issued by the IDSA and ATS recommend either a fluoroquinolone or macrolide as targeted therapy for LD.[64] If concern for persistent fever is noted in *Legionella* CAP, a quinolone is preferred to older macrolides for its more rapid clinical response.[87] The length of therapy is typically 7 to 14 days in uncomplicated patients; however, therapy for immunocompromised patients often requires 21 days for adequate resolution of symptoms. Of importance, any significant delay in initiating antimicrobial therapy increases the mortality associated with LD.[88] Despite the ease with which many organisms develop resistance to quinolones, to date resistance is not a significant concern in LD, possibly because of the sporadic, environmentally derived nature of the outbreaks.

Resistance to β-lactams is a significant concern for *S pneumoniae* infections. Directed therapy, therefore, depends on knowing whether the causative organism is penicillin resistant or susceptible. Directed therapy is a β-lactam; however, many clinical/epidemiologic variables need to be considered and are beyond the scope of this work. The reader is referred to the IDSA/ATS guidelines for each specific recommendation.[64]

Treatment of Histoplasma

Treatment of histoplasmosis is intimately linked to the site of infection and presentation (localized disease vs disseminated disease). Traditional options include lipid versions of amphotericin B as induction (depending on severity) with consolidation regimens of itraconazole. Disseminated disease requires reduction in

Table 4
Treatment of *Histoplasma capsulatum* infection by disease manifestation[a]

Disease Manifestation	Treatment
Acute localized pulmonary	Itraconazole 12 wk[b]
Chronic cavitary (pulmonary)	Itraconazole 12 mo
Disseminated	Lipid formulation of amphotericin B followed by 12 mo itraconazole[c]
Histoplasmosis of central nervous system	Lipid formulation of amphotericin B 4–6 wk followed by 12 mo itraconazole
Pericarditis, mediastinal lymphadenopathy, pulmonary nodules, rheumatologic syndromes, broncholithiasis	No antifungal treatment indicated; may consider anti-inflammatory medicine in select cases

[a] Taken from the 2007 Infectious Disease Society of America guidelines.[89]
[b] Treatment indicated if illness present >1 month or if severe symptoms present.
[c] For milder disease, treatment is begun with itraconazole.

immunosuppression and addition of combined antiretroviral therapy in patients with acquired immunodeficiency syndrome. Newer triazoles (posaconazole, voriconazole) are reserved for refractory instances.[89] Treatment guidelines for histoplasmosis are summarized in **Table 4**.

SUMMARY AND DISCUSSION

Urinary antigen tests for LD and pneumococcal CAP are rapid and readily available methods of laboratory testing that should be incorporated into all testing algorithms for CAP. Use of these methods as front-end diagnostic tools can provide important early recognition of the pneumonia-causing agent, and provide early and appropriate administration of pathogen-targeted antimicrobial therapy. Despite the very high clinical specificity of urinary antigen tests for LD and pneumococcal CAP, the comparatively lower clinical sensitivity of these assays cannot effectively exclude disease.

Although urine antigen testing provides diagnostic benefit, culture remains a necessary epidemiologic tool for the interrogation of LD and pneumococcal CAP. Cultured isolates provide invaluable information for outbreak investigations and, in the case of *Pneumococcus*, surveying localized rates of antimicrobial resistance and associated serotypes. For this reason, culture and antigen detection are an ideal diagnostic combination for comprehensive clinical investigation of these diseases.

Urine and serum antigen testing for histoplasmosis has revolutionized the diagnosis of this disease, particularly if disseminated, and effectively supplants serologic testing in particular in such a setting, owing to concomitant immunosuppression. A caveat is that urine and serum antigen performance is much less robust in more focal respiratory disease, where additional investigation including serology, culture, and histopathology is still recommended. Ostensibly, while the MVista EIA maintains the preponderance of evidence supporting use, it is not as readily available as the polyclonal IMMY ALPHA EIA. Finally, the monoclonal IMMY ASR assay, also available commercially, shows promise, but requires further scrutiny before widespread implementation.

REFERENCES

1. She RC, Billetdeaux E, Phansalkar AR, et al. Limited applicability of direct fluorescent-antibody testing for *Bordetella* sp. and *Legionella* sp. specimens for the clinical microbiology laboratory. J Clin Microbiol 2007;45(7):2212–4.

2. Rowbotham TJ. Preliminary report on the pathogenicity of *Legionella pneumophila* for freshwater and soil amoebae. J Clin Pathol 1980;33(12):1179–83.
3. Edelstein PH, Cianciotto NP. Legionella. In: Mandell GL, Bennett JE, Dolin R, editors. Principles and practice of infectious diseases. 7th edition. Philadelphia: Churchill Livingstone/Elsevier; 2010. p. 2967–84.
4. van der Poll T, Opal SM. Pathogenesis, treatment, and prevention of pneumococcal pneumonia. Lancet 2009;374(9700):1543–56.
5. Kim JO, Weiser JN. Association of intrastrain phase variation in quantity of capsular polysaccharide and teichoic acid with the virulence of *Streptococcus pneumoniae*. J Infect Dis 1998;177(2):368–77.
6. Yother J. Capsules of *Streptococcus pneumoniae* and other bacteria: paradigms for polysaccharide biosynthesis and regulation. Annu Rev Microbiol 2011;65:563–81.
7. Lijek RS, Luque SL, Liu Q, et al. Protection from the acquisition of *Staphylococcus aureus* nasal carriage by cross-reactive antibody to a pneumococcal dehydrogenase. Proc Natl Acad Sci U S A 2012;109(34):13823–8.
8. Lijek RS, Weiser JN. Co-infection subverts mucosal immunity in the upper respiratory tract. Curr Opin Immunol 2012;24(4):417–23.
9. Bradsher RW. Histoplasmosis and blastomycosis. Clin Infect Dis 1996;22(Suppl 2):S102–11.
10. Kwon-Chung KJ, Weeks RJ, Larsh HW. Studies on *Emmonsiella capsulata* (*Histoplasma capsulatum*). II. Distribution of the two mating types in 13 endemic states of the United States. Am J Epidemiol 1974;99(1):44–9.
11. Swanson MS, Hammer BK. *Legionella pneumophila* pathogenesis: a fateful journey from amoebae to macrophages. Annu Rev Microbiol 2000;54:567–613.
12. Tsai TF, Finn DR, Plikaytis BD, et al. Legionnaires' disease: clinical features of the epidemic in Philadelphia. Ann Intern Med 1979;90(4):509–17.
13. Diederen BM. *Legionella* spp. and Legionnaires' disease. J Infect 2008;56(1):1–12.
14. Den Boer JW, Yzerman EP, Schellekens J, et al. A large outbreak of Legionnaires' disease at a flower show, the Netherlands, 1999. Emerg Infect Dis 2002;8(1):37–43.
15. Burnsed LJ, Hicks LA, Smithee LM, et al. A large, travel-associated outbreak of legionellosis among hotel guests: utility of the urine antigen assay in confirming Pontiac fever. Clin Infect Dis 2007;44(2):222–8.
16. Edelstein PH. Urine antigen tests positive for Pontiac fever: implications for diagnosis and pathogenesis. Clin Infect Dis 2007;44(2):229–31.
17. Tossa P, Deloge-Abarkan M, Zmirou-Navier D, et al. Pontiac fever: an operational definition for epidemiological studies. BMC Public Health 2006;6:112.
18. Vives M, Garcia ME, Saenz P, et al. Nasopharyngeal colonization in Costa Rican children during the first year of life. Pediatr Infect Dis J 1997;16(9):852–8.
19. Gray BM, Converse GM 3rd, Dillon HC Jr. Epidemiologic studies of *Streptococcus pneumoniae* in infants: acquisition, carriage, and infection during the first 24 months of life. J Infect Dis 1980;142(6):923–33.
20. Hill PC, Townend J, Antonio M, et al. Transmission of *Streptococcus pneumoniae* in rural Gambian villages: a longitudinal study. Clin Infect Dis 2010;50(11):1468–76.
21. Abdullahi O, Karani A, Tigoi CC, et al. Rates of acquisition and clearance of pneumococcal serotypes in the nasopharynges of children in Kilifi District, Kenya. J Infect Dis 2012;206(7):1020–9.

22. Spijkerman J, Prevaes SM, van Gils EJ, et al. Long-term effects of pneumo-coccal conjugate vaccine on nasopharyngeal carriage of *S. pneumoniae*, *S. aureus*, *H. influenzae* and *M. catarrhalis*. PLoS One 2012;7(6):e39730.

23. Talbot TR, Poehling KA, Hartert TV, et al. Reduction in high rates of antibiotic-nonsusceptible invasive pneumococcal disease in Tennessee after introduc-tion of the pneumococcal conjugate vaccine. Clin Infect Dis 2004;39(5): 641–8.

24. Simell B, Auranen K, Kayhty H, et al. The fundamental link between pneumo-coccal carriage and disease. Expert Rev Vaccines 2012;11(7):841–55.

25. van Gils EJ, Veenhoven RH, Hak E, et al. Effect of reduced-dose schedules with 7-valent pneumococcal conjugate vaccine on nasopharyngeal pneumo-coccal carriage in children: a randomized controlled trial. JAMA 2009;302(2): 159–67.

26. Jacobs MR, Good CE, Bajaksouzian S, et al. Emergence of *Streptococcus pneumoniae* serotypes 19A, 6C, and 22F and serogroup 15 in Cleveland, Ohio, in relation to introduction of the protein-conjugated pneumococcal vac-cine. Clin Infect Dis 2008;47(11):1388–95.

27. Johansson N, Kalin M, Tiveljung-Lindell A, et al. Etiology of community-acquired pneumonia: increased microbiological yield with new diagnostic methods. Clin Infect Dis 2010;50(2):202–9.

28. Honkinen M, Lahti E, Osterback R, et al. Viruses and bacteria in sputum sam-ples of children with community-acquired pneumonia. Clin Microbiol Infect 2012;18(3):300–7.

29. Walker CL, Rudan I, Liu L, et al. Global burden of childhood pneumonia and diarrhoea. Lancet 2013;381(9875):1405–16.

30. Thigpen MC, Whitney CG, Messonnier NE, et al. Bacterial meningitis in the United States, 1998-2007. N Engl J Med 2011;364(21):2016–25.

31. McIntyre PB, O'Brien KL, Greenwood B, et al. Effect of vaccines on bacterial meningitis worldwide. Lancet 2012;380(9854):1703–11.

32. Baddley JW, Winthrop KL, Patkar NM, et al. Geographic distribution of endemic fungal infections among older persons, United States. Emerg Infect Dis 2011; 17(9):1664–9.

33. Kasuga T, Taylor JW, White TJ. Phylogenetic relationships of varieties and geographical groups of the human pathogenic fungus *Histoplasma capsulatum* Darling. J Clin Microbiol 1999;37(3):653–63.

34. Kasuga T, White TJ, Koenig G, et al. Phylogeography of the fungal pathogen *Histoplasma capsulatum*. Mol Ecol 2003;12(12):3383–401.

35. Loulergue P, Bastides F, Baudouin V, et al. Literature review and case histories of *Histoplasma capsulatum* var. *duboisii* infections in HIV-infected patients. Emerg Infect Dis 2007;13(11):1647–52.

36. Goldani LZ, Aquino VR, Lunardi LW, et al. Two specific strains of *Histoplasma capsulatum* causing mucocutaneous manifestations of histoplasmosis: prelimi-nary analysis of a frequent manifestation of histoplasmosis in southern Brazil. Mycopathologia 2009;167(4):181–6.

37. Monforte R, Estruch R, Vidal J, et al. Delayed seroconversion in Legionnaire's disease. Lancet 1988;2(8609):513.

38. Edelstein PH. Chapter 45: Legionella. In: Versalovic J, Carroll KC, Funke G, edi-tors. Manual of Clinical Microbiology. 10th edition. Washington, DC: ASM Press; 2011. p. 770–85.

39. Kohler RB, Winn WC Jr, Wheat LJ. Onset and duration of urinary antigen excre-tion in Legionnaires disease. J Clin Microbiol 1984;20(4):605–7.

40. Yzerman EP, den Boer JW, Lettinga KD, et al. Sensitivity of three urinary antigen tests associated with clinical severity in a large outbreak of Legionnaires' disease in The Netherlands. J Clin Microbiol 2002;40(9):3232–6.

41. Helbig JH, Uldum SA, Luck PC, et al. Detection of *Legionella pneumophila* antigen in urine samples by the BinaxNOW immunochromatographic assay and comparison with both Binax Legionella Urinary Enzyme Immunoassay (EIA) and Biotest Legionella Urin Antigen EIA. J Med Microbiol 2001;50(6): 509–16.

42. Shimada T, Noguchi Y, Jackson JL, et al. Systematic review and metaanalysis: urinary antigen tests for Legionellosis. Chest 2009;136(6):1576–85.

43. Fields BS, Benson RF, Besser RE. Legionella and Legionnaires' disease: 25 years of investigation. Clin Microbiol Rev 2002;15(3):506–26.

44. Svarrer CW, Luck C, Elverdal PL, et al. Immunochromatic kits Xpect Legionella and BinaxNOW Legionella for detection of *Legionella pneumophila* urinary antigen have low sensitivities for the diagnosis of Legionnaires' disease. J Med Microbiol 2012;61(Pt 2):213–7.

45. Bruin JP, Diederen BM. Evaluation of Meridian TRU *Legionella*(R), a new rapid test for detection of *Legionella pneumophila* serogroup 1 antigen in urine samples. Eur J Clin Microbiol Infect Dis 2013;32(3):333–4.

46. Diederen BM, Peeters MF. Evaluation of the SAS Legionella Test, a new immunochromatographic assay for the detection of *Legionella pneumophila* serogroup 1 antigen in urine. Clin Microbiol Infect 2007;13(1):86–8.

47. Guerrero C, Toldos CM, Yague G, et al. Comparison of diagnostic sensitivities of three assays (Bartels enzyme immunoassay [EIA], Biotest EIA, and Binax NOW immunochromatographic test) for detection of *Legionella pneumophila* serogroup 1 antigen in urine. J Clin Microbiol 2004;42(1):467–8.

48. Dominguez JA, Manterola JM, Blavia R, et al. Detection of *Legionella pneumophila* serogroup 1 antigen in nonconcentrated urine and urine concentrated by selective ultrafiltration. J Clin Microbiol 1996;34(9):2334–6.

49. de Ory F. Evaluation of a new ELISA (Bartels) for detection of *Legionella pneumophila* antigen in urine. Enferm Infecc Microbiol Clin 2002;20(3):106–9 [in Spanish].

50. Dominguez J, Gali N, Blanco S, et al. Assessment of a new test to detect Legionella urinary antigen for the diagnosis of Legionnaires' disease. Diagn Microbiol Infect Dis 2001;41(4):199–203.

51. Briones ML, Blanquer J, Ferrando D, et al. Assessment of analysis of urinary pneumococcal antigen by immunochromatography for etiologic diagnosis of community-acquired pneumonia in adults. Clin Vaccine Immunol 2006;13(10): 1092–7.

52. Dominguez J, Gali N, Blanco S, et al. Detection of *Streptococcus pneumoniae* antigen by a rapid immunochromatographic assay in urine samples. Chest 2001;119(1):243–9.

53. Gutierrez F, Masia M, Rodriguez JC, et al. Evaluation of the immunochromatographic Binax NOW assay for detection of *Streptococcus pneumoniae* urinary antigen in a prospective study of community-acquired pneumonia in Spain. Clin Infect Dis 2003;36(3):286–92.

54. Marcos MA, Jimenez de Anta MT, de la Bellacasa JP, et al. Rapid urinary antigen test for diagnosis of pneumococcal community-acquired pneumonia in adults. Eur Respir J 2003;21(2):209–14.

55. Murdoch DR, Laing RT, Mills GD, et al. Evaluation of a rapid immunochromatographic test for detection of *Streptococcus pneumoniae* antigen in urine

samples from adults with community-acquired pneumonia. J Clin Microbiol 2001;39(10):3495–8.

56. Smith MD, Sheppard CL, Hogan A, et al. Diagnosis of *Streptococcus pneumoniae* infections in adults with bacteremia and community-acquired pneumonia: clinical comparison of pneumococcal PCR and urinary antigen detection. J Clin Microbiol 2009;47(4):1046–9.

57. Sorde R, Falco V, Lowak M, et al. Current and potential usefulness of pneumococcal urinary antigen detection in hospitalized patients with community-acquired pneumonia to guide antimicrobial therapy. Arch Intern Med 2011; 171(2):166–72.

58. Stralin K, Kaltoft MS, Konradsen HB, et al. Comparison of two urinary antigen tests for establishment of pneumococcal etiology of adult community-acquired pneumonia. J Clin Microbiol 2004;42(8):3620–5.

59. Boulware DR, Daley CL, Merrifield C, et al. Rapid diagnosis of pneumococcal pneumonia among HIV-infected adults with urine antigen detection. J Infect 2007;55(4):300–9.

60. Guchev IA, Yu VL, Sinopalnikov A, et al. Management of nonsevere pneumonia in military trainees with the urinary antigen test for *Streptococcus pneumoniae*: an innovative approach to targeted therapy. Clin Infect Dis 2005;40(11):1608–16.

61. Roson B, Fernandez-Sabe N, Carratala J, et al. Contribution of a urinary antigen assay (Binax NOW) to the early diagnosis of pneumococcal pneumonia. Clin Infect Dis 2004;38(2):222–6.

62. Genne D, Siegrist HH, Lienhard R. Enhancing the etiologic diagnosis of community-acquired pneumonia in adults using the urinary antigen assay (Binax NOW). Int J Infect Dis 2006;10(2):124–8.

63. Smith MD, Derrington P, Evans R, et al. Rapid diagnosis of bacteremic pneumococcal infections in adults by using the Binax NOW *Streptococcus pneumoniae* urinary antigen test: a prospective, controlled clinical evaluation. J Clin Microbiol 2003;41(7):2810–3.

64. Mandell LA, Wunderink RG, Anzueto A, et al. Infectious Diseases Society of America/American Thoracic Society consensus guidelines on the management of community-acquired pneumonia in adults. Clin Infect Dis 2007;44(Suppl 2): S27–72.

65. Hamer DH, Egas J, Estrella B, et al. Assessment of the Binax NOW *Streptococcus pneumoniae* urinary antigen test in children with nasopharyngeal pneumococcal carriage. Clin Infect Dis 2002;34(7):1025–8.

66. Dowell SF, Garman RL, Liu G, et al. Evaluation of Binax NOW, an assay for the detection of pneumococcal antigen in urine samples, performed among pediatric patients. Clin Infect Dis 2001;32(5):824–5.

67. Wheat LJ, Kohler RB, Tewari RP. Diagnosis of disseminated histoplasmosis by detection of *Histoplasma capsulatum* antigen in serum and urine specimens. N Engl J Med 1986;314(2):83–8.

68. Fojtasek MF, Kleiman MB, Connolly-Stringfield P, et al. The *Histoplasma capsulatum* antigen assay in disseminated histoplasmosis in children. Pediatr Infect Dis J 1994;13(9):801–5.

69. Wheat LJ, Connolly-Stringfield P, Kohler RB, et al. *Histoplasma capsulatum* polysaccharide antigen detection in diagnosis and management of disseminated histoplasmosis in patients with acquired immunodeficiency syndrome. Am J Med 1989;87(4):396–400.

70. Zimmerman SE, Stringfield PC, Wheat LJ, et al. Comparison of sandwich solid-phase radioimmunoassay and two enzyme-linked immunosorbent assays for

detection of *Histoplasma capsulatum* polysaccharide antigen. J Infect Dis 1989; 160(4):678–85.

71. Durkin MM, Connolly PA, Wheat LJ. Comparison of radioimmunoassay and enzyme-linked immunoassay methods for detection of *Histoplasma capsulatum var. capsulatum* antigen. J Clin Microbiol 1997;35(9):2252–5.

72. Swartzentruber S, LeMonte A, Witt J, et al. Improved detection of *Histoplasma* antigenemia following dissociation of immune complexes. Clin Vaccine Immunol 2009;16(3):320–2.

73. Egan L, Connolly PA, Fuller D, et al. Detection of *Histoplasma capsulatum* antigenuria by ultrafiltration of samples with false-negative results. Clin Vaccine Immunol 2008;15(4):726–8.

74. Wheat LJ, Witt J 3rd, Durkin M, et al. Reduction in false antigenemia in the second generation *Histoplasma* antigen assay. Med Mycol 2007;45(2): 169–71.

75. Connolly PA, Durkin MM, Lemonte AM, et al. Detection of histoplasma antigen by a quantitative enzyme immunoassay. Clin Vaccine Immunol 2007;14(12): 1587–91.

76. Wheat L. MVista *Histoplasma capsulatum* quantitative antigen EIA. 2013. Available at: http://www.miravistalabs.com/medical-testing/histoplasmosis/. Accessed December 15, 2014.

77. Wheat J, Wheat H, Connolly P, et al. Cross-reactivity in *Histoplasma capsulatum* variety capsulatum antigen assays of urine samples from patients with endemic mycoses. Clin Infect Dis 1997;24(6):1169–71.

78. Wheat LJ, Kohler RB, Tewari RP, et al. Significance of *Histoplasma* antigen in the cerebrospinal fluid of patients with meningitis. Arch Intern Med 1989;149(2): 302–4.

79. Hage CA, Davis TE, Fuller D, et al. Diagnosis of histoplasmosis by antigen detection in BAL fluid. Chest 2010;137(3):623–8.

80. Williams BJ, Connolly-Stringfield P, Bartlett M, et al. Correlation of *Histoplasma capsulatum* polysaccharide antigen with the severity of infection in murine histoplasmosis. J Clin Lab Anal 1991;5(2):121–6.

81. Wheat LJ, Connolly-Stringfield P, Blair R, et al. Histoplasmosis relapse in patients with AIDS: detection using *Histoplasma capsulatum* variety capsulatum antigen levels. Ann Intern Med 1991;115(12):936–41.

82. Cloud JL, Bauman SK, Neary BP, et al. Performance characteristics of a polyclonal enzyme immunoassay for the quantitation of *Histoplasma* antigen in human urine samples. Am J Clin Pathol 2007;128(1):18–22.

83. LeMonte A, Egan L, Connolly P, et al. Evaluation of the IMMY ALPHA *Histoplasma* antigen enzyme immunoassay for diagnosis of histoplasmosis marked by antigenuria. Clin Vaccine Immunol 2007;14(6):802–3.

84. Cloud JL, Bauman SK, Pelfrey JM, et al. Biased report on the IMMY ALPHA *Histoplasma* antigen enzyme immunoassay for diagnosis of histoplasmosis. Clin Vaccine Immunol 2007;14(10):1389–90 [author reply: 1390–1].

85. Theel ES, Jespersen DJ, Harring J, et al. Evaluation of an enzyme immunoassay for detection of *Histoplasma capsulatum* antigen from urine specimens. J Clin Microbiol 2013;51(11):3555–9.

86. Zhang X, Gibson B Jr, Daly TM. Evaluation of commercially available reagents for the diagnosis of histoplasmosis infection in immunocompromised patients. J Clin Microbiol 2013;51(12):4095–101.

87. Sabria M, Pedro-Botet ML, Gomez J, et al. Fluoroquinolones vs macrolides in the treatment of Legionnaires disease. Chest 2005;128(3):1401–5.

88. Heath CH, Grove DI, Looke DF. Delay in appropriate therapy of *Legionella* pneumonia associated with increased mortality. Eur J Clin Microbiol Infect Dis 1996; 15(4):286–90.
89. Wheat LJ, Freifeld AG, Kleiman MB, et al. Clinical practice guidelines for the management of patients with histoplasmosis: 2007 update by the Infectious Diseases Society of America. Clin Infect Dis 2007;45(7):807–25.

Pertussis
Relevant Species and Diagnostic Update

Amy L. Leber, PhD, D(ABMM)

KEYWORDS

- Pertussis laboratory diagnosis • *Bordetella* epidemiology • *Bordetella pertussis* PCR
- Pertussis serology • *Bordetella holmesii* infection • *Bordetella parapertussis* infection

KEY POINTS

- Pertussis cases are increasing as a result of multiple factors, including increasing awareness by clinicians, decreased effectiveness of acellular vaccines, and improved detection with molecular methods.
- *Bordetella pertussis* is the causative agent of pertussis but other *Bordetella* species such as *B parapertussis*, and more recently, *B holmesii*, have been associated with pertussislike illness.
- Laboratory diagnosis of pertussis is made using various test methods, with molecular methods supplanting culture in many settings because of their increased sensitivity. Serology is useful particularly in diagnosis of prolonged cough, but standardized methods that are commercially available are needed.
- The targets used for molecular detection are varied. Laboratorians must consider if detection and differentiation of various species, such as *B pertussis*, *B parapertussis*, and *B holmesii*, is necessary for the patient population when choosing a particular amplified testing approach.

INTRODUCTION

Bordetella pertussis is the causative agent of pertussis, also called whooping cough or the cough of 100 days. Infection can result in significant morbidity and mortality, particularly in young infants. Our understanding of the epidemiology of pertussis and pertussislike illness is expanding, in part based on molecular-based diagnostic testing. The role of other *Bordetella* species, such as *B parapertussis*, in causing illness has been appreciated for some time. More recently, *B holmesii* has emerged as a potentially significant pathogen in respiratory illness.

Despite widespread vaccination, pertussis is still present, with peaks occurring every 3 to 5 years, and the number of cases has been increasing. Evidence is mounting that the use of current acellular vaccines for control of *B pertussis* infection

Department of Pathology and Laboratory Medicine, Nationwide Children's Hospital, The Ohio State University College of Medicine, 700 Children's Drive, Columbus, OH 43205, USA
E-mail address: amy.leber@nationwidechildrens.org

Clin Lab Med 34 (2014) 237–255
http://dx.doi.org/10.1016/j.cll.2014.02.003
0272-2712/14/$ – see front matter © 2014 Elsevier Inc. All rights reserved.

may not provide strong or lasting immunity. Efforts to increase immunity through booster vaccination and also to improve the clinical and laboratory diagnosis of the disease are important to prevent outbreaks of disease.

The use of sensitive diagnostic tests, such as polymerase chain reaction (PCR), has become standard of care in many settings. Culture, although highly specific, presents significant challenges, including reduced sensitivity and increased time to result compared with PCR. In contrast to the advantages of molecular testing mentioned, there are potential problems related to specificity and cross-reactions that complicate the interpretation of test results for pertussis diagnosis. The complexity of molecular targets used for diagnosis must be understood fully, with an eye toward judicious use of resources balanced against a desire to better understand the epidemiology of pertussis.

Serology can plan a significant role in detecting individuals infected with *B pertussis*. The specific antigens used in testing and the cutoff values must be well understood to interpret the meaning of serologic results, particularly in those previously vaccinated against pertussis.

In this article, the laboratory diagnosis of pertussis is discussed, including the pros and cons of various test methods, including PCR and serology. Because *B parapertussis* causes a clinically similar, although often milder, respiratory infection than *B pertussis*, detection and differentiation of the two bacteria are often desirable. Recent data related to the detection of *B holmesii* in individuals with respiratory symptoms suggest that detection of this organism may be important. The other *Bordetella* species are not discussed in detail, except as they relate to diagnostic problems caused by cross-reactions in laboratory tests. The reader is referred to comprehensive reviews by others for a full discussion of all diagnostic testing for *Bordetella*.[1–4]

MICROBIOLOGY

Bordetella species are gram-negative coccobacilli that grow aerobically at optimal temperatures between 35°C and 37°C. They are all closely related genetically and grouped within the family Alcaligenaceae. They are differentiated into species based primarily on phenotypic traits such as growth characteristic and biochemical reactions (catalase, oxidase, urease production, and motility). Molecular methods such as 16S ribosomal RNA gene sequencing do not adequately differentiate among all species of *Bordetella*, because of their close genetic relatedness.[5] There are currently 10 reported species in the genus: *B pertussis*, *B parapertussis*, bovine-associated *B parapertussis*, *B brochiseptica*, *B avium*, *B hinzii*, *B holmesii*, *B trematum*, *B petri*, and *B ansorpii*.

B pertussis is a nonmotile, oxidase-positive, catalase-positive organism, with a fastidious growth requirement for culture (see section on culture). The organism is a strict aerobe and is relatively inert biochemically. *B parapertussis* is similar to *B pertussis* in that it is catalase positive and nonmotile; however, it is oxidase negative and less fastidious in culture. It can be differentiated from *B pertussis* by being urease positive and producing a soluble brown pigment on peptone agars such as Mueller Hinton or heart infusion agar.[6] *B holmesii* and *B bronchiseptica* also are not fastidious and grow on routine microbiological media. *B holmesii* is urease negative, whereas *B bronchiseptica* produces a rapid urease reaction.

EPIDEMIOLOGY

Before the availability of effective vaccines, pertussis was a major cause of childhood disease. With the advent of vaccines, the incidence of disease declined dramatically into the 1970s. However, pertussis is still present, with peaks occurring every 3 to

5 years. The number of reported cases has been increasing in the United States since the 1980s, despite widespread vaccination. **Fig. 1** shows the incidence of disease by age group for 1990 to 2009. The highest rates are in infants younger than 1 year, but adolescents and young adults have contributed a growing proportion of cases over the last several years.[7]

With reports of numerous outbreaks of pertussis across the United States, there is heightened interest in the control and diagnosis of the disease. A documented pertussis outbreak in California during 2010 (the largest outbreak in California in more than 60 years) resulted in more than 5900 reported cases from January to October 19, 2010 including 10 deaths in infants, all younger than 3 months.[8] More than 48,000 cases were reported in the United States in 2012. Multiple factors may influence the increased numbers of reported cases, including heightened physician awareness, more sensitive testing methods, waning immunity, and other vaccine-related phenomena, such as poor immunogenicity, antigen variation, and loss of expression of key antigens.[9–12]

The impact of other *Bordetella* species on our understanding of the epidemiology of pertussis illness is emerging as an import area of research. Parapertussis is estimated to represent 2% to 20% of pertussis cases in various settings, with infection most common during the first 5 years of life.[2,13] It has also been associated with bacteremia in children.[14]

B holmseii was believed to be a rare isolate in humans, with some reports of septicemia in immunocompromised patients.[15,16] In respiratory specimens, it has been reported in some populations (prevalence ranging from 0.3% to <4% of cultured specimens in a Massachusetts study)[17,18]; however, it has also been reported to be absent in others.[19,20] As is detailed later, the use of targets for PCR has significant implications on the ability to detect and recognizing the role of *B holmesii*.

Several recent studies have provided convincing evidence that *B holmesii* can cause pertussislike illness. The first documented mixed outbreak of *B pertussis* and

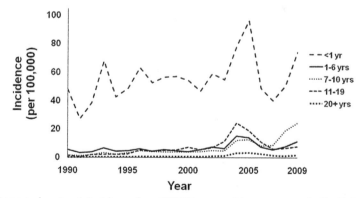

Fig. 1. Reported pertussis incidence (per 100,000 persons) by age group in the United States from 1990 to 2009. Infants younger than 6 months, who are at greatest risk for severe disease and death, continue to have the highest reported rate of pertussis, with a 60% increase in incidence observed between 2008 and 2009 (79.4/100,000 in 2008; 127/100,000 in 2009). Although adolescents (aged 11–19 years) and adults (aged >20 years) accounted for approximately 40% of reported cases in 2009, persons aged 7 to 10 years have contributed an increasing proportion of cases over the last several years (23% of cases in 2009, 23.5% of cases in 2008, 13% in 2007, 9% in 2006). (*From* Centers for Disease Control and Protection. Pertussis (whooping cough) surveillance and reporting. Available at: http://www.cdc.gov/pertussis/surv-reporting.html#trends. Accessed December 15, 2013.)

B holmesii infections was reported in central Ohio during 2010 to 2011, with most cases being tested in the author's own laboratory.[21] Additional analysis of this outbreak revealed that B parapertussis was also circulating during this same period. The PCR results used for initial diagnosis were confirmed by isolation of the three species in culture.[22] B holmesii particularly affected older children; among 48 patients with B holmesii infections, 63% were aged 11 to 18 years, compared with 35% of 112 patients with B pertussis infections.[21] Symptoms were similar among B holmesii-infected and B pertussis-infected patients.

In a retrospective analysis of samples tested for pertussis, a group in France also reported a significant number of cases of B holmesii (20.3% of 177 samples) in adolescent and adult patients.[23] Workers in Japan reported on infections with B holmesii among adolescents and adults identified in a laboratory-based active surveillance.[24] These investigators provide some evidence of human-to-human transmission among students and a teacher at a junior high school.[24]

B brochiseptica is a known respiratory pathogen in mammals, such as dogs and pigs. It has been detected in humans, most often in association with immunocompromise, or close links to infected animals.[2] However, others have stated that this organism has little or no relevance to human upper respiratory infections.[25]

CLINICAL PRESENTATIONS

Classic pertussis has a characteristic, if not always pathognomonic, clinical presentation, involving 3 stages:

- The catarrhal or prodromal stage is characterized by a mild coldlike presentation lasting 1 to 3 weeks.
- The paroxysmal stage is next and is characterized by spasms of uncontrollable coughing, often followed by an inspiratory whoop. Vomiting may also be seen at the end of the paroxysms. This stage may last up to 6 weeks or more.
- The convalescent stage is last, in which recovery begins and the cough lessens in intensity and duration. Symptoms may persist for up to 6 months.

Systemic manifestations, such as significant fever, are not common with the infection although leukocytosis with lymphocytosis is seen in most unvaccinated children related to the action of pertussis toxin.[2] B parapertussis infection can present much like B pertussis, although it is often less severe, and lymphocytosis is uncommon.[26]

The clinical picture of pertussis described earlier is more often seen in immunologically naive individuals, particularly in children aged 1 to 10 years. Infections in infants less than 1 year are often severe, with pulmonary hypertension, cyanosis, apnea, and seizures, and may lead to death; the highest morbidity and mortality are seen in infants. Immunization and previous infection can modify the disease, resulting in atypical presentations, ranging from prolonged and repetitive cough to milder respiratory disease. In adults and adolescents with prolonged cough, B pertussis is common, although it might often remain undiagnosed,[2] and although there is no evidence of a chronic carrier state, there is substantial evidence for mild or subclinical infections in adults and adolescents.[27,28]

PATHOGENESIS, IMMUNITY, AND VACCINATION

B pertussis transmission occurs by inhalation of droplets from other infected individuals. Once inhaled, the organisms attach to the ciliated epithelium in the upper respiratory tract. There, they evade the host immune system, leading to local tissue

systemic manifestations. Attack rates are high (>70%), and trans-
st earlier in the illness.

ces numerous virulence factors, including filamentous hemagglu-
, pertactin, adenylate cyclase dermonecrotic toxin, and tracheal
B pertussis is the production of pertussis toxin. Although believed
r many of the symptoms associated with disease, the exact role of
is still unclear.[2] Other Bordetella species such as B parapertussis,
ochiseptica do not produce toxin; although they contain the gene,
, because of lack of a functional promoter region.

ely a human pathogen, whereas B parapertussis has been isolated
heep. B brochiseptica is found in the respiratory tract of many an-
ly from humans. The isolation of B holmesii in humans had been
th disease but recent evidence suggests it is an agent of pertussis-

tussis after natural infection or vaccination is reported to last for 6
immunity wanes, reinfection can occur. Although disease may be
, transmission of the bacterium to other susceptible individuals is
are particularly vulnerable to infection, because the vaccination
t until 2 months of age and there may be no transplacental immu-
he mother. The use of immunization for young children is firmly
United States and was highly effective in reducing the incidence
until recently.

able vaccines contain acellular pertussis components combined
ohtheria. The childhood series is given in 5 doses at ages 2, 4, 5,
booster at age 4 to 6 years. Another booster dose of a combination
and acellular pertussis vaccine with reduced antigenicity (Tdap)
as of 2006 for use in 11-year-olds to 64-year-olds to supplement
nation series.[35,36] The goal of these newer recommendations is
immunity after the initial childhood series. Data derived from the
in 2010 suggest that immunity after the fifth booster may wane
native vaccines or different schedules may be warranted.[37]

tions with both B parapertussis and B holmesii may falsely
ent clinical vaccine failures, because current pertussis vaccines
ss-protection.[21]

ation, or cocooning, is a vaccination strategy to target mothers
ving close contact with an infant. The Centers for Disease Control
)) updated its guidance for pregnant mothers to recommend acel-
ne (Tdap) not only before and immediately after pregnancy but
cy after 20 weeks' gestation[38] and more recently recommended
each subsequent pregnancy.[39] The maternal antibodies are
ctive for the infant. The data on the effectiveness of this strategy
research is needed.[40,41]

ta suggest that the booster vaccine is effective in preventing dis-

ɔsis of classic pertussis may be made by a physician on clinical grounds
conjunction with laboratory testing. Assessment of clinical symptoms alone
ɔem to be highly reliable,[45] particularly because atypical presentations of
ʻe common and can mimic other infections. Laboratory testing often serves
the diagnosis of pertussis. Testing may include culture, PCR, and serology.
e and PCR are more sensitive earlier in the disease process and in younger
ʻhereas serology is more sensitive later in disease.[46] The optimal timing of
ɔds for diagnosis of pertussis is shown in **Fig. 2**.

⅃ITIONS

ɘrtussis is one of the nationally notifiable infectious diseases in the United
  Council of State and Territorial Epidemiologists and the CDC have pub-
ɔ criteria that define both probable and confirmed cases in terms of clinical
  and laboratory testing.[47] These definitions are instructive, because they
cal criteria and also reflect the perceptions about reliability of certain labo-
ʒ for detection of B pertussis. The clinical criteria for a case of pertussis in a
ɪk situation include a cough illness lasting at least 2 weeks with one of the
ɔaroxysms of coughing, inspiratory whoop, or posttussive vomiting, without
ɪrent cause. During outbreaks, a case may be defined as a cough illness
least 2 weeks. For the laboratory diagnosis of pertussis, isolation of
ʒ in culture or detection of B pertussis nucleic acid by PCR are the recom-
ʒsts. Culture is considered definitive and assumed to have absolute speci-
ʒociation with any cough illness, whereas PCR must be linked to the
ic clinical symptoms of pertussis. Serology is not currently included in these
tions; however, the state of Massachusetts does include a pertussis toxin-
ʒ serology for enhanced surveillance.[35] Also, the World Health Organization
de paired serology as part of the criteria for laboratory confirmation of
[8] The changing methods used for confirmation of pertussis using laboratory
ɔlogic evidence are shown in **Fig. 3**. These data from the CDC clearly show
ard PCR for diagnosis.
ɘfinitions do not take into account the impact of other Bordetella species,
ʻy account for the variability in disease presentations at various ages. It
ʒuggested that this is not a 1-size-fits-all situation and that alternative or
definitions are needed to recognize infections in adolescents, adults, and
ʒ. Toward that end, the report from the 2011 Global Pertussis Initiative Con-
ɘsents age-specific algorithms, which may be useful.[49]

:ough Onset

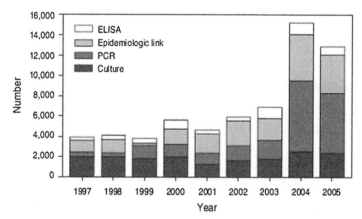

* Some cases were confirmed by more than one method. Cases were classified as follows: 1) all cases with a positive culture result were classified as culture confirmed; 2) cases with polymerase chain reaction (PCR) confirmation but no positive culture result were classified as PCR confirmed; 3) cases with confirmation by epidemiologic link but no positive culture or PCR results were classified as confirmed by epidemiologic link; 4) cases diagnosed in Massachusetts using the state-validated serologic assay by enzyme-linked immunosorbent assay (ELISA) with no positive culture or PCR result and no epidemiologic link were classified as ELISA confirmed.

Fig. 3. Number of confirmed pertussis cases, by confirmation method* (National Notifiable Disease Surveillance System and Supplemental Pertussis Surveillance System, United States, 1997 to 2005). ELISA, enzyme-linked immunosorbent assay. (*From* CDC. Outbreaks of Respiratory Illness Mistakenly Attributed to Pertussis–New Hampshire, Massachusetts, and Tennessee, 2004–2006. MMWR Recomm Rep 2007;56:837–42.)

LABORATORY TESTING
Specimens

The specimens of choice for detection of *B pertussis* by PCR or culture are nasopharyngeal (NP) swab, nasal wash, or nasal aspirate. These samples should contain ciliated epithelial cells from the upper respiratory tract, for which the bacterium is tropic. The use of other sample types such as throat swabs, although not acceptable for culture, have not been so thoroughly evaluated for use in amplified methods, but may be acceptable for PCR.[50] Use of Dacron-tipped or rayon-tipped swabs has been recommended; use of calcium alginate and aluminum shafts has been reported to be inhibitory to PCR,[51,52] but this may not be true with use of newer extraction techniques.

For PCR, the transport medium does not necessarily need to maintain organism viability; therefore, samples collected on NP swabs may be sent dry or in solutions such as sterile saline. If viability is of interest, then solutions such as casamino acids, Regan-Lowe or Amies medium (with antimicrobials) may be considered.[53] Specimens should be collected as soon as possible in disease and preferably before antibiotic therapy. Sensitivity decreases with patient age and length of symptoms.

Test Methods

The usefulness of various tests for diagnosis of pertussis is summarized in **Table 1** and discussed in the next sections.

Table 1
Laboratory testing for diagnosis of pertussis

Test	Sensitivity (%)	Specificity (%)	Advantages	Disadvantages
Culture[a,b]	12–60	100	• Assumed to have absolute specificity • Able to detect other *Bordetella* species such as *B parapertussis* and *B holmesii* • Isolate available for further testing (ie, antimicrobial susceptibility testing)	• Requires special transport and media • Lacks sensitivity; sensitivity affected by patient age, vaccination status, and length of illness • Long time to results
Direct fluorescent antibody[b]	11–68	99–100	• Rapid results	• Lack of sensitivity and specificity • CDC does not recommend use for diagnosis
PCR[a,b]	70–99	86–100	• Increased sensitivity vs other methods • Rapid results • More sensitive late in disease and with atypical presentations than culture • One FDA-cleared test currently available, with more in development	• No standardized protocols for testing and interpretation • Specificity adversely affected by presence of certain targets in multiple *Bordetella* species • Prone to environmental contamination, particularly with multicopy targets such as IS481 • May not reflect active infections; detects dead organisms
Serology: PT antibodies	50–99 by >3 wk after cough onset	>90	• PT IgG shows high sensitivity and specificity, PT IgA shows good specificity • Can help distinguish infection from vaccine response, depending on antibody isotype(s) and level detected Knowledge of vaccine history is necessary for proper interpretation	• No FDA-cleared tests • PT IgA only 50% sensitive at >3 wk after cough onset • Neither PT IgG nor IgA sensitive during first 2 wk after cough onset

Abbreviations: FDA, US Food and Drug Administration; PT, *B pertussis* toxin.
[a] Test included in CDC case definitions of pertussis.
[b] Based on Ref.[58]
Data from Leber A, Salamon D, Prince P. Pertussis diagnosis in the 21st century: progress and pitfall, part II. Clin Microbiol Newsl 2011;33:119–26.

Direct fluorescent antibody
Direct fluorescent antibody (DFA) staining is not considered useful or reliable for routine diagnosis of B pertussis. Although it is rapid, its performance characteristics are poor.

Culture
The growth characteristics of the Bordetella species commonly found in the respiratory tract are varied. B pertussis in culture requires special supplements in transport and culture media to facilitate initial isolation. Specialized media, such as Bordet-Gengou or Regan-Lowe, with and without antibiotics, in addition to bedside inoculation, may be used to maximize isolation rates.[1] Cultures should be incubated at 35°C in moist air without CO_2. Most colonies of B pertussis are detected in 5 to 7 days, but some may take as long as 12 days.[6] B parapertussis, B holmesii, and B bronchiseptica are not as fastidious and grow on sheep blood or chocolate agar usually within 3 to 5 days. The identification of isolates of Bordetella is based on phenotypic and biochemical tests.[6] Use of a confirmatory antibody for fluorescent staining or agglutination can be helpful for rapid identification of culture isolates.

The isolation of B pertussis is considered definitive and assumed to have absolute specificity for diagnosis of pertussis. It is most sensitive in unvaccinated infants and in samples collected soon after the onset of symptoms. Culture is prone to sensitivity problems associated with specimen collection/transport and culture conditions. Culture may still be useful in cases of outbreak investigation, quality assurance studies, and in individual cases in which treatment failure as a result of resistance is under consideration.[54] It also allows detection of other Bordetella species if protocols are in place to look for nonpertussis isolates.

Nucleic acid amplification tests
The most commonly used nucleic acid amplification test (NAAT) for detection of B pertussis and B parapertussis is PCR and it has become a standard of care test in many laboratories. PCR has several advantages over culture and DFA. It has been clearly shown to have better sensitivity, and results are available faster than culture; the drawback of PCR relates to issues with specificity and concerns for false-positive results.

There are numerous published protocols for PCR, leading to great variety in sample types accepted, extraction methods used, primer and probe chemistries, and interpretation and reporting of results. Most testing in clinical laboratories is performed using laboratory-developed tests using a real-time PCR format. Analyte specific reagents are available from several companies, and some of these are approved by regulatory agencies outside the United States. At time of writing, there is one test cleared by the US Food and Drug Administration (FDA) that detects B pertussis as part of a multiplex real-time PCR test (FilmArray Respiratory Panel, Biofire Diagnostics, Salt Lake City, UT). This test is reportedly specific for B pertussis and does not detect B parapertussis or B holmesii.

Pretreatment and extraction
Crude sample treatments, such as boiling or proteinase K treatment before amplification, have largely been replaced by commercial kits for nucleic acid extraction.[20] These commercial kits include both manual and automated techniques. Many laboratories continue to use manual methods, such as spin-columns (Qiagen, Valencia, CA), whereas others have moved to automated systems, such as the EZ1 (Qiagen), MagNA Pure, (Roche Applied Science, Indianapolis, IN), or easyMag (bioMerieux, Durham, NC).

Targets for PCR

Finding targets with absolute specificity is difficult and requires comprehensive analysis of known sequence data and testing with clinical isolates. Ideally, any target region selected is both sensitive and specific. Several chromosomal regions have been used as targets for PCR-based detection of B pertussis, including single copy genes, such as pertussis toxin promoter region, adenylate cyclase, pertactin, porin, and rec A.[2,19,55–58] A multicopy target, insertion sequence, IS481, has also been widely used as a target for B pertussis.[20,59] For detection of B parapertussis, the multicopy insertion sequence IS1001 region is most commonly used.[60] Several publications include use of both IS481 and IS1001 for detection of B pertussis and B parapertussis DNA.[46,61,62] This is a common strategy used by clinical laboratories in the United States.

Single-copy targets are believed to have better specificity for B pertussis than multicopy ones such as IS481, but sensitivity may be lower. Therefore, a sample with very low bacterial load, which has been shown to occur in older patients as well as in samples collected late in the disease, could be falsely negative.[63] In addition, cross-reactions with single-copy targets have also been reported, which may also affect specificity.[64,65]

IS481 is arguably the most commonly used target for the detection of B pertussis in clinical samples. It is advantageous in that it is present in high copies, from 50 up to 238 copies per cell, adding to the analytical sensitivity of this PCR over single-copy targets.[66] The IS481 target has been estimated to detect 0.3 to 0.5 colony forming units (CFU)/reaction[67] and would be expected to be about 2 logs more sensitive in the detection of B pertussis than a single-copy target PCR.[68] Because all strains of Bordetella are prone to containing IS481 as a result of horizontal or vertical transmission,[69] specificity can be compromised. In B holmseii, IS481 is found in up to 10 copies per genome; for B brochiseptica, the sequence has been detected from some human isolates.[70,71] Thus, clinical assays targeting IS481 for B pertussis may be falsely positive, because of presence of other Bordetella species. The IS1001 sequence is present in all B parapertussis isolates and in some B brochiseptica strains, but not in B pertussis.[69]

Use of the pertussis toxin promoter region along with IS481 and IS1001 targets in a triplex assay has been reported for detection and differentiation of B pertussis and B parapertussis.[72,73] Use of a B pertussis–specific target such as the toxin promoter region, either as part of a multiplex or a confirmatory assay, affords a check on specificity of the IS481 positive samples. If a specimen is positive for both IS481 and toxin promoter, it is interpreted as positive for B pertussis; if it is positive for IS481 but not toxin promoter, it is a Bordetella species, most likely B holmesii. However, it is possible that a specimen containing low levels of B pertussis DNA would amplify with IS481, but not toxin promoter based on sensitivity differences. A positive result with IS1001 is assumed to be B parapertussis. For further confirmation of the presence of B holmesii, a specific PCR test can be performed either as a part of a multiplex assay or a reflex test from IS481 positive specimens.[19,74]

Such a strategy was used to confirm B holmesii during the outbreak documenting cocirculation of B pertussis, B parapertussis, and B holmesii species.[22] A multiplex assay combining IS481 and IS1001 was used for routine diagnostic testing. For further investigation of the outbreak, retrospective testing using a B pertussis–specific, toxin promoter region target, and a B holmesii–specific insertion sequence target (IS1001-like) were used. **Table 2** shows the interpretation of results associated with the 4 targets.

Tatti and colleagues[75] also reported a multitarget strategy to differentiate among the Bordetella species, using a total of 4 targets and 2 separate assays. IS481 and IS1001

Table 2
Differentiation of *Bordetella* species by using multiple PCR targets

Species	Results of PCR Assay[a]			
	IS481/IS1001 Multiplex			
	IS481	IS1001	ptxA-PR	IS1001-like
B pertussis	+	−	+	−
B parapertussis	−	+	−	−
B holmesii	+	−	−	+
Bordetella species[b]	+	−	−	−

[a] IS481/IS1001 performed as a multiplex real-time PCR. Single-copy targets: ptxA-PR = pertussis toxin, specific for *B pertussis*; IS1001-like, insertion sequence found specifically in *B holmesii* performed as singleplex real-time PCR.
[b] Detection of IS481 without confirmation with single-copy targets for *B pertussis* or *B holmesii*. This situation could be caused by low copy number of *B pertussis*, which is not detected in the single-copy PCR assays for confirmation of *B pertussis* or *B holmesii*.
   Data from Spicer KB, Salamon D, Cummins C, et al. Occurrence of three Bordetella species during an outbreak of cough illness in Ohio: epidemiology, clinical features, laboratory findings, and antimicrobial susceptibility. Pediatr Infect Dis J 2014 Jan 17. [Epub ahead of print].

were combined with the *B holmseii*–specific IS1001 target as a triplex assay. The second assay contained a pertussis toxin subunit target common to *B pertussis* and *B parapertussis*. This algorithm and the one mentioned earlier do not include differentiation of *B bronchiseptica*, based on the belief that this species is a rare human pathogen.

Low copy number and high C_T values
Less than a single organism can theoretically be detected in an IS481 assay, and therefore, a high crossing threshold (C_T) value in a real-time PCR assay could represent low bacterial load of *B pertussis*. A study using quantitative IS481 PCR reported lower bacterial loads in NP swab specimens from adults versus children with pertussis with a mean C_T value of 34.9 for adults versus 27.1 in children.[63] However, the clinical meaning of detection of very low levels of bacteria (<1 CFU per reaction) is uncertain.[76] The exact values vary with each particular assay, but C_T values greater than 35 have been cited as correlating with less than 1 CFU/mL and may be a reasonable cutoff value for a positive result in clinical specimens.[67,77]

Higher C_T values would also be expected if other *Bordetella* species such as *B holmesii* were present, because of the lower copy number of IS481 in these species versus *B pertussis*.[61,71] Templeton and colleagues[61] found that IS481 PCR had a sensitivity of 10 CFU/mL for *B holmesii* versus 1 CFU/mL for *B pertussis*, reflective of the lower copy number present.

NAATs other than PCR
Other amplification techniques have been used for detection of *Bordetella* species in clinical samples.[78,79] Loop-mediated isothermal amplification (LAMP) is a technique using multiple primers and a polymerase enzyme. It does not require thermocycling; the reactions are carried out at a single temperature and product can be detected visually (with turbidity or fluorescence) or on an instrument. At time of writing, a LAMP-based test for detection of *B pertussis* was under development for commercial distribution (Illumigene, Meridian Diagnostics, Cincinnati, OH). This assay uses the IS481 target, so would be expected to also detect *B holmesii* and rare IS481-positive strains of *B bronchiseptica* in addition to *B pertussis*.

Contamination

There have been multiple reports of pseudo-outbreaks associated with false-positive PCR results.[80] False-positive results can be caused by several conditions, including contamination of specimens with either the native organism or an amplicon created from a previous reaction.[81] A multicopy target such as IS481 is more prone than a single-copy target to these contamination problems. To avoid laboratory-based contamination, use of various strategies such as unidirectional workflow, chemical and physical controls, and careful quality control are all necessary.

Contamination can also occur during sample collection. Gloves and mask should be worn during collection to prevent spread of organism to staff, other patients, and other specimens. Both whole cell and certain acellular vaccines have amplifiable IS481 target DNA. During vaccine administration in a physician office, DNA from the vaccine may contaminate the office environment and subsequently the samples collected.[81–83] Ideally, specimens should be collected and vaccines administered in separate areas using careful technique and decontamination of surfaces. It is also paramount to only test patients who are symptomatic.

Interpretation

Reporting a false-positive PCR result has undesired consequences, such as missing the true diagnosis, unnecessary treatment or contact prophylaxis, and inappropriate furlough from work or school. Every effort should be made to minimize environmental causes of false-positive results in the laboratory or physician office. However, the detrimental effect of misidentification of other *Bordetella* species that are truly present in the specimen is less clear. Determination of the exact *Bordetella* species does have implications, in that some control measures, such as vaccination with acellular pertussis vaccine, are effective against only *B pertussis*. However, antimicrobial prophylaxis with a macrolide would be effective against most *Bordetella* species. Clearly, more work is needed to answer these questions. In the meantime, laboratories may choose to address these issues in several ways, including:

- Optimize sensitivity by using IS481 and accept the possible decrease in specificity. Add a disclaimer to the results about possible cross-reactions or the need for confirmation.
- Optimize specificity with a single-copy target such as the toxin promoter region and accept a possible decrease in sensitivity.
- Adopt a multitarget algorithm using IS481 coupled with a single-copy target, such as toxin promoter region to increase specificity. This procedure may include additional targets to identify other species such as *B parapertussis* and *B holmesii*.

Serology

Serology is a useful tool for diagnosis of pertussis illness related to infections with *B pertussis*, particularly late in cough illness, when the organism itself is no longer detectable.[4] However, it is not widely used in the United States, because of the lack of standardized, FDA-cleared testing, need for paired sera to optimize performance, and the problems associated with interpretation, as discussed later. Serology is not a useful diagnostic tool in neonates or young infants.

The most meaningful serologic results are obtained using enzyme-linked immunosorbent assay (ELISA)-based formats with purified antigens, such as *B pertussis* toxin (PT) and FHA. Because PT is produced only by *B pertussis*, detection of PT antibodies constitutes the most specific serologic indicator of pertussis infection.[53,84–88] FHA, like other antigens, such as pertactin and fimbrial protein, is found in *B parapertussis* and other *Bordetella* species, as well as *B pertussis*. This factor limits the specificity for pertussis diagnosis. Mixtures of antigens or whole organism lysates are not recommended, because of poor specificity.[89]

Complicating serologic diagnosis is that PT is contained in substantial amounts in all acellular vaccines. Therefore, antibody generated to infection or vaccination cannot be clearly distinguished for at least 6 months after vaccination.[90] Because of a continuous circulation of *Bordetella* in the population, IgG-anti-PT may be detectable in most adolescent and adult populations, so establishing a cutoff value correlating with recent infection is important. Therefore, accurate interpretation of serologic results requires knowledge of vaccination history and possible exposures to determine the reason for detectable antibody responses to *B pertussis*.

The use of antibody isotypes may also be valuable for distinguishing infection from vaccine responses. Both IgG and IgA responses can be informative. For example, PT IgG is increased after either vaccination or natural infection; in contrast, PT IgA is increased after natural infection only, and not in response to vaccination.[86,91–93] This IgA response occurs in only about 50% of infected individuals, so it is not always helpful.[53,86,91,94] IgM response is not generally useful, in that the level of IgM generated in an amnestic response is low and does not increase diagnostic yield over testing for IgG and IgA.[4,94–96]

The CDC has reported the use of a single serum ELISA using purified PT as antigen designed for detection of late infections.[97] Such a single-point test would obviate parried acute and convalescent sera. A single serum test would be useful both for epidemiologic and clinical purposes; however, the assay is not yet available to private or commercial laboratories. At time of writing, there are no FDA-cleared serologic tests using purified PT as the antigen. Clinicians and laboratorians should understand the details of the testing, such as antigen formulations and cutoff values used. There are significant differences in testing offered by the major reference laboratories in the United States, some of which use mixtures of pertussis antigens, thus having lower specificity for active disease.

TREATMENT

The treatment of pertussis and also postexposure prophylaxis are considered standard of care, and help control the spread of infection. The usefulness of antimicrobials to treat an individual patient is controversial, in that it does not prevent symptoms from developing but may lessen their severity and duration. It is most effective when given early in the course of disease, ideally before the onset of the paroxysmal coughing. The macrolides are the treatment of choice for *B pertussis*, with erythromycin, azithromycin, and clarithromycin all being effective. Alternatively, a 14-day course of trimethoprim/sulfamethoxazole can be used.[98] There have been limited reports of resistance to macrolides in *B pertussis* isolates.[99,100] For the treatment of *B parapertussis* or *B holmesii*, there is less known about the effectiveness of antimicrobial therapy, but some in vitro data suggest that macrolides would be effective.[22]

SUMMARY/DISCUSSION

The control of pertussis must include multiple approaches, including increasing clinician awareness, improving vaccination strategies, and optimizing laboratory-based diagnostics. The goal is to reduce the number of reported cases and the associated morbidity and mortality, particularly in infants. For the clinical laboratory, real-time PCR has become the mainstay of diagnosis, largely replacing culture. Serology has an important role, particularly late in the course of a chronic cough disease in adolescents and adults. However, a standardized test is available only in the public health setting. Once this test is more widely available, a multitest approach including both PCR and serology may help to increase diagnostic yield.

Recognizing the complexities associated with PCR, such as cross-reactions among *Bordetella* species and contamination associated with vaccine, allows each laboratory to decide which type of PCR testing best fits their population and work flow. As more tests are being developed by commercial manufacturers, they too need to make these determinations. The identification and differentiation of species such as *B pertussis*, *B parapertussis*, and *B holmesii* are important for the increased understanding of the epidemiology of these organisms. The data supporting the role of *B holmesii* as a potential pathogen are growing. So the question becomes: does the laboratory need to differentiate between *B pertussis* and *B holmesii*? Some may say yes; we need to understand how these organisms present, and their full clinical impact. Others may say no; all 3 seem to produce pertussislike illness and are susceptible to macrolide therapy. Therefore, resources of the laboratory may be better used elsewhere. The decision lies with each laboratory based on their abilities and needs.

REFERENCES

1. Loeffelholz MJ, Sanden GN. Manual of clinical microbiology, vol. 1. Washington, DC: ASM Press; 2007.
2. Mattoo S, Cherry JD. Molecular pathogenesis, epidemiology, and clinical manifestations of respiratory infections due to *Bordetella pertussis* and other *Bordetella* subspecies. Clin Microbiol Rev 2005;18:326–82.
3. Leber A, Salamon D, Prince P. Pertussis diagnosis in the 21st century: progress and pitfalls, part 1. Clin Microbiol Newsl 2011;33:111–5.
4. Leber A, Salamon D, Prince P. Pertussis diagnosis in the 21st century: progress and pitfalls, part II. Clin Microbiol Newsl 2011;33:119–26.
5. Clinical and Laboratory Standards Institute. Interpretive criteria for identification of bacteria and fungi by DNA target sequencing; approved guideline, MM18-A. 2008; 28. Available at: http://www.clsi.org/standards/
6. McGowan K. *Bordetella* cultures. In: Garcia LS, editor. Clinical microbiology procedures handbook, vol. 1, 3rd edition. Washington, DC: ASM Press; 2007. p. 1–14.
7. Guris D, Strebel PM, Bardenheier B, et al. Changing epidemiology of pertussis in the United States: increasing reported incidence among adolescents and adults, 1990-1996. Clin Infect Dis 1999;28:1230–7.
8. Centers for Disease Control and Prevention. Notes from the field: pertussis–California, January–June 2010. Available at: http://www.cdc.gov/mmwr/preview/mmwrhtml/mm5926a5.htm?s_cid=mm5926a5_e%0d%0a. Accessed November 13, 2010.
9. Litt DJ, Neal SE, Fry NK. Changes in genetic diversity of the *Bordetella pertussis* population in the United Kingdom between 1920 and 2006 reflect vaccination coverage and emergence of a single dominant clonal type. J Clin Microbiol 2009;47:680–8.
10. Cherry JD. Epidemiology of pertussis. Pediatr Infect Dis J 2006;25:361–2.
11. Bouchez V, Brun D, Cantinelli T, et al. First report and detailed characterization of *B. pertussis* isolates not expressing pertussis toxin or pertactin. Vaccine 2009;27:6034–41.
12. Pawloski LC, Queenan AM, Cassiday PK, et al. Prevalence and molecular characterization of pertactin-deficient *Bordetella pertussis* in the US. Clin Vaccine Immunol 2014;21(2):119–25.

13. Cherry JD, Seaton BL. Patterns of *Bordetella parapertussis* respiratory illnesses: 2008-2010. Clin Infect Dis 2012;54:534–7.
14. Wallihan R, Selvarangan R, Marcon M, et al. *Bordetella parapertussis* bacteremia: two case reports. Pediatr Infect Dis J 2013;32:796–8.
15. Njamkepo E, Delisle F, Hagege I, et al. *Bordetella holmesii* isolated from a patient with sickle cell anemia: analysis and comparison with other *Bordetella holmesii* isolates. Clin Microbiol Infect 2000;6:131–6.
16. Weyant RS, Hollis DG, Weaver RE, et al. *Bordetella holmesii* sp. nov., a new gram-negative species associated with septicemia. J Clin Microbiol 1995;33: 1–7.
17. Yih WK, Silva EA, Ida J, et al. *Bordetella holmesii*-like organisms isolated from Massachusetts patients with pertussis-like symptoms. Emerg Infect Dis 1999; 5:441–3.
18. Mazengia E, Silva EA, Peppe JA, et al. Recovery of *Bordetella holmesii* from patients with pertussis-like symptoms: use of pulsed-field gel electrophoresis to characterize circulating strains. J Clin Microbiol 2000;38:2330–3.
19. Antila M, He Q, de Jong C, et al. *Bordetella holmesii* DNA is not detected in nasopharyngeal swabs from Finnish and Dutch patients with suspected pertussis. J Med Microbiol 2006;55:1043–51.
20. Riffelmann M, Wirsing von Konig CH, Caro V, et al. Nucleic acid amplification tests for diagnosis of *Bordetella* infections. J Clin Microbiol 2005;43:4925–9.
21. Rodgers L, Martin SW, Cohn A, et al. Epidemiologic and laboratory features of a large outbreak of pertussis-like illnesses associated with cocirculating *Bordetella holmesii* and *Bordetella pertussis*-Ohio, 2010-2011. Clin Infect Dis 2013; 56:322–31.
22. Spicer KB, Salamon D, Cummins C, et al. Occurrence of three *Bordetella* species during an outbreak of cough illness in Ohio: epidemiology, clinical features, laboratory findings, and antimicrobial susceptibility. Pediatr Infect Dis J 2014 Jan 17. [Epub ahead of print].
23. Njamkepo E, Bonacorsi S, Debruyne M, et al. Significant finding of *Bordetella holmesii* DNA in nasopharyngeal samples from French patients with suspected pertussis. J Clin Microbiol 2011;49:4347–8.
24. Kamiya H, Otsuka N, Ando Y, et al. Transmission of *Bordetella holmesii* during pertussis outbreak, Japan. Emerg Infect Dis 2012;18:1166–9.
25. Tatti KM, Wu KH, Tondella ML, et al. Development and evaluation of dual-target real-time polymerase chain reaction assays to detect *Bordetella* spp. Diagn Microbiol Infect Dis 2008;61:264–72.
26. Heininger U, Stehr K, Schmitt-Grohe S, et al. Clinical characteristics of illness caused by *Bordetella parapertussis* compared with illness caused by *Bordetella pertussis*. Pediatr Infect Dis J 1994;13:306–9.
27. Long SS, Welkon CJ, Clark JL. Widespread silent transmission of pertussis in families: antibody correlates of infection and symptomatology. J Infect Dis 1990;161:480–6.
28. Mink CM, Cherry JD, Christenson P, et al. A search for *Bordetella pertussis* infection in university students. Clin Infect Dis 1992;14:464–71.
29. Hallander HO, Ljungman M, Storsaeter J, et al. Kinetics and sensitivity of ELISA IgG pertussis antitoxin after infection and vaccination with *Bordetella pertussis* in young children. APMIS 2009;117:797–807.
30. Le T, Cherry JD, Chang SJ, et al. Immune responses and antibody decay after immunization of adolescents and adults with an acellular pertussis vaccine: the APERT Study. J Infect Dis 2004;190:535–44.

31. Heininger U, Cherry JD, Stehr K. Serologic response and antibody-titer decay in adults with pertussis. Clin Infect Dis 2004;38:591–4.
32. Forsyth KD, Campins-Marti M, Caro J, et al. New pertussis vaccination strategies beyond infancy: recommendations by the global pertussis initiative. Clin Infect Dis 2004;39:1802–9.
33. Edelman K, He Q, Makinen J, et al. Immunity to pertussis 5 years after booster immunization during adolescence. Clin Infect Dis 2007;44:1271–7.
34. Sin MA, Zenke R, Ronckendorf R, et al. Pertussis outbreak in primary and secondary schools in Ludwigslust, Germany demonstrating the role of waning immunity. Pediatr Infect Dis J 2009;28:242–4.
35. Broder KR, Cortese MM, Iskander JK, et al. Preventing tetanus, diphtheria, and pertussis among adolescents: use of tetanus toxoid, reduced diphtheria toxoid and acellular pertussis vaccines recommendations of the Advisory Committee on Immunization Practices (ACIP). MMWR Recomm Rep 2006; 55:1–34.
36. Kretsinger K, Broder KR, Cortese MM, et al. Preventing tetanus, diphtheria, and pertussis among adults: use of tetanus toxoid, reduced diphtheria toxoid and acellular pertussis vaccine recommendations of the Advisory Committee on Immunization Practices (ACIP) and recommendation of ACIP, supported by the Healthcare Infection Control Practices Advisory Committee (HICPAC), for use of Tdap among health-care personnel. MMWR Recomm Rep 2006; 55:1–37.
37. Klein NP, Bartlett J, Rowhani-Rahbar A, et al. Waning protection after fifth dose of acellular pertussis vaccine in children. N Engl J Med 2012;367:1012–9.
38. Centers for Disease Control and Prevention. Updated recommendations for use of tetanus toxoid, reduced diphtheria toxoid and acellular pertussis vaccine (Tdap) in pregnant women and persons who have or anticipate having close contact with an infant aged <12 months–Advisory Committee on Immunization Practices (ACIP), 2011. MMWR Recomm Rep 2011;60:1424–6.
39. Centers for Disease Control and Prevention. Updated recommendations for use of tetanus toxoid, reduced diphtheria toxoid, and acellular pertussis vaccine (Tdap) in pregnant women–Advisory Committee on Immunization Practices (ACIP), 2012. MMWR Recomm Rep 2013;62:131–5.
40. Halperin BA, Morris A, Mackinnon-Cameron D, et al. Kinetics of the antibody response to tetanus-diphtheria-acellular pertussis vaccine in women of child-bearing age and postpartum women. Clin Infect Dis 2011;53:885–92.
41. Mooi FR, de Greeff SC. The case for maternal vaccination against pertussis. Lancet Infect Dis 2007;7:614–24.
42. Wei SC, Tatti K, Cushing K, et al. Effectiveness of adolescent and adult tetanus, reduced-dose diphtheria, and acellular pertussis vaccine against pertussis. Clin Infect Dis 2010;51:315–21.
43. Kallonen T, He Q. Bordetella pertussis strain variation and evolution postvaccination. Expert Review Vaccines 2009;8:863–75.
44. Queenan AM, Cassiday PK, Evangelista A. Pertactin-negative variants of Bordetella pertussis in the United States. N Engl J Med 2013;368:583–4.
45. Cornia PB, Hersh AL, Lipsky BA, et al. Does this coughing adolescent or adult patient have pertussis? JAMA 2010;304:890–6.
46. van der Zee A, Agterberg C, Peeters M, et al. A clinical validation of Bordetella pertussis and Bordetella parapertussis polymerase chain reaction: comparison with culture and serology using samples from patients with suspected whooping cough from a highly immunized population. J Infect Dis 1996;174:89–96.

47. Centers for Disease Control and Prevention. Pertussis (*Bordetella pertussis*) (whooping cough) 2010 Case Definition CSTE Position Statement Number: 09-ID-51. Available at: http://www.cdc.gov/ncphi/disss/nndss/print/pertussis_current.htm. Accessed November 18, 2010.

48. World Health Organization. WHO-recommended standards for surveillance of selected vaccine-preventable diseases. 2003; WHO/V&B/03.01. Available at: http://whqlibdoc.who.int/hq/2003/who_v&b_03.01.pdf.

49. Cherry JD, Tan T, Wirsing von Konig CH, et al. Clinical definitions of pertussis: summary of a Global Pertussis Initiative roundtable meeting, February 2011. Clin Infect Dis 2012;54:1756–64.

50. Farrell DJ, Daggard G, Mukkur TK. Nested duplex PCR to detect *Bordetella pertussis* and *Bordetella parapertussis* and its application in diagnosis of pertussis in nonmetropolitan Southeast Queensland, Australia. J Clin Microbiol 1999;37:606–10.

51. Cloud JL, Hymas W, Carroll KC. Impact of nasopharyngeal swab types on detection of *Bordetella pertussis* by PCR and culture. J Clin Microbiol 2002;40:3838–40.

52. Wadowsky RM, Laus S, Libert T, et al. Inhibition of PCR-based assay for *Bordetella pertussis* by using calcium alginate fiber and aluminum shaft components of a nasopharyngeal swab. J Clin Microbiol 1994;32:1054–7.

53. Muller FM, Hoppe JE, Wirsing von Konig CH. Laboratory diagnosis of pertussis: state of the art in 1997. J Clin Microbiol 1997;35:2435–43.

54. Sotir MJ, Cappozzo DL, Warshauer DM, et al. Evaluation of polymerase chain reaction and culture for diagnosis of pertussis in the control of a county-wide outbreak focused among adolescents and adults. Clin Infect Dis 2007;44:1216–9.

55. Houard S, Hackel C, Herzog A, et al. Specific identification of *Bordetella pertussis* by the polymerase chain reaction. Res Microbiol 1989;140:477–87.

56. Douglas E, Coote JG, Parton R, et al. Identification of *Bordetella* pertussis in nasopharyngeal swabs by PCR amplification of a region of the adenylate cyclase gene. J Med Microbiol 1993;38:140–4.

57. Vincart B, De Mendonca R, Rottiers S, et al. A specific real-time PCR assay for the detection of *Bordetella pertussis*. J Med Microbiol 2007;56:918–20.

58. Wendelboe AM, Van Rie A. Diagnosis of pertussis: a historical review and recent developments. Expert Rev Mol Diagn 2006;6:857–64.

59. Glare EM, Paton JC, Premier RR, et al. Analysis of a repetitive DNA sequence from *Bordetella pertussis* and its application to the diagnosis of pertussis using the polymerase chain reaction. J Clin Microbiol 1990;28:1982–7.

60. van der Zee A, Agterberg C, van Agterveld M, et al. Characterization of IS1001, an insertion sequence element of *Bordetella parapertussis*. J Bacteriol 1993; 175:141–7.

61. Templeton KE, Scheltinga SA, van der Zee A, et al. Evaluation of real-time PCR for detection of and discrimination between *Bordetella pertussis*, *Bordetella parapertussis*, and *Bordetella holmesii* for clinical diagnosis. J Clin Microbiol 2003; 41:4121–6.

62. Sloan LM, Hopkins MK, Mitchell PS, et al. Multiplex LightCycler PCR assay for detection and differentiation of *Bordetella pertussis* and *Bordetella parapertussis* in nasopharyngeal specimens. J Clin Microbiol 2002;40:96–100.

63. Nakamura Y, Kamachi K, Toyoizumi-Ajisaka H, et al. Marked difference between adults and children in *Bordetella pertussis* DNA load in nasopharyngeal swabs. Clin Microbiol Infect 2010;17(3):365–70.

64. Register KB, Nicholson TL. Misidentification of *Bordetella bronchiseptica* as *Bordetella pertussis* using a newly described real-time PCR targeting the pertactin gene. J Med Microbiol 2007;56:1608–10.

65. Register KB, Nicholson TL, Guthrie JL. Evaluation of specificity of BP3385 for *Bordetella pertussis* detection. J Clin Microbiol 2010;48:3334–7.
66. Parkhill J, Sebaihia M, Preston A, et al. Comparative analysis of the genome sequences of *Bordetella pertussis*, *Bordetella parapertussis* and *Bordetella bronchiseptica*. Nat Genet 2003;35:32–40.
67. Loeffelholz MJ, Thompson CJ, Long KS, et al. Comparison of PCR, culture, and direct fluorescent-antibody testing for detection of *Bordetella pertussis*. J Clin Microbiol 1999;37:2872–6.
68. Koidl C, Bozic M, Burmeister A, et al. Detection and differentiation of *Bordetella* spp. by real-time PCR. J Clin Microbiol 2007;45:347–50.
69. Diavatopoulos DA, Cummings CA, Schouls LM, et al. *Bordetella pertussis*, the causative agent of whooping cough, evolved from a distinct, human-associated lineage of *B. bronchiseptica*. PLoS Pathog 2005;1:e45.
70. Register KB, Sanden GN. Prevalence and sequence variants of IS481 in *Bordetella bronchiseptica*: implications for IS481-based detection of *Bordetella pertussis*. J Clin Microbiol 2006;44:4577–83.
71. Reischl U, Lehn N, Sanden GN, et al. Real-time PCR assay targeting IS481 of *Bordetella pertussis* and molecular basis for detecting *Bordetella holmesii*. J Clin Microbiol 2001;39:1963–6.
72. Dragsted DM, Dohn B, Madsen J, et al. Comparison of culture and PCR for detection of *Bordetella pertussis* and *Bordetella parapertussis* under routine laboratory conditions. J Med Microbiol 2004;53:749–54.
73. Xu Y, Hou Q, Yang R, et al. Triplex real-time PCR assay for detection and differentiation of *Bordetella pertussis* and *Bordetella parapertussis*. APMIS 2010;118:685–91.
74. Guthrie JL, Robertson AV, Tang P, et al. Novel duplex real-time PCR assay detects *Bordetella holmesii* in specimens from patients with pertussis-like symptoms in Ontario, Canada. J Clin Microbiol 2010;48:1435–7.
75. Tatti KM, Sparks KN, Boney KO, et al. Novel multitarget real-time PCR assay for rapid detection of *Bordetella* species in clinical specimens. J Clin Microbiol 2011;49:4059–66.
76. Papenburg J, Fontela P. What is the significance of a high cycle threshold positive IS481 PCR for *Bordetella pertussis*? Pediatr Infect Dis J 2009;28:1143 [author reply: 1143–4].
77. Guthrie JL, Seah C, Brown S, et al. Use of *Bordetella pertussis* BP3385 to establish a cutoff value for an IS481-targeted real-time PCR assay. J Clin Microbiol 2008;46:3798–9.
78. Otsuka N, Yoshino S, Kawano K, et al. Simple and specific detection of *Bordetella holmesii* by using a loop-mediated isothermal amplification assay. Microbiol Immunol 2012;56:486–9.
79. Kamachi K, Toyoizumi-Ajisaka H, Toda K, et al. Development and evaluation of a loop-mediated isothermal amplification method for rapid diagnosis of *Bordetella pertussis* infection. J Clin Microbiol 2006;44:1899–902.
80. Centers for Disease Control and Prevention. Outbreaks or respiratory illness mistakenly attributed to pertussis–New Hampshire, Massachusetts, and Tennessee, 2004-2006. MMWR Morb Mortal Wkly Rep 2007;56:837–42.
81. Taranger J, Trollfors B, Lind L, et al. Environmental contamination leading to false-positive polymerase chain reaction for pertussis. Pediatr Infect Dis J 1994;13:936–7.
82. Tatti KM, Slade B, Patel M, et al. Real-time polymerase chain reaction detection of *Bordetella pertussis* DNA in acellular pertussis vaccines. Pediatr Infect Dis J 2008;27:73–4.

83. Leber A, Salamon D, Cummins C, et al. Detection of *Bordetella pertussis* DNA in acellular vaccines and in environmental samples from pediatric physician offices. Abstract number D-149. In: Interscience Conference on Antimicrobial Agents and Chemotherapeutics. Boston (MA).

84. Cherry JD, Grimprel E, Guiso N, et al. Defining pertussis epidemiology: clinical, microbiologic and serologic perspectives. Pediatr Infect Dis J 2005;24: S25–34.

85. Isacson J, Trollfors B, Hedvall G, et al. Response and decline of serum IgG antibodies to pertussis toxin, filamentous hemagglutinin and pertactin in children with pertussis. Scand J Infect Dis 1995;27:273–7.

86. Hallander HO. Microbiological and serological diagnosis of pertussis. Clin Infect Dis 1999;28(Suppl 2):S99–106.

87. Greenberg DP. Pertussis in adolescents: increasing incidence brings attention to the need for booster immunization of adolescents. Pediatr Infect Dis J 2005;24:721–8.

88. Ward JI, Cherry JD, Chang SJ, et al. *Bordetella pertussis* infections in vaccinated and unvaccinated adolescents and adults, as assessed in a national prospective randomized Acellular Pertussis Vaccine Trial (APERT). Clin Infect Dis 2006;43:151–7.

89. Xing D, Markey K, Newland P, et al. EUVAC.NET collaborative study: evaluation and standardisation of serology for diagnosis of pertussis. J Immunol Methods 2011;372:137–45.

90. Pawloski LC, Kirkland KB, Baughman AL, et al. Does tetanus-diphtheria-acellular pertussis vaccination interfere with serodiagnosis of pertussis infection? Clin Vaccine Immunol 2012;19:875–80.

91. Hoppe JE. Update of epidemiology, diagnosis, and treatment of pertussis. Eur J Clin Microbiol Infect Dis 1996;15:189–93.

92. Burstyn DG, Baraff LJ, Peppler MS, et al. Serological response to filamentous hemagglutinin and lymphocytosis-promoting toxin of *Bordetella pertussis*. Infect Immun 1983;41:1150–6.

93. Cherry JD. Pertussis in adults. Ann Intern Med 1998;128:64–6.

94. Granstrom G, Wretlind B, Salenstedt CR, et al. Evaluation of serologic assays for diagnosis of whooping cough. J Clin Microbiol 1988;26:1818–23.

95. Steketee RW, Burstyn DG, Wassilak SG, et al. A comparison of laboratory and clinical methods for diagnosing pertussis in an outbreak in a facility for the developmentally disabled. J Infect Dis 1988;157:441–9.

96. Klement E, Kagan N, Hagain L, et al. Correlation of IgA, IgM and IgG antibody-detecting assays based on filamentous haemagglutinin, pertussis toxin and *Bordetella pertussis* sonicate in a strictly adult population. Epidemiol Infect 2005; 133:149–58.

97. Menzies SL, Kadwad V, Pawloski LC, et al. Development and analytical validation of an immunoassay for quantifying serum anti-pertussis toxin antibodies resulting from *Bordetella pertussis* infection. Clin Vaccine Immunol 2009;16:1781–8.

98. Tiwari T, Murphy TV, Moran J. Recommended antimicrobial agents for the treatment and postexposure prophylaxis of pertussis: 2005 CDC Guidelines. MMWR Recomm Rep 2005;54:1–16.

99. Bartkus JM, Juni BA, Ehresmann K, et al. Identification of a mutation associated with erythromycin resistance in *Bordetella pertussis*: implications for surveillance of antimicrobial resistance. J Clin Microbiol 2003;41:1167–72.

100. Guillot S, Descours G, Gillet Y, et al. Macrolide-resistant *Bordetella pertussis* infection in newborn girl, France. Emerg Infect Dis 2012;18:966–8.

Antibiotic Resistance in Nosocomial Respiratory Infections

Gerald A. Denys, PhD, D(ABMM)*, Ryan F. Relich, PhD, MLS(ASCP)CM

KEYWORDS

- Health care–associated infections • Hospital-acquired pneumonia
- Ventilator-associated pneumonia • Nosocomial • Multidrug resistant pathogens

KEY POINTS

- Nosocomial respiratory infections are the most common acquired infections in patients with severe underlying conditions and are responsible for high morbidity and mortality in this patient population.
- Multidrug-resistant (MDR) pathogens are associated with hospital-acquired pneumonia (HAP) and ventilator-associated pneumonia (VAP).
- Empiric treatment of HAP and VAP is based on onset of disease and presence or absence of risk factors associated with multidrug-resistant pathogens.
- Molecular assays directly applicable to respiratory specimen testing have the potential to improve adequacy of empiric therapy and spare use of broad-spectrum antibiotics.
- Effective strategies for the prevention of HAP and VAP and newer antimicrobial agents are needed to combat MDR pathogens.

INTRODUCTION

The emergence of multidrug resistance among bacterial species is a worldwide public health threat that is evolving at an alarming rate. Pathogens, including extended-spectrum beta-lactamase (ESBL)-producing and carbapenem-resistant Enterobacteriaceae (CRE), methicillin-resistant *Staphylococcus aureus* (MRSA), vancomycin-resistant *Enterococcus* species, and multidrug-resistant *Acinetobacter baumannii*, are associated with both hospital-acquired and community-acquired infections.[1] Antimicrobial-resistant pathogens that are associated with nosocomial infections, or health care–associated infections (HAI) pose an ongoing challenge to hospitals, both in terms of patient treatment and in the prevention of transmission of resistant pathogens from patient to patient.[1,2]

Disclosures: The authors have no potential conflicts of interest to report.
Division of Clinical Microbiology, Department of Pathology and Laboratory Medicine, Indiana University School of Medicine, 350 West 11th Street, Room 6027B, Indianapolis, IN 46202, USA
* Corresponding author.
E-mail address: gdenys@iupui.edu

Clin Lab Med 34 (2014) 257–270
http://dx.doi.org/10.1016/j.cll.2014.02.004
0272-2712/14/$ – see front matter © 2014 Elsevier Inc. All rights reserved.

Of the HAIs, lower respiratory tract (LRT) infections are among the most frequently acquired, particularly among patients in the intensive care unit (ICU).[3] Because of the unique combination of critically ill, and often immunosuppressed, hosts and chronically high antibiotic selective pressures, the ICU is an important environment for the emergence of antimicrobial drug resistance and the spread of drug-resistant organisms. Despite advances in antimicrobial therapy, supportive care, and infection control measures, hospital-acquired pneumonia (HAP) and ventilator-associated pneumonia (VAP) cause considerable morbidity and mortality. In addition, these infections are associated with increased costs to health care systems.[1,4,5] The incidence of HAP ranges from 5 to more than 20 cases per 1000 hospital admissions.[6,7] In patients not in the ICU, the highest rates are seen in the elderly, the immunosuppressed, surgical patients, and those receiving enteral feeding through a nasogastric tube.[6] Approximately one-third of HAPs are ICU-acquired, with VAP accounting for approximately 90% of the cases. VAP occurs in 9% to 40% of intubated and mechanically ventilated individuals, which represents the most frequent ICU-acquired infection.[8,9] The current incidence of VAP ranges from 2 to 16 cases per 1000 ventilator days, with a mortality rate ranging from of 3% to 17%.[7] The estimated cost per HAP or VAP infection is in excess of $40,000, with a mortality rate ranging from 10% to 50%.[10] This article describes the etiology, epidemiology, pathogenesis, diagnosis, and treatment of HAP and VAP associated with antibiotic-resistant bacterial pathogens.

ETIOLOGY

The etiology of HAP and VAP depends on whether the patient has risk factors for the acquisition of multidrug-resistant (MDR) pathogens. Factors, including the duration of mechanical ventilation, length of hospital and ICU stay, previous exposure to antibiotics, and local endemic pathogens in a given ICU, influence the likelihood of MDR pathogen infection.[1,11] A summary of the risk factors for infection with MDR pathogens is presented in **Box 1**.[10,12] The frequency of specific MDR pathogens varies among

---

Box 1
Risk factors associated with multidrug-resistant (MDR) pathogens causing hospital-acquired pneumonia and ventilator-associated pneumonia

- Antibiotic use in previous 3 months
- Hospitalization in the previous 3 months or ≥5 days
- Exposure to the intensive care unit
- Exposure to specific hospital unit with high frequency of antibiotic resistance
- Previous residence in nursing home or long-term care facility
- Home infusion therapy (including antibiotics)
- Hemodialysis
- Home wound care in past 30 days
- Family member with MDR pathogen
- Immunosuppression

Data from Sydnor ER, Perl TM. Hospital epidemiology and infection control in acute-care settings. Clin Microbiol Rev 2011;24:141–73; and Papazian L, Donati SY. Hospital-acquired pneumonia. In: Cohen J, Powderly WG, Opel SM, editors. van der Meer JWM, Didier, Sobel JD, section editors. Cohen, Powderly and Opal's infectious diseases. 3rd edition. Philadelphia: Mosby Elsevier; 2010. p. 294–9.

hospitals, specific hospital units, and patient populations (eg, medical, surgical, or trauma), including those patients who have recently been exposed to antibiotics. These pathogens may originate from the patient's endogenous flora, other patients, hospital staff, contaminated medical devices, or the environment.[13]

Guidelines for the treatment of nosocomial pneumonia defines HAP into early-onset pneumonia, which occurs within the first 5 days of admission, and those who develop late-onset nosocomial pneumonia, which occurs 5 days or more after admission.[1] Late-onset HAP mostly involves hospital-acquired MDR pathogens, a result of antibiotic selective pressure, cross-transmission, and colonization from ICU environmental sources.[1,11,14] However, MDR pathogens may be isolated in early-onset HAP when risk factors exist before ICU admission.[14] **Table 1** lists the predominant bacterial agents causing nosocomial pneumonia. In general, organisms causing early-onset HAP reflect antibiotic-susceptible community isolates, such as Streptococcus pneumoniae, Haemophilus influenzae, Moraxella catarrhalis, S aureus, nonresistant Enterobacteriaceae, anaerobic bacteria, and Legionella pneumophila. Patients who develop late-onset pneumonia are more likely to be infected with MDR organisms, including Pseudomonas aeruginosa, A baumannii, ESBL-producing and carbapenemase-producing Enterobacteriaceae, and MRSA.

EPIDEMIOLOGY

More than 60% of reported HAP and VAP are caused by gram-negative bacilli; however, 20% to 40% are now caused by S aureus, most of which are methicillin-resistant strains.[6] Pneumonia due to hospital-acquired MRSA has been increasing worldwide for the past 10 years; reports indicate that community-acquired MRSA clones (eg, US300/400) emerging in hospitals cause HAP and VAP.[15] Increasing resistance to vancomycin (minimum inhibitory concentration [MIC] 2 μg/mL) or vancomycin intermediate-resistant S aureus (MIC 4–8 μg/mL) have been seen worldwide and are associated with poor clinical outcomes.[16,17] In addition, recent reports of linezolid resistance in MRSA isolates is a significant concern.[18,19] Among the Enterobacteriaceae, resistance to third-generation and fourth-generation cephalosporins is expressed by acquired ESBLs and/or AmpC β-lactamases. Another emerging resistance concern is the increase of carbapenemase-producing strains associated with

Table 1
Predominant bacterial agents causing nosocomial pneumonia

Early-Onset HAP (<5 d Hospitalization) Non-MDR Pathogens[a]	Late-Onset HAP and VAP (≥5 d Hospitalization) MDR Pathogens
Streptococcus pneumoniae	Methicillin-resistant S aureus (MRSA)
Haemophilus influenzae	Pseudomonas aeruginosa
Moraxella catarrhalis	Acinetobacter species
Staphylococcus aureus	ESBL-producing Klebsiella pneumoniae, Escherichia coli, or Enterobacter species
Anaerobic bacteria Legionella pneumophila	Carbapenemase-producing K pneumoniae, or E coli, or Enterobacter species

Abbreviations: ESBL, extended-spectrum beta-lactamase; HAP, hospital-acquired pneumonia; MDR, multidrug resistant; VAP, ventilator-associated pneumonia.
[a] Antimicrobial susceptibility testing warranted due to the threat of resistance.
Data from Spellberg B, Blaser M, Guidos RJ, et al. Combating antimicrobial resistance: policy recommendations to save lives. Clin Infect Dis 2011;52(Suppl 5):S397–428.

health care exposures.[20,21] Many of these enzymes are encoded by genes that are present on transmissible plasmids, and have been identified in several species of CREs.[22] *P aeruginosa* is the most common MDR pathogen causing VAP and is associated with increased mortality.[23] *A baumannii* is a frequent cause of outbreaks in the hospital setting. A growing number of *A baumannii* strains are MDR, and are difficult to control and eradicate.[6] An increasing prevalence of MDR *P aeruginosa* and *A baumannii* strains causing VAP are carbapenem-resistant, leaving the polymyxins (eg, colistin) as the last therapeutic option to treat infections caused by these organisms.[9,24,25] Colistin resistance is also reported to be on the rise in ICUs, with a high prevalence of carbapenem resistance and heavy usage of colistin.[26,27] Newer antimicrobial agents are needed to target MDR gram-negative bacteria in the current nosocomial setting.[28]

CLINICAL PRESENTATION

HAP is currently defined as pneumonia that develops in patients who have been admitted for more than 48 hours and in whom no antecedent signs or symptoms of infection were evident at the time of hospital admission.[6,29,30] For intubated and mechanically ventilated patients, pneumonia developing more than 48 hours but less than 72 hours after endotracheal tube placement is consistent with VAP.[29] In these patients, clinical signs and symptoms often overlap and usually include a new or progressive pulmonary infiltrate, as demonstrated by chest radiography, as well as the onset of fever, decreased oxygenation, production of purulent sputum, and either leukopenia (<4000 white blood cells [WBC]/mL) or leukocytosis (>12,000 WBC/mL).[29,30] In addition, some patient populations, including those 70 years and older, may experience mental status change, which can be an important sign used to facilitate diagnosis.[29] MDR pathogen–associated HAP and VAP are typically refractory to treatment with many antimicrobial drugs, including many broad-spectrum agents,[31] so when deciding on empiric antimicrobial treatment regimens, consideration of these organisms as causes of a patient's lower airway disease is imperative.

PATHOGENESIS

Several factors can influence the outcome of nosocomial pneumonia, including the immunologic fitness of the host and the types, quantities, and virulence of pathogens introduced into the LRT. To successfully colonize the tissues of the lower airway, pathogens must first circumvent physical barriers and evade cells and effector molecules of the innate and adaptive immune defenses. Because patients who are at risk for developing nosocomial pneumonia typically have compromised defenses, pathogens that colonize the lower airway can often quickly overwhelm this already weakened site, leading to infection. Predisposing conditions include one or more underlying disease processes; receipt of immunosuppressive chemotherapy, antibiotics, or other medications that modulate the immune system or enrich for drug-resistant microorganisms; and invasive medical procedures, such as placement of respiratory devices and surgery.[29]

In cases of HAP, most often, pathogens colonizing sites in the upper airway bypass physical barriers, such as the mucociliary escalator, via aspiration of contaminated upper respiratory tract secretions. Factors that increase the risk of aspiration include dysphagia, emesis, intubation, and sedation.[6,30] In a very small subset of cases, microorganisms that colonize other sites, including the gastrointestinal tract, can be translocated to the lower airway. For VAP, pathogens can access the LRT directly through the endotracheal tube via inhalation of infectious aerosols and reflux of contaminated endotracheal tube condensate, or through leakage of pathogen-laden upper respiratory secretions around the endotracheal tube cuff.[30]

Both endogenous and exogenous sources of nosocomial pneumonia–associated pathogens, including MDR bacterial pathogens, exist. Opportunistic members of the patient's normal microbiota can be involved in these infections; however, pathogens are often acquired from exogenous sources, including health care devices, health care personnel, other patients, and environmental reservoirs.[6,29] Because of the MDR pathogen-selecting environment of the ICU, many of these pathogens could persist in these environments, especially in the absence of appropriate disinfection and hygienic standards.[32]

DIAGNOSIS

The clinical diagnosis of HAP and VAP is difficult because the clinical findings are often nonspecific. Guidelines on the management of adults with HAP, VAP, and health care–associated pneumonia by the American Thoracic Society and Infectious Diseases Society of America (ATS/IDSA) provide specific criteria for diagnosis.[6] Similar guidelines by the Association of Medical Microbiology and Infectious Disease Canada and the Canadian Thoracic Society (AMMI/CTS) are provided for the management of HAP and VAP.[33] The presence of new or progressive radiographic infiltrates plus 2 or more other clinical characteristics, such as purulent LRT secretions, leukocytosis or leukopenia, fever higher than 38°C, and decreased partial pressure of oxygen in arterial blood, represent clinically relevant criteria to start empiric antimicrobial therapy. Once VAP is considered, cultures must be obtained immediately and empiric therapy must be initiated without delay.

To distinguish colonization of the lower airway with microorganisms from infection with etiologic agents of nosocomial pneumonia, specimen collection is best achieved by bronchoscope-assisted bronchoalveolar lavage (BAL) or protected brush specimens (PBS) in combination with quantitative culture of the material obtained. Endotracheal aspirates, nonbronchoscopic BAL specimens, or PBS in combination with quantitative culture is an alternative in patients suspected of having VAP. Specimens that are likely to contain saliva should be avoided, because they are likely to be heavily contaminated with upper respiratory tract microbiota. Ideally, specimens should be transported to the laboratory immediately after collection.[34] Care should be taken to avoid excess time between specimen collection and inoculation of culture media, as prolongation of processing is often associated with a loss of organism viability.[34] Blood cultures also may be helpful, but they are seldom positive, except in the cases of pneumococcal and *S aureus* pneumonia.

A carefully prepared Gram stain of specimens can often provide a clue as to the number and types of bacteria present, as well as the number and types of host cells, including polymorphonuclear leukocytes and macrophages, which are suggestive of inflammation and infection. The initial Gram stain should be meticulously examined, because the data provided by this examination are often used as a guide for the interpretation of cultures. For isolation of bacterial pathogens, inoculation of nonselective blood-containing media (eg, tryptic soy agar plus 5% sheep's blood), chocolate agar, and a gram-negative selective and differential medium, such as MacConkey agar or eosin-methylene blue agar, is typically sufficient to recover most clinically relevant bacterial pathogens.[34] Plates should be incubated at 35 to 37°C in an atmosphere containing 5% CO_2 and examined at 24 hours and then reincubated for an additional 24 to 48 hours to permit the growth of slower-growing pathogens.[34] Altogether, current methods for isolation, identification, and antimicrobial susceptibility testing of bacterial pathogens usually takes no less than 48 to 72 hours. **Fig. 1** outlines the clinical and bacteriologic strategies in patients suspected of HAP. The decision to discontinue antibiotics may differ based on the type of sample collected (PSB, BAL, endotracheal aspirate) and whether results are reported as quantitative or semiquantitative colony counts. In the future, inclusion of selective and differential chromogenic agars in the primary isolation media battery may facilitate quicker pathogen identification, which could lead to faster implementation of targeted antimicrobial chemotherapy. A number of these media are already commercially available for the detection of MDR pathogens, including ESBL-producing gram-negative bacilli and MRSA, among others. However, there is a paucity of reported data regarding the utility of these media for detection of MDR pathogens from LRT specimens from patients with suspected HAP or VAP.

There is currently a high demand for rapid tests that can be used for the detection of microorganisms, including MDR pathogens, directly from patient specimens. This need has arisen especially as a result of the emergence of an ever-growing list of resistant bacterial pathogens. Because of their relatively rapid time to result, high sensitivity, and high specificity, molecular methods, such as nucleic acid amplification assays, are appealing alternatives or adjuncts to conventional cultivation-based diagnostic approaches.[35] **Table 2** lists potential targets that would be clinically informative if they could be identified by nucleic acid amplification assays in patients with suspected HAP and VAP.[36,37] Presently, there are a number of rapid molecular methods developed that can detect bacterial pathogens directly from patient specimens, or

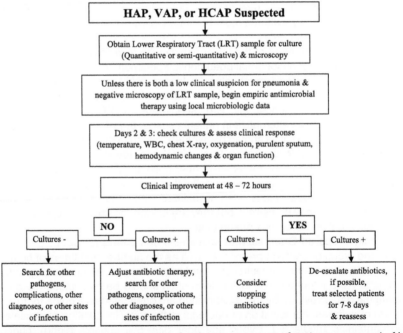

Fig. 1. Clinical and bacteriologic strategy for the management of patients suspected of having HAP, VAP, or health care–associated pneumonia. (*Reprinted* with permission of the American Thoracic Society. Copyright © 2014 American Thoracic Society. Niederman MS, Craven DE, Bonten MJ. American Thoracic Society and Infectious Disease Society of America (ATS/IDSA): guidelines for the management of adults with hospital-acquired, ventilator-associated, and healthcare-associated pneumonia. Am J Respir Crit Care Med 2005;171:388–416. Official Journal of the American Thoracic Society.)

Table 2
Potential targets for molecular amplification assays in patients with HAP and VAP

Pathogen	Target Gene	Mediates Resistance to or Important Feature
Staphylococcus aureus	mecA	All β-lactams, except ceftaroline
	Panton-Valentine leukocidin	PVL gene that encodes for cytotoxin
Pseudomonas aeruginosa	bla_{VIM}, bla_{IMP}	All β-lactams
Acinetobacter spp	bla_{OxA}	Penicillins; extended-spectrum cephalosporins; carbapenems
Enterobacteriaceae	bla_{KPC}	All β-lactams

Abbreviations: HAP, hospital-acquired pneumonia; VAP, ventilator-associated pneumonia.
   Data from Tenover FC. Developing molecular amplification methods for rapid diagnosis of respiratory tract infections caused by bacterial pathogens. Clin Infect Dis 2011;52(Suppl 4):S338–45.

identify cultivated bacterial isolates, and the presence of antimicrobial resistance genes.[38] Most of these assays are polymerase chain reaction (PCR) based and developed to detect S aureus and MRSA. PCR-based assays include the GeneXpert system (Cepheid, Sunnyvale, CA), the GeneOhm MRSA assay (Becton Dickenson, Sparks, MD), the StaphPlex and ResPlex systems (Qiagen, Venlo, Netherlands), the Light Cycler (Roche, Pleasanton, CA), and FilmArray systems (Biofire Diagnostics, Inc, Salt lake City, UT). Methods applied to cultivated bacterial isolates include AccuProbe (Hologic Gen-Probe, San Diego, CA) and matrix-assisted laser desorption ionization time-to flight mass spectrometry (Brucker Daltonics, Inc, Billerica, MA, and Biomerieux, Durham, NC). The T5000 and PLEX-ID Biosensors (Ibis Biosciences, a subsidiary of Abbott Molecular, Inc, Carlsbad, CA, and Abbott Park, IL) combines PCR with electrospray ionization mass spectrometry (PCR/ESI-MS). To date, PCR/ESI-MS has been has been applied for the detection of resistance genes gyrA, parC, mecA, and bla_{KPC}. Microarray technology has been used to detect and identify bla genes belonging to the TEM, SHV, CTX-M, and KPC β-lactamases. The Check KPC/ESBL microarray system (Check-Points Health BV, Wageningen, Netherlands) detects β-lactamase genes conferring resistance to cephalosporins and carbapenems.[39] Card and colleagues[40] described an expanded microarray assay capable of detecting antibiotic resistance genes to a broad range of gram-negative pathogens. In their study, microarray detected 75 clinically important acquired resistance genes encompassing 19 different antimicrobial classes. Microarray-positive results were highly predictive of resistance compared with phenotypic MIC and disk diffusion testing. Despite the advances made in developing these molecular assays, application to bacterial pneumonia and/or point-of-care testing remains undetermined. In a preclinical study, the Cepheid Xpert MRSA/SA SSTI assay compared favorably with quantitative culture for the rapid detection of MRSA and methicillin-susceptible S aureus (MSSA) directly from LRT secretions from patients suspected of VAP.[41] The Xpert PCR assay detects 3 amplified targets: spa, mecA, and staphylococcal cassette chromosome mec element. The specificity of the assay could be improved, however, if samples from patients with a higher clinical suspicion of S aureus pneumonia were tested. Technologies such as the Food and Drug Administration–cleared BioFire Diagnostics, Inc., Salt lake City, Utah, USA. FilmArray Respiratory Panel, a multiplex nucleic acid amplification–based array for detection of 17 respiratory viruses and 3 bacterial pathogens, shows promise that such assays for direct specimen application will eventually be available. Clinical studies are needed, however, to determine the

Table 3
Guidelines for initial therapy for HAP and VAP in patients with late-onset disease or risk factors for MDR pathogens

MDR Pathogens	Antibiotic Therapy	Dosage	Comments
HA-MRSA	Vancomycin or Linezolid	15 mg/kg q12h 600 mg q12h IV/PO	• VRSA/VISA associated with poor outcomes and may not be detected by current susceptibility test methods • High-dose vancomycin is recommended due to treatment failure • Linezolid safe alternative option
Pseudomonas aeruginosa	Cefepime or Ceftazidime or Carbapenem: Imipenem or meropenem *or* PIP/TAZ *plus* AMG: Amikacin Gentamicin, or tobramycin *or* Anti-pseudomonal FQ: Ciprofloxacin Levofloxacin	2 g q8-12h IV 2 g q8h IV 1g q8h 4.5 g q6h IV or 3.375 g 6 h over 4-h infusion 15 mg/kg/d IV 5-7 mg/kg/d IV 400 mg q8h IV 750 mg qd IV	• Automated susceptibility test methods for β-lactams antibiotics may have high rate of false S or R compared to disk diffusion and Etest® (antimicrobial susceptibility test reagent strip to determine on-scale MICs [bioMerieux Clinical Diagnostics, Marcy l'Etoile, France]) • Extended infusion of PIP/TAZ improves time above MIC and reduces mortality • *P aeruginosa* has enhanced capacity to develop resistance • Combination therapy (β-lactam + AMG) should be used until susceptibility results are available • Empiric use of FQ may contribute to greater resistance and risk of MRSA
Acinetobacter spp	Carbapenem *plus* Aminoglycoside or Polymyxin E (Colistin)	See doses above See doses above See Ref.[48] for loading dose and maintenance dose. Inhalation 50-75 mg in 3-4 mL saline via nebulizer 2-3×/d	• Treatment options limited for VAP due to widespread resistance • In vitro susceptibility and clinical response to carbapenems and other drugs may not correlate • Treatment for highly resistant isolates may be limited to Colistin + AMG or RIF • Aerosolized polymyxin useful as adjunct therapy in VAP with MDR

| ESBL-producing Enterobacteriaceae | Carbapenem ± Aminoglycoside | See doses above See doses above | • In vitro testing may not detect all ESBLs
• If ESBL *Klebsiella* or *Acinetobacter* is suspected use carbapenem
• Avoid use of 3rd- and 4th- generation cephalosporins as monotherapy
• Avoid use of 3rd- and 4th- generation cephalosporins for treatment of *Enterobacter* spp VAP
• Most reliable empiric therapy: Carbapenen + AMG |
| Carbapenemase-producing gram-negative organisms | Polymyxin E (Colistin) *plus* Carbapenem (high-dose meropenem)

or RIF *or* Tigecycline | See doses above See doses above 300 mg IV q12h or 600 mg IV q24h
10 mg/kg IV q12h
100 mg IV initially, then 50 mg IV q12h | • Cabepenem resistance is beginning to increase
• Combination therapy recommended
• Colistin resistance reported in ICUs with heavy usage |

Abbreviations: AMG, aminoglycoside; ESBL, extended-spectrum beta-lactamase; FQ, fluoroquinolone; HA-MRSA, hospital-acquired-MRSA; HAP, hospital-acquired pneumonia; ICU, intensive care unit; IV, intravenous; MDR, multidrug resistant; MIC, minimum inhibitory concentration; MRSA, methicillin-resistant *S aureus*; PIP/TAZ, piperacillin-tazobactam; PO, by mouth; q, every; R, resistant; RIF, rifampin; S, susceptible; VAP, ventilator-associated pneumonia; VRSA/VISA, vancomycin-resistant *S aureus*/vancomycin-intermediate *S aureus*.

Data from Craven DE, Chroneou A. Chapter 303, nosocomial pneumonia. In: Mandell GL, Bennett JE, Dolin R, editors. Mandell, Douglas, and Bennett's principles and practices of infectious diseases. 7th edition. Philadelphia: Churchill Livingstone Elsevier; 2010. p. 3717–24; and Petrosillo N, Giannella M, Russel L, et al. Treatment of carbapenem-resistant *Klebsiella pneumoniae*. Expert Rev Anti Infect Ther 2013;11(2):159-77.

most relevant methods for diagnosis of HAP and VAP and the significance of detecting bacterial DNA, especially in the absence of positive culture.

In addition to the obvious benefit of quicker diagnosis and sooner initiation of targeted antimicrobial therapy, detection of MDR pathogens or their antimicrobial drug resistance determinants by rapid molecular tests could also usher in improved infection control practices. For example, patients could potentially be screened for MDR pathogens either before, or on, admission to a health care institution and, when testing is complete, they could be isolated from general patient populations if the assays identify markers of MDR pathogens in their specimen(s).

Another avenue that is being explored is the identification of host-produced biomarkers of HAP and/or VAP. As an adjunct to directly identifying pathogens within clinical samples, the detection of host biomarkers produced in response to microbial pathogens could potentially prove useful for making decisions regarding treatment of patients. However, as summarized by Fagon,[42] recent research into biomarkers assayed directly from BAL specimens, including procalcitonin,[43] C-reactive protein,[44] and soluble triggering receptor expressed on myeloid cells-1,[45] among others, appear to add little in the way of diagnostic value for VAP.[44,46]

TREATMENT

Evidence-based guidelines by ATS/IDSA and by the AMMI/CTS for the management of HAP and VAP recommend rapid diagnosis, immediate empiric antibiotic therapy, avoiding unnecessary antibiotics by de-escalation, and shortening the duration of therapy to the minimum effective period.[6,33] Early clinical diagnosis of HAP and laboratory-based identification of its etiology are critical in guiding empiric antimicrobial therapy. Inappropriate antibiotic use can be the strongest determinant of clinical outcome. The treatment and initial management of HAP and VAP are based on the time of onset of disease and the presence or absence of risk factors for MDR pathogens (see **Box 1** and **Table 1**). Delays in the administration of appropriate antimicrobial therapy for VAP have been associated with excess mortality.[47]

In the absence of risk factors for MDR pathogens, the recommended initial therapy for early-onset HAP caused by S pneumoniae, H influenzae, MSSA, and antibiotic susceptible gram-negative enteric organisms include ceftriaxone, quinolones (levofloxacin, moxifloxacin, or ciprofloxacin), ampicillin/sulbactam, or ertapenem.[6] If L pneumophila is suspected, the use of a fluoroquinolone or azithromycin is recommended. For aerobic coverage, moxifloxicin and ampicillin-sulbactam are recommended.

When the risk factors for MDR pathogens are present, the initial therapy for late-onset HAP or VAP should be broadened for additional coverage of suspected pathogens endemic in the ICUs, such as MRSA, P aeruginosa, A baumannii, and ESBL-producing and carbapenemase-producing Enterobacteriaceae (eg, Klebsiella spp, Escherichia coli, Enterobacter spp, and Serratia spp). Initial empiric therapy in this patient population should include either an antipseudomonal cephalosporin (cefepime or ceftazadime), an antipseudomonal carbapenem (imipenem or meropenem), or a β-lactam/β-lactamase inhibitor combination (piperacillin-tazobactam) plus an antipseudomonal fluoroquinolone (ciprofloxacin or levofloxacin) or an aminoglycoside (amikacin, gentamicin, or tobramycin) plus linezolid or vancomycin is recommend for 48 hours until culture and antimicrobial susceptibility results are available.[14] New clinical evidence supports combination empiric therapy for carbapenem-resistant Klebsiella pneumoniae.[48] The initial therapy and dosing for HAP and VAP in patients with late-onset disease or risk factors for MDR pathogens is summarized in **Table 3**. Although controversial, initiating combination therapy is recommended in patients infected with MDR pathogens. Aerosolized antibiotics may be considered as an adjunct therapy in patients with MDR gram-negative organisms who are not responding to systemic therapy. Based on the patient's clinical assessment (fever, oxygenation, leukocyte count, and vital signs) and microbiologic data (Gram stain, culture, and antimicrobial susceptibility data) 24 to 48 hours after empiric therapy, the initial antibiotic regimen should be deescalated, if possible. In patients responding to treatment, the ATS/IDSA recommends that antibiotics be discontinued after 7 days of therapy for uncomplicated HAP and VAP with close follow-up for relapse in patients with *P aeruginosa*. Effective strategies for the prevention and risk reduction of HAP and VAP include the use of strict infection control, hand hygiene, microbiological surveillance studies, monitoring the early removal of invasive devices, and programs to reduce or alter antibiotic-prescribing practices. Several excellent review articles are available to address these prevention strategies.[10,32,49,50]

SUMMARY

Nosocomial respiratory infections are among the most common conditions affecting hospitalized patients (HAP), particularly in mechanically ventilated patients in the ICU (VAP). HAP and VAP are caused by a variety of MDR pathogens and are the leading cause of death associated with hospital-acquired infections. The frequency of MDR pathogens as the etiologic agents of HAP and VAP in patients in the ICU and patients with risk factors is increasing. Evidence-based guidelines to identify patients at increased risk of MDR pathogens and management of HAP and VAP are published by ATS/IDSA. The challenge for clinicians is to identify patients who can benefit from empiric therapy with broad-spectrum antibiotics with activity against MDR pathogens. The diagnosis of HAP and VAP should be suspected in patients with new or progressive lung infiltrates on radiographic images and other clinical characteristics of pneumonia. Culture specimens should be obtained immediately by endotracheal tube or quantitative BAL and appropriate antibiotics should be started without delay. Despite its current limitation, rapid molecular methods have the potential to identify microorganisms and antimicrobial resistance targets directly from unprocessed specimens. The development of new diagnostic tools and therapeutic agents is urgently needed to face the epidemic of MDR pathogens.

REFERENCES

1. Spellberg B, Blaser M, Guidos RJ, et al. Combating antimicrobial resistance: policy recommendations to save lives. Clin Infect Dis 2011;52(Suppl 5): S397–428.
2. Sievert DM, Ricks P, Edwards JR, et al. Antimicrobial-resistant pathogens associated with healthcare-associated infections: summary of data reported to the National Healthcare Safety Network at the Centers for Disease Control and Prevention, 2009-2010. Infect Control Hosp Epidemiol 2013;34(1):1–14.
3. National Nosocomial Infections Surveillance (NNIS) System. National Nosocomial Infections Surveillance (NNIS) system report, data summary from January 1992 through June 2004, issued October 2004. Am J Infect Control 2004;32: 470–85.
4. Cosgrove SE. The relationship between antimicrobial resistance and patient outcomes: mortality, length of hospital stay, and health care cost. Clin Infect Dis 2006;42(Suppl 2):S82–9.
5. Holmberg SD, Solomon SL, Blake PA. Health and economic impacts of antimicrobial resistance. Rev Infect Dis 1987;9:1065–78.

6. Niederman MS, Craven DE, Bonten MJ. American Thoracic Society and Infectious Disease Society of America (ATS/IDSA): guidelines for the management of adults with hospital-acquired, ventilator-associated, and healthcare-associated pneumonia. Am J Respir Crit Care Med 2005;171:388–416.

7. Barbier F, Andremont A, Wolff M, et al. Hospital-acquired pneumonia and ventilator-associated pneumonia: recent advances in epidemiology and management. Curr Opin Pulm Med 2013;19(3):216–28.

8. Vincent JL, Rello J, Marshall J, et al. International study of the prevalence and outcomes of infection in intensive care units. JAMA 2009;302:2323–9.

9. Rosenthal VD, Bijie H, Maki DG, et al. International Nosocomial Infection Control Consortium (INICC) report, data summary of 36 countries, for 2004-2009. Am J Infect Control 2012;40:396–407.

10. Sydnor ER, Perl TM. Hospital epidemiology and infection control in acute-care settings. Clin Microbiol Rev 2011;24:141–73.

11. Jones RN. Microbial etiologies of hospital-acquired bacterial pneumonia and ventilator-associated bacterial pneumonia. Clin Infect Dis 2010;51(Suppl 1): S81–7.

12. Papazian L, Donati SY. Hospital-acquired pneumonia. In: Cohen J, Powderly WG, Opel SM, editors. van der Meer JWM, Didier, Sobel JD, section editors. Cohen, Powderly and Opal's infectious diseases. 3rd edition. Philadelphia: Mosby Elsevier; 2010. p. 294–9.

13. Safder N, Crnich CJ, Maki DG. The pathogenesis of ventilator-associated pneumonia: its relevance to developing effective strategies for prevention. Respir Care 2005;50:725–39.

14. Ferrer M, Liapikou A, Valencia M, et al. Validation of the American Thoracic Society-Infectious Diseases Society of America guidelines for hospital-acquired pneumonia in the intensive care unit. Clin Infect Dis 2010;50:945–52.

15. Popovich KJ, Weinstein RA, Hota B. Are community-associated methicillin-resistant *Staphylococcus aureus* (MRSA) strains replacing traditional nosocomial MRSA strains? Clin Infect Dis 2008;46:787–94.

16. De Lassence A, Hidri N, Timsit JF, et al. Control and outcome of a large outbreak of colonization and infection with glycopeptides-intermediate *Staphylococcus aureus* in an intensive care unit. Clin Infect Dis 2006;42:170–8.

17. Deresinski S. Counterpoint: vancomycin and *Staphylococcus aureus*—an antibiotic enters obsolescence. Clin Infect Dis 2007;44:1543–8.

18. Morales G, Picazo JJ, Baos E, et al. Resistance to linezolid is mediated by the cfr gene in the first report of an outbreak of linezolid-resistant *Staphylococcus aureus*. Clin Infect Dis 2010;50:821–5.

19. Sánchez Garcia M, De la Torre MA, Morales G, et al. Clinical outbreak of linezolid-resistant *Staphylococcus aureus* in an intensive care unit. JAMA 2010;303:2260–4.

20. Nordmann P, Naas T, Poirel L. Global spread of carbapenemase-producing Enterobacteriaceae. Emerg Infect Dis 2011;17:1791–8.

21. Centers for Disease Control and Prevention (CDC). Vital signs: carbapenem-resistant Enterobacteriaceae. MMWR Morb Mortal Wkly Rep 2013;62:165–70.

22. Tzouvelekis LS, Markogiannakis A, Psichogiou M, et al. Carbapenemases in *Klebsiella pneumoniae* and other Enterobacteriaceae: an evolving crisis of global dimensions. Clin Microbiol Rev 2012;25(4):682–707.

23. Roy-Burman A, Savel RH, Racine S, et al. Type III protein secretion is associated with death in lower respiratory and systemic *Pseudomonas aeruginosa* infections. J Infect Dis 2001;183:1767–74.

24. Chung DR, Song JH, Kim SH, et al. High prevalence of multidrug-resistant non-fermenters in hospital-acquired pneumonia in Asia. Am J Respir Crit Care Med 2011;184:1409–17.

25. Livermore DM. Has the era of untreatable infections arrived? J Antimicrob Chemother 2009;64(Suppl 1):i29–36.

26. Antoniadou A, Kontopidou F, Poulakou G, et al. Colistin-resistant isolates of *Klebsiella pneumoniae* emerging in intensive care unit patients: first report of a multiclonal cluster. J Antimicrob Chemother 2007;59:786–90.

27. Bogdanovich T, Adams-Haduch JM, Tian GB, et al. Colistin-resistant, *Klebsiella pneumoniae* carbapenemase (KPC)-producing *Klebsiella pneumoniae* belonging to the international epidemic clone ST258. Clin Infect Dis 2011;53:373–6.

28. Pucci MJ, Bush K. Investigational antimicrobial agents of 2013. Clin Microbiol Rev 2013;26(4):792–821.

29. Kieninger AN, Lipsett PA. Hospital-acquired pneumonia: pathophysiology, diagnosis, and treatment. Surg Clin North Am 2009;89:439–61.

30. Craven DE, Chroneou A. Chapter 303, nosocomial pneumonia. In: Mandell GL, Bennett JE, Dolin R, editors. Mandell, Douglas, and Bennett's principles and practices of infectious diseases. 7th edition. Philadelphia: Churchill Livingstone Elsevier; 2010. p. 3717–24.

31. Jean SS, Hsueh PR. Current review of antimicrobial treatment of nosocomial pneumonia caused by multidrug-resistant pathogens. Expert Opin Pharmacother 2011;12(14):2145–8.

32. Joseph NM, Sistla S, Dutta TK, et al. Role of intensive care unit environment and health-care workers in transmission of ventilator-associated pneumonia. J Infect Dev Ctries 2010;4(5):282–91.

33. Rotstein C, Evans G, Born A, et al. Clinical practice guidelines for hospital-acquired pneumonia and ventilator-associated pneumonia in adults. Can J Infect Dis Med Microbiol 2008;19(1):19–53.

34. Garcia LS, editor. 2007 update: clinical microbiology procedures handbook. 2nd edition. Washington, DC: ASM Press; 2007.

35. Gilbert DN, Spellberg B, Bartlett G. An unmet medical need: rapid molecular diagnostic tests for respiratory tract infections. Clin Infect Dis 2011;52(Suppl 4):S386–95.

36. Lung M, Codina G. Molecular diagnosis in HAP/VAP. Curr Opin Crit Care 2012; 18(5):487–94.

37. Tenover FC. Developing molecular amplification methods for rapid diagnosis of respiratory tract infections caused by bacterial pathogens. Clin Infect Dis 2011; 52(Suppl 4):S338–45.

38. Endimiani A, Hujer KM, Hujer AM, et al. Are we ready for novel detection methods to treat respiratory pathogens in hospital-acquired pneumonia? Clin Infect Dis 2011;52(Suppl 4):S373–83.

39. Endimiani A, Hujer AM, Hujer KM, et al. Evaluation of a commercial microarray system for detection of SHV-, TEM-, CTX-M-, and KPC-type beta-lactamase genes in Gram-negative isolates. J Clin Microbiol 2010;48:2618–22.

40. Card R, Zhang J, Das P, et al. Evaluation of an expanded microarray for detecting antibiotic resistance genes in a broad range of gram-negative bacterial pathogens. Antimicrob Agents Chemother 2013;57:458–65.

41. Cercenado E, Marin M, Burillo A, et al. Rapid detection of *Staphylococcus aureus* in lower respiratory tract secretions from patients with suspected ventilator-associated pneumonia: evaluation of the Cepheid Xpert MRSA/SA SSTI assay. J Clin Microbiol 2012;50:4095–7.

42. Fagon JY. Biological markers and diagnosis of ventilator-associated pneumonia. Crit Care 2011;15:130.
43. Luyt CE, Combes A, Reynaud C, et al. Usefulness of procalcitonin for the diagnosis of ventilator-associated pneumonia. Intensive Care Med 2008;34: 1434–40.
44. Linssen CF, Bekers O, Drent M, et al. C-reactive protein and procalcitonin concentrations in bronchoalveolar lavage fluid as a predictor of ventilator-associated pneumonia. Ann Clin Biochem 2008;45:293–8.
45. Gibot S, Kolopp-Sarda MN, Béné MC, et al. Plasma level of a triggering expressed on myeloid cells-1: its diagnostic accuracy in patients with suspected sepsis. Ann Intern Med 2004;141(1):9–15.
46. Anand NJ, Zuick S, Klesney-Tait J, et al. Diagnostic implications of soluble triggering receptor expressed on myeloid cells-1 in BAL fluid of patients with pulmonary patients in the ICU. Chest 2009;135:641–7.
47. Iregui M, Ward S, Sherman G, et al. Clinical importance of delays in the initiation of appropriate antibiotic treatment for ventilator-associated pneumonia. Chest 2002;122:262–8.
48. Petrosillo N, Giannella M, Russel L, et al. Treatment of carbapenem-resistant *Klebsiella pneumoniae*. Expert Rev Anti Infect Ther 2013;11(2):159–77.
49. Tablan OC, Anderson LJ, Besser R, et al. Guidelines for preventing health-care associated pneumonia, 2003: recommendations of CDC and the Healthcare Infection Control Practices Advisory Committee. MMWR Recomm Rep 2004; 53:1–36.
50. Koenig SM, Jonathon DT. Ventilator-associated pneumonia: diagnosis, treatment, and prevention. Clin Microbiol Rev 2006;19(4):637–57.

Nontuberculous Mycobacteria in Respiratory Infections
Advances in Diagnosis and Identification

Akos Somoskovi, MD, PhD, DSc[a], Max Salfinger, MD[b],*

KEYWORDS

- Nontuberculous mycobacteria • NTM • Mycobacterium • Identification
- Antimicrobial susceptibility testing

KEY POINTS

- Among adults 65 years or older, from 1997 to 2007, the annual prevalence of pulmonary NTM disease significantly increased from 20 to 47 cases per 100,000 persons, or 8.2% per year. Women were 1.4 times more likely to be a pulmonary NTM case than men. Relative to white individuals, Asian/Pacific Islander individuals were twice as likely to be a case, whereas black individuals were half as likely.
- For optimal recovery of mycobacteria, clinical specimens from nonsterile body sites must be subjected to digestion, decontamination, and concentration. This procedure aims to eradicate more rapidly growing contaminants, such as normal flora (other bacteria and fungi), while not seriously affecting the viability of the mycobacteria.
- One of the most urgent questions that needs to be addressed rapidly by the mycobacteriology laboratory is whether *Mycobacterium tuberculosis* complex or NTM is involved. NAA assays are excellent tools for the purpose, and can be used directly on the clinical specimens of patients suspected of having mycobacterial disease, allowing same-day reporting of results. However, these tests are usually evaluated primarily with respiratory specimens and adequate information of their performance on nonrespiratory specimens stratified to different body compartments is often lacking.
- The Centers for Disease Control and Prevention recommends the use of both liquid and solid media for the growth detection of mycobacteria to decrease the time to detection and to increase the yield of growth detection.
- With the recent advances in chemistry and automation of instrumentation, DNA sequencing of variable genomic regions offers a rapid, accurate, and relatively inexpensive method for the identification of mycobacteria. The most routinely used and reliable method of this kind is the amplification and sequence analysis of hypervariable regions of the gene encoding 16S rRNA.

[a] Institute of Medical Microbiology, Swiss National Reference Center for Mycobacteriology, University of Zuirch, Gloriastrasse 30/32, CH-8006, Zurich, Switzerland; [b] Department of Medicine, National Jewish Health, K420, 1400 Jackson Street, Denver, CO 80206, USA
* Corresponding author.
E-mail address: salfingerm@njhealth.org

Clin Lab Med 34 (2014) 271–295
http://dx.doi.org/10.1016/j.cll.2014.03.001
0272-2712/14/$ – see front matter © 2014 Elsevier Inc. All rights reserved.

MICROBIOLOGY

Together with the genera *Corynebacterium* and *Nocardia*, the genus *Mycobacterium* forms a monophyletic taxon, the so-called CMN group, within the phylum Actinobacteria. The genus *Mycobacterium* is highly diverse, thanks to its ancient origin and years of evolution in multiple habitats. Historically, the species within the genus *Mycobacterium* have been classified based on their growth rate in a subculture as rapid (visible growth in <7 days) and slow growers (growth detection >7 days), and on their pigment production as scotochromogenic (pigment production in dark), photochromogenic (pigment production after exposure to light), or nonchromogenic.[1–5]

Previously, the identification of mycobacteria used a panel of cultural characteristics and biochemical tests; however, these assays are not only unacceptably time consuming, but also often inaccurate, laborious, or not capable of identifying the mycobacterium species at all. In addition, some fastidious species (eg, *Mycobacterium haemophilum* or *Mycobacterium genavense*) require special growth conditions (hemin source or unusually acidic pH), necessitating rarely used and special media, as well as an exquisite collaboration between the clinician requesting the test and the laboratory professional performing the test.[1–5]

The plethora of newly described species seen in the past decades (**Table 1**) is in part the consequence of the availability and increased reliability of new DNA-sequencing methods that are capable of differentiating even closely related species and an increased frequency of isolation of mycobacteria. The latter may be the result of newly emerging manmade reservoirs for certain species. From 41 valid species in 1980, currently this genus encompasses 169 recognized species and 13 subspecies (**Fig. 1**) (http://www.bacterio.net/mycobacterium.html).[1–5]

The *Mycobacterium* genus includes strict pathogens, potentially or opportunistic pathogens, and nonpathogenic saprophytic species. According to the presently prevailing terminology, the mycobacteria species that earlier were referred to as atypical mycobacteria or mycobacteria other than tuberculosis are now called nontuberculous mycobacteria (NTM). Gene sequence similarities within the genus sequences (>94.3% for 16S rRNA gene) and robust phylogenetic reconstructions using concatenated sequences of housekeeping genes have confirmed the natural division among slow-grower and rapid-grower mycobacteria, and also have demonstrated that all slow growers belong to a single evolutionary branch that emerged from the rapidly growing mycobacteria.[2–5] This feature is intrinsically linked to their pathogenic ability to infect humans and, therefore, all obligatory pathogens and most opportunistic pathogens belong the slow-growing evolutionary branch.[5]

EPIDEMIOLOGY

NTM are ubiquitous environmental microorganisms that can be recovered from soil and fresh water and seawater (natural and treated).[1–5] Until recently there was no evidence of human-to-human or animal-to-human transmission of NTM. However, 2 recent findings investigating outbreaks in patients with cystic fibrosis using thorough conventional epidemiologic and state-of-the-art molecular typing investigations, such as whole-genome sequencing, have challenged the dogma of person-to-person transmission indicating potential transmission of *Mycobacterium abscessus* subspecies *massiliense* and *M abscessus* between these patients.[6,7] Because NTM may be found in both natural and manmade reservoirs, human infections are suspected of being acquired from these environmental sources. However, the identification of the specific source of infection is usually not possible. NTM diseases are usually not

Table 1
List of novel nontuberculous mycobacteria species since 2004 causing pulmonary disease or were isolated from respiratory specimens

Novel Species	Year	Growth	Closely Related to
M abscessus ssp abscessus	2011	Rapid	M abscessus
M abscessus ssp bolletii	2011	Rapid	M abscessus
M alsiense*	2007	Slow	M szulgai/M malmoense
M arosiense	2008	Slow	M avium/M intracellulare
M arupense	2006	Slow	M nonchromogenicum
M aubagnense	2006	Rapid	M mucogenicum
M barrassiae*	2006	Rapid	M moriokaense
M boenickei	2004	Rapid	M porcinum
M bouchedurhonense	2009	Slow	M avium
M chimaera	2004	Slow	M avium/M intracellulare
M colombiense	2006	Slow	M avium
M conceptionense	2006	Rapid	M fortuitum
M cosmeticum	2004	Rapid	M smegmatis
M europaeum	2011	Slow	M simiae
M florentinum	2005	Slow	M lentiflavum/M triplex
M fragae	2013	Slow	M celatum
M fukienense**	2013	Rapid	M chelonae/M abscessus
M houstonense	2004	Rapid	M fortuitum
M insubricum	2009	Rapid	M farcinogenes/M houstonense/M senegalense
M iranicum	2013	Rapid	M gilvum
M koreense	2012	Slow	M triviale
M kyorinense	2009	Slow	M celatum
M mantenii	2009	Slow	M scrofulaceum
M marseillense	2009	Slow	M avium
M massiliense	2004	Rapid	M abscessus ssp bolletii
M monacense	2006	Rapid	M doricum
M nebraskense	2004	Slow	M scrofulaceum
M noviomagense	2009	Slow	M xeopi
M paragordonae	2014	Slow	M gordonae
M parakoreense	2013	Slow	M koreense
M paraseoulense	2010	Slow	M seoulense
M paraterrae*	2010	Slow	M terrae
M parascrofulaceum	2004	Slow	M scrofulaceum
M phocaicum	2006	Rapid	M mucogenicum
M riyadhense	2009	Slow	M szulgai
M saskatchewanense	2004	Slow	M interjectum
M senuense	2008	Slow	M terrae
M seoulense	2007	Slow	M scrofulaceum
M sherrisii	2004	Slow	M simiae
M shinjukuense	2011	Slow	M tuberculosis H37Rv/M marinum/M ulcerans
M timonense	2009	Slow	M avium
M yongonense	2013	Slow	M intracellulare

* List of prokaryotic names without standing in nomenclature.
** Biomed Environ Sci 2013;26:894-901.
   Data from List of prokaryotic names with standing in nomenclature. Available at: http://www.bacterio.net/mycobacterium.html. Accessed March 4, 2014.

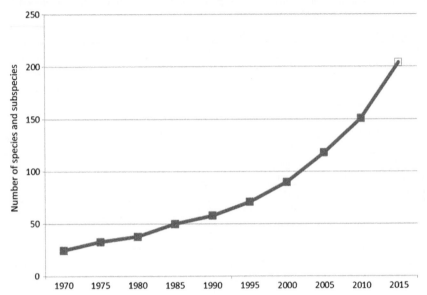

Fig. 1. Newly described species and subspecies: *Mycobacterium*. (*Data from* List of prokaryotic names with standing in nomenclature. Available at: http://www.bacterio.net/mycobacterium. html. Accessed March 4, 2014.)

mandatory to report, as they are not communicable, and surveillance data are not only limited but also unreliable.[1,8]

The average annual (2004–2006) site-specific prevalence among 4 integrated health care delivery systems ranged from 1.4 to 6.6 per 100,000. Prevalence was 1.1-fold to 1.6-fold higher among women relative to men across sites. Among persons aged 60 years or older, annual prevalence increased from 19.6 per 100,000 from 1994 to 1996, to 26.7 per 100,000 from 2004 to 2006.[9]

Marras and colleagues[10] reported an increase in the number of pulmonary NTM isolates in Ontario, Canada, from 9.1 per 100,000 in 1997 to 14.1 per 100,000 in 2003. In a follow-up study, the same research group measured the prevalence and temporal trends of pulmonary NTM disease among residents of Ontario from 1998 to 2010. Five-year prevalence increased from 29.3 cases per 100,000 persons from 1998 to 2002, to 41.3 per 100,000 in 2006 to 2010.[11]

The prevalence and trends of pulmonary NTM-associated hospitalizations in the United States were estimated using national hospital discharge data from 11 states with continuous data available from 1998 through 2005. Pulmonary NTM hospitalizations increased significantly with age among both sexes: relative prevalence for persons 70 to 79 years of age compared with those 40 to 49 years of age was 15 per 100,000 for women (9.4 vs 0.6) and 9 per 100,000 for men (7.6 vs 0.83). Annual prevalence increased significantly among men and women in Florida (3.2%/year and 6.5%/year, respectively) and among women in New York (4.6%/year), with no significant changes in California.[12]

Adjemian and colleagues[13] described the prevalence and trends of pulmonary NTM disease among adults aged 65 years or older throughout the United States in a nationally representative 5% sample of Medicare Part B beneficiaries from 1997 to 2007. From 1997 to 2007, the annual prevalence significantly increased from 20 to 47 cases per 100,000 persons, or 8.2% per year. Women were 1.4 times more likely to be a pulmonary NTM case than men. Relative to white individuals, Asian/Pacific Islander individuals were twice as likely to be a case, whereas black individuals were half as likely (**Figs. 2** and **3**).

PATHOGENESIS AND CLINICAL SIGNIFICANCE

NTM may result in colonization, infection, and disease.[1,8] NTM that are also called opportunistic mycobacteria may become pathogenic in certain conditions (**Box 1**), whereas other so-called saprophytic NTM never or very rarely cause diseases. Colonization can be defined by the absence of host immune reaction, whereas in the event of infection, the host may respond with skin test reaction or antibody production but without disease manifestation. Colonization and infection can be transient, intermittent, and prolonged. Because humans are in regular contact with NTM in the environment, NTM can be detected in the respiratory and gastrointestinal tract or on the skin in healthy individuals.

NTM may occur in natural and manmade environments, such as treated urban water and sewage systems, swimming pools, hot tubs, pedicure foot baths and showers, tattoo inks, fish tanks, or medical devices, such as endoscopes and their washing machines, ice machines used to refrigerate surgical solutions, or inadequately sterilized surgical equipment or solutions.[1,8] Certain NTM, such as *Mycobacterium avium*, *Mycobacterium chelonae*, or *Mycobacterium marinum,* are more commonly recoverable in artificial sources, whereas the natural reservoir of *Mycobacterium kansasii* and *Mycobacterium xenopi* is unknown. Other species, such as *Mycobacterium gordonae*, are common in both natural and artificial sources. NTM can form a biofilm on a wide range of organic (plastic, silicone, rubber, PVC) and inorganic material (glass and

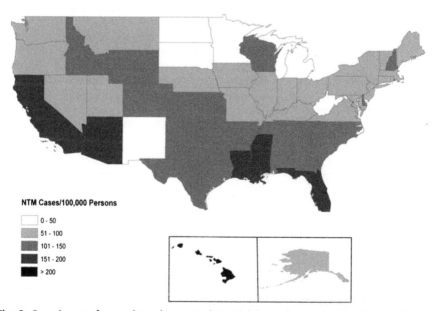

Fig. 2. Prevalence of nontuberculous mycobacterial lung disease in US Medicare beneficiaries. (*Reprinted* with permission of the American Thoracic Society. Copyright © 2014 American Thoracic Society. Adjemian J, Olivier KN, Seitz AE, et al. Prevalence of nontuberculous mycobacterial lung disease in U.S. Medicare beneficiaries. Am J Respir Crit Care Med 2012;185:881–6. Official Journal of the American Thoracic Society.)

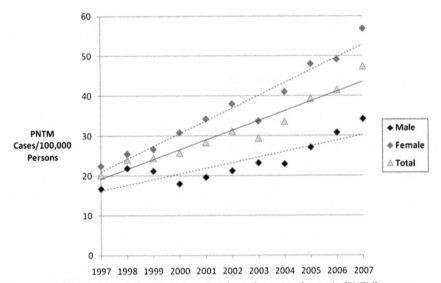

Fig. 3. Annual prevalence of pulmonary nontuberculous mycobacteria (PNTM) cases among a sample of US Medicare part B enrollees by sex from 1997 to 2007. (*Reprinted* with permission of the American Thoracic Society. Copyright © 2014 American Thoracic Society. Adjemian J, Olivier KN, Seitz AE, et al. Prevalence of nontuberculous mycobacterial lung disease in U.S. Medicare beneficiaries. Am J Respir Crit Care Med 2012;185:881–6. Official Journal of the American Thoracic Society.)

metals, metallic fluids of machines) due to their hydrophobic cell wall, and their resistance to disinfectants, antibiotics, or heavy metals. Both in natural and manmade environments, biofilms may have an important role in protecting NTM against aggressive external factors and in promoting their colonization. This colonization of NTM in biofilms may lead to contaminations that can be source of pseudoinfections or NTM diseases. Pseudoinfections may be the result of contamination during collection of specimens (eg, biofilms in improperly cleaned endoscopes) or contamination during laboratory testing (contaminated water source for reagent preparation). Although pseudoinfections do not necessarily cause disease, they may create difficult diagnostic confusion.[1,2,8]

Box 1
Underlying conditions predispose to nontuberculous mycobacteria (NTM) lung disease

- Bronchiectasis
- Chronic obstructive pulmonary disease
- Alpha-1-antitrypsin anomalies
- Pneumoconiosis
- Pulmonary alveolar proteinosis
- Immunosuppressive states (ie, use of anti–tumor necrosis factor-alpha biologics, posttransplantation immunosuppression, HIV infection)

From Chan ED, Iseman MD. Underlying host risk factors for nontuberculous mycobacterial lung disease. Semin Respir Crit Care Med 2013;34:110–23.

Therefore, when NTM are suspected as the etiologic agent of disease (called a mycobacteriosis), the definitive diagnosis should always be supported by repeated isolation of the NTM from several specimens of the patient or a single specimen if collected aseptically from a closed lesion (**Box 2**).[1,8] However, laboratory identification of potentially pathogenic or saprophytic NTM alone are not enough to dictate patient care, and laboratory results should always be correlated with the individual's clinical presentation and radiologic and histologic findings (**Table 2**) to determine the clinical significance of the specimen and make the correct diagnosis. This requires a partnership and ongoing consultation between the laboratory and clinicians.

DIAGNOSIS

Accurate, rapid microbiological diagnosis of tuberculosis (TB) and other mycobacterial infections begins with proper specimen collection and rapid transport to the laboratory. To ensure collection of the best possible specimen, the health care worker has to be properly trained and the patient provided with clearly presented and fully understood instructions for sputum and other specimen collection to obtain a quality specimen with adequate volume and to avoid contamination with NTM. Improper specimen

---

Box 2
Clinical and microbiological criteria for diagnosing NTM

Clinical (both required)

1. Pulmonary symptoms, nodular or cavitary opacities on chest radiograph, or a high-resolution computed tomography scan that shows multifocal bronchiectasis with multiple small nodules and

2. Appropriate exclusion of other diagnoses

Microbiologic

1. Positive culture results from at least 2 separate expectorated sputum samples. If the results from (1) are nondiagnostic, consider repeat sputum acid-fast bacilli (AFB) smears and cultures

or

2. Positive culture result from at least 1 bronchial wash or lavage

or

3. Transbronchial or other lung biopsy with mycobacterial histopathologic features (granulomatous inflammation or AFB) and positive culture for NTM or biopsy showing mycobacterial histopathologic features (granulomatous inflammation or AFB) and one or more sputum or bronchial washings that are culture-positive for NTM

4. Expert consultation should be obtained when NTM are recovered that are either infrequently encountered or that usually represent environmental contamination

5. Patients who are suspected of having NTM lung disease but do not meet the diagnostic criteria should be followed until the diagnosis is firmly established or excluded

6. Making the diagnosis of NTM lung disease does not, per se, necessitate the institution of therapy, which is a decision based on potential risks and benefits of therapy for individual patients

Reprinted with permission of the American Thoracic Society. Copyright © 2014 American Thoracic Society. Griffith DE, Aksamit T, Brown-Elliott BA, et al. An official ATS/IDSA statement: diagnosis, treatment, and prevention of nontuberculous mycobacterial diseases. Am J Respir Crit Care Med 2007;175:367–416. Official Journal of the American Thoracic Society.

Table 2
Clinical and radiologic findings in pulmonary nontuberculous mycobacteria infections

Signs and Symptoms	Radiology
Cough (chronic)	Fibrocavitary: *M avium* complex
Fatigue	Nodular and interstitial nodular infiltrates: *M avium* complex
Weight loss	Fibrocavitary: *M kansasii*
Hemoptysis	Multilobar, reticulonodular, or mixed reticulonodular-alveolar
Dyspnea	Opacities: *M abscessus* complex

Data from Daley CL. Nontuberculous mycobacterial infections. Eur Respir Mon 2011;52:115–29.

collection and contamination of specimens with NTM, especially in tap water, can seriously hamper the determination of clinical significance of specimens. The best example of this significant problem is the use of nonsterile bronchoscopes (rinsed with nonsterile or nonfiltered water that contained NTM).[14–16] To avoid false-positive culture or nucleic acid amplification (NAA)-related pseudo-outbreaks due to "mycobacterium-contaminated" bronchoscopes, these researchers recommend rinsing the instrument with sterile or filtered water, and for amplification tests, a sterile prewash of the bronchoscopes be performed and analyzed along with the actual clinical specimen.[15,16] However, the use of routine environmental microbiological testing of bronchoscopes for quality assurance has not yet been established, although the implementation of an effective pathogen surveillance program is recommended by the American College of Chest Physicians and American Association for Bronchology.[17]

To provide the best results, collect multiple specimens (especially respiratory), if possible, and the volume of a sputum specimen should exceed 5 mL.[18] Histologic parameters also can provide useful information regarding specimen sampling. There is evidence that biopsy specimens that show necrotizing granulomas, non-necrotizing granulomas, poorly formed granulomas, or acute inflammation are optimal for mycobacterial growth detection. However, biopsy specimens showing only fibrotic or hyalinized granulomas, nonspecific chronic inflammation, reactive or reparative changes, malignancy, or no significant abnormalities are less appropriate for mycobacterial culture and staining.[19]

Most respiratory specimens will contain microorganisms other than mycobacteria. Therefore, the specimen should be refrigerated if transportation is delayed more than 1 hour, or otherwise overgrowth of more rapidly growing contaminants may occur.[20]

SPECIMEN PROCESSING

For optimal recovery of mycobacteria, clinical specimens from nonsterile body sites must be subjected to digestion, decontamination, and concentration. This procedure aims to eradicate more rapidly growing contaminants, such as normal flora (other bacteria and fungi), while not seriously affecting the viability of the mycobacteria.[18] Biopsy samples or body fluids from normally sterile sites do not require pretreatment and can be directly inoculated onto culture media. The efficacy of decontamination procedures is highly influenced by the time of exposure to the reagent used for decontamination, the toxicity of that reagent, the efficiency of centrifugation, and the killing effect of heat buildup during centrifugation.[18] NTM, in particular rapidly growing mycobacteria (RGM), are more vulnerable to decontamination than *Mycobacterium tuberculosis*. Therefore, it is important to keep in mind that even the mildest decontamination methods, such as the widely used N-acetyl-L-cysteine/NaOH method, can kill approximately 33% of the mycobacteria in a clinical specimen, whereas more overzealous methods can kill up to 70%.[18] In addition, samples from particular patient populations might need special attention regarding the homogenization and decontamination method to be used. This is especially true for respiratory specimens from patients with bronchiectasis or cystic fibrosis, as NTM are being recovered from these patients with increasing frequency. Because oftentimes specimens of these patients may also contain Gram-negative rods, such as *Pseudomonas aeruginosa*, which can overgrow the culture medium and thus prevent the isolation of NTM, it was recommended that the N-acetyl-L-cysteine/NaOH decontamination method should be followed by a 5% oxalic acid treatment. This extra decontamination step can sufficiently reduce the potential overgrowth by *P aeruginosa* and may well improve the recovery rate of clinically significant NTM.[18,21] However, certain NTM may also be susceptible to oxalic acid, resulting in a reduced growth detection yield; therefore, double-processing by oxalic acid may be restricted to only those specimens from patients who show contamination either by prescreening on a nutrient agar or on cultures for mycobacteria.

A recent study has shown that decontamination by chlorhexidine yielded the isolation of more NTM than the N-acetyl-L-cysteine/NaOH with oxalic acid on solid culture.[22] However, chlorhexidine cannot be used with broth-based culture systems and its improved recovery rate on solid culture was balanced by the higher yield of liquid culture when that was used with N-acetyl-L-cysteine/NaOH and oxalic acid.

ACID-FAST MICROSCOPY

Acid-fast microscopy is the fastest, easiest, and least-expensive tool for the rapid identification of patients with mycobacterial infections,[23] and semiquantitative results of smear examinations may be an important aid in determining the clinical significance of specimens with NTM isolates. However, microscopy is unable to distinguish within the *Mycobacterium* genus and between viable and nonviable mycobacteria. The sensitivity of microscopy is influenced by numerous factors, such as the prevalence and severity of tuberculosis or NTM disease, the type of specimen, the quality of specimen collection, the number of mycobacteria present in the specimen, the method of processing (direct or concentrated), the method of centrifugation, and, most importantly, by the staining technique and the quality of the examination.[2] To facilitate proper patient management, all results should be reported to the physician within 24 hours of specimen collection or, if an off-site laboratory is used, within 24 hours after receipt of the specimen.[18,21,24]

It is generally accepted that, owing to an average of 10% higher sensitivity, the fluorescent method should be given preference over the carbol fuchsin–based (Ziehl-Neelsen [ZN]) or Kinyoun staining methods.[25] However, it is often forgotten that fluorochrome stains may stain other bacteria damaged by antituberculous drugs at a higher rate than carbol fuchsin, and lead to a false-positive result.[26,27] This possibility should be considered when the specimen is from a patient on therapy. Recently, it has been shown that vital staining with fluorescent diacetate may serve as a reliable method to microscopically visualize only viable mycobacteria and to rapidly confirm therapeutic failure before culture results are available.[28] It also has been shown that with the application of simple small-membrane filters directly on clinical specimens, the sensitivity of smear microscopy could be well increased above the level of that with centrifugation-based sample preparation methods in paucibacillary HIV-infected individuals as well. Because extrapulmonary specimens of NTM diseases may often contain low amounts of detectable mycobacteria, this approach may warrant further validation on specimens from different body compartments as well.[29,30]

It is noteworthy that NTM, especially RGM, may be more sensitive to the decoloriza-tion procedure with acid alcohol during staining. Indeed, several studies have indi-cated a clear trend toward less detection of NTM compared with *M tuberculosis* complex by fluorescent microscopy regardless of the source of light (traditional fluo-rescent lamp or light-emitting diode light source).[31,32] Because of a tendency toward false-positivity with fluorochrome staining, good laboratory practice requires that any doubtful and smear-positive results should be confirmed. This can be accomplished by a second observer, restaining of the slide using ZN or Kinyoun stain, or by initially preparing 2 smears, one for the fluorescent stain and the other for ZN or Kinyoun in the event of a positive with fluorochrome staining.[18,23,25,33]

DIRECT NAA ASSAYS

One of the most urgent questions that needs to be addressed rapidly by the mycobac-teriology laboratory is whether *M tuberculosis* complex or NTM is involved. NAA as-says are excellent tools for the purpose, and can be used directly on the clinical specimens of patients suspected of having mycobacterial disease, allowing same-day reporting of results.[34] However, these tests are usually evaluated primarily with respiratory specimens and adequate information of their performance on nonrespira-tory specimens stratified to different body compartments is often lacking.

The LightCycler Mycobacterium Detection Kit (Roche Products Ltd, Randburg, South Africa) that was developed for use on respiratory specimens was reported to be an accurate tool for the direct detection of *M tuberculosis*, *M avium*, and *M kansasii* within 90 minutes.[35] The assay targets the 16S rRNA gene and uses fluorogenic hy-bridization probes for species identification by melting curve analysis on the LightCy-cler 2.0 platform. An internal control also has been integrated in the assay and the platform enables a high-throughput testing capacity.

The Genotype Mycobacteria Direct test (Hain Lifescience GmbH, Nehren, Germany) is based on the amplification of the 23S rRNA gene in an isothermal reaction. Subse-quently biotinylated amplicons are hybridized to oligonucleotide probes anchored on a strip. The assay detects the *M tuberculosis* complex, *M avium*, *Mycobacterium intra-cellulare*, *M kansasii*, and *Mycobacterium malmoense* directly from processed respira-tory specimens; however, further studies are needed to determine assay performance for NTM.[36,37]

Recently, a new polymerase chain reaction (PCR) and line probe assay–based test was developed by Nipro Co (Osaka, Japan) for the rapid detection of *M tuberculosis* complex and rifampin and isoniazid resistance-associated mutations along with the rapid detection and identification of 3 NTM (*M avium*, *M intracellulare*, and *M kansasii*) directly in clinical specimens. The assay was evaluated directly on 163 processed sputum samples and showed a sensitivity of 90.2% for the *M tuberculosis* complex, 84.6% for *M avium*, 54.5% for *M intracellulare*, and 80.0% for *M kansasii*.[38]

GROWTH DETECTION

The Centers for Disease Control and Prevention recommends the use of both liquid and solid media for the growth detection of mycobacteria to decrease the time to detection and to increase the yield of growth detection.[39] Growth detection is still indispensable for the following reasons: (1) culture is more sensitive for the detection of mycobacteria than acid-fast microscopy or NAA (especially in paucibacillary dis-ease or in certain extrapulmonary specimens); (2) semiquantitative results of NTM colony counts on solid media may be useful to determine clinical significance or assess response to therapy; (3) growth is necessary for precise identification

d M abscessus complex, M marinum and Mycobacterium ulcer-
d M gastri); (4) phenotypic antimicrobial susceptibility tests (AST)
isms, whereas detection of particular resistance-associated mo-
s require pure culture and large biomass; and (5) genotyping of
NTM (ie, M avium, M abscessus, M chelonae) can be used for
oses.

ure systems have the potential to significantly decrease turn-
owth detection of mycobacteria.[25] These systems include the
ria Growth Indicator Tube (MGIT; Becton-Dickinson Diagnostic
s, Sparks, MD) and fully automated systems, such as the
(Becton-Dickinson Diagnostic Instrument Systems), the BACTEC
Dickinson Diagnostic Instrument Systems), the MB/BacT 3D
m, NC), and the ESPII (Trek Diagnostic Systems, Oakwood
With the exception of the BACTEC 9000 MB systems, these
stems cannot be used for direct inoculation of blood. Blood sam-
ted into these systems only after lysis and centrifugation steps.[45]
ature of NTM infections of certain organs or body sites or the dif-
specimen collection from particular extrapulmonary compart-
hamper the growth detection and laboratory confirmation of
ently, it has been shown that both the mycobacterial yield and
f growth detection in the MGIT 960 system could significantly
e addition of a simple nutrient broth (modified Dubos liquid me-
ary pediatric samples.[46]

h-based systems have decreased the time to detection to 1 to
edium should be used for those strains that may not grow well
particular, this holds true for M haemophilum, which will grow
a (supplemented with hemin or hemoglobin as an iron source).[47]
: M avium subsp paratuberculosis also requires additional nutri-
he siderophore mycobactin J) in both liquid and solid media for
ereas M ulcerans may be optimally recovered with egg yolk
8

ecies like M genavense show a better recovery rate in liquid me-
acidic pH (pH 5.5).[1,49] Similar to liquid media, the pH of solid me-
antly influence the growth of mycobacteria. It has been shown
ing mycobacteria, based on the testing of 16 different species,
öwenstein-Jensen (LJ) medium was between 5.8 and 6.5.[50] As
al pH was between 7.0 and 7.4, with the exception of M chelo-
d an acidic pH.[50] These findings indicate that the routinely
with pH 7.0 is not optimal for the isolation of all mycobacteria.
endemic for lung or other diseases caused by NTM, inoculation
slant with an acidic pH, or to Ogawa medium (pH 6), is

e for culturing mycobacteria on solid media is that growth can be

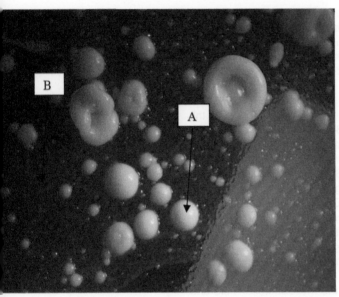

...vium (smooth [A] and translucent [B]).

...cultures of all skin, joint fluid, and bone specimens should be incubated at 30°C and 35 to 37°C.[1,2]

...TION
...d Hybridization Methods

...ercially available AccuProbe (Hologic Gen-Probe Inc, San Diego, CA) ...d hybridization assay allows the rapid identification of the *M tuberculosis* ...he *M avium* complex, *M avium*, *M intracellulare*, *M gordonae*, and *M kansasii* ...ours following growth detection in culture, as they do not include an

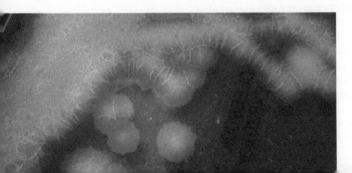

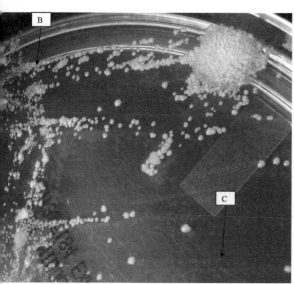

M abscessus (rough [A] and smooth [B]) and *M avium* (translucent [C]).

Cross-reaction has been reported with AccuProbe MTB complex
er *Mycobacterium celatum* types 1 and 3 or *Mycobacterium terrae*
performed at the proper hybridization temperature (between 60 and
± 1°C).[51] It has been reported that, in rare circumstances, some
iae and *M kansasii* may be falsely negative with AccuProbe.[52,53]
be considered when other assays lead to the identification of an
gordonae or *M kansasii*. DNA/RNA probes are usually capable of
cteria in contaminated liquid cultures depending on the extent of
because they have a sensitivity and specificity of nearly 100%
ganisms are present.[54]
agues[55] pointed out the potential inadequacies of nonsequencing
ds, such as hybridization DNA probe assays, 16S rRNA gene
CR restriction fragment length polymorphism analysis (PRA), for
1 species, such as *M intracellulare* and *M chimaera*. Their study
that lumping mycobacteria into groups or complexes will obscure
cs, such as their ecology, epidemiology, virulence, and even sus-
icrobial agents.
y (Third Wave Technologies, Madison, WI) also was shown to be a
n method to rapidly identify mycobacteria isolates.[56] This assay
criminate single-base differences and can measure directly on
ut prior amplification by using isothermal conditions. The assay

is aided with automated fluorescence capillary electrophoresis offers the
of higher accuracy and rapidity. Alternative diagnostic algorithms also
ped based on the PRA of the *dnaJ* gene, the 16S-23S DNA spacer region,
poB gene of mycobacteria.[61–63] The first method identified 48 species, 40
, and 4 subtypes, whereas the second method identified 50 species and 13
drawback of PRA is misidentification due to intraspecies genetic vari-
PRA pattern is not distinct).

Assays

nercially available (except in the United States) line probe assay–based
the Inno-LiPA Mycobacteria assay (Innogenetics N.V., Ghent, Belgium)
notype Mycobacterium CM and AS assays (Hain Lifescience GmbH, Neh-
ny) target the 16S-23S rDNA spacer region and the 23S rDNA for identifi-
nycobacteria.[64–68] These LPAs are based on the solid phase reverse
n of biotinylated PCR amplicons of the target region to oligonucleotide
anged on a membrane strip. The Inno-LiPA test is capable of detecting
ing the *M tuberculosis* complex and an additional 15 NTM, the GenoType
rium CM test is capable of identifying the *M tuberculosis* complex and an
4 NTM, and the GenoType Mycobacterium AS test is capable of identifying
onal 19 NTM from solid and liquid media. LPAs also may enable the simul-
tection of species in mixed cultures.[64–68] The Inno-Lipa Mycobacteria
was used for the direct detection of NTM in respiratory samples, with an
cal sensitivity and specificity of 79.5% and 84.6%, respectively.[69] The
roduced Speed-oligo Mycobacteria test (Vircell, Cordoba, Spain) is also
-based assay to rapidly differentiate the most frequently isolated myco-
clinical isolates. It is a PCR-based test targeting the 16S rRNA (for genus
and 16S-23S rRNA (for species identification) regions. The kit consists of
dly lyophilized PCR mix with a noncompetitive internal amplification con-
roducts are detected by a dipstick device and the entire test can be
within 2 hours. The assay is intended for the rapid detection of *Mycobac-
Mycobacterium fortuitum*, *M avium-intracellulare*, *M tuberculosis* complex,
M gordonae, and *M abscessus-chelonae* complex.[70] The test provided
results for these species in 177 of 182 isolates (including 61 *M tuberculosis*
olates).[70] Following a simple purification test of the PCR amplicon, direct
equencing of a *Mycobacterium* genus–positive specimen also may be per-
4 hours for rapid identification of additional NTMs.

ncing

ecent advances in chemistry and automation of instrumentation, DNA
of variable genomic regions offers a rapid, accurate, and relatively inex-
thod for the identification of mycobacteria. The most routinely used and
thod of this kind is the amplification and sequence analysis of hypervariable
the gene encoding 16S rRNA.[71–73] For taxonomic and phylogenetic pur-

that clear-cut results with DNA sequencing are not the rule, as public or commercial databases may be inaccurate or may not include all established species.[83]

Accurate and unambiguous identification at the species and even subspecies level may be clinically important because of differences in susceptibilities against antimicrobial agents, virulence, epidemiology, and ecology.[55,84,85] However, the use of a single DNA-sequencing target may not always provide this necessary answer, as it was shown in the case of identification of different members of the *M abscessus* complex. The taxonomic definition of the *M abscessus* complex is controversial. Based on their *rpoB* sequences earlier, 2 new species, *Mycobacterium massiliense* and *Mycobacterium bolletii*, were proposed. However, recent studies have shown that these new species cannot be distinguished by biochemical and mycolic acid pattern testing and indicated less genomic divergence expected for distinct species using *rpoB* sequencing alone, suggesting an intergroup lateral transfer of the gene.[76,86,87] Therefore, it has been proposed to unite *M massiliense* and *M bolletii* as *M abscessus* subsp *bolletii* and identify a new taxon *M abscessus* subsp *abscessus*.[86] However, a recent whole-genome sequencing–based phylogenetic investigation gave additional support to subgroup the *M abscessus* complex into 3 subspecies.[7] More recently, a multilocus DNA sequence analysis approach involving 8 housekeeping genes, a multispacer sequence typing, and simple and robust PCR-based typing scheme targeting 4 discriminatory locations identified from array-based comparative genomic hybridization was reported to be an effective tool to identify members of the *M abscessus* group.[76,80,87,88]

The advantage of simultaneous amplification, sequencing, and analysis of 16S rRNA and *rpoB* genes also was highlighted by a recent study that applied the RipSeq dual locus identification system (iSentio, Bergen, Norway).[89]

MALDI-TOF MS

Whole-cell matrix-assisted laser desorption ionization-time-of-flight mass spectrometry (MALDI-TOF MS) can be used in the identification of mycobacteria. This technology is designed to provide a protein "fingerprint" based on the desorbed ions from the cell surfaces. Bacterial cells are applied to a target plate after inactivation and extraction, and overlaid with a matrix solution. After analysis, the instrument software automatically acquires and analyzes the data and generates a profile for comparison to a database of reference spectra composed of previously well-characterized isolates with an algorithm that can analyze mixed electropherograms obtained by sequencing of 2 different gene targets in one step.[90] The integration of the 16S rRNA gene and *rpoB* sequencing allowed the identification of 50 additional organisms to the species level compared with identification using the 16S rRNA gene alone. In addition, this approach allowed the same step distinction of members of the *M abscessus-chelonae* complex or *M kansasii* from *M gastri*. The dual-locus algorithm was able to identify closely related 16S rRNA gene reference sequences for 138 of 139 samples and closely related *rpoB* gene reference sequences for 134 of 139 samples without manual inspection of the mixed electropherograms or database scrutiny.

In a recent study from the University of Washington, rapidly growing mycobacteria were extracted after 3 to 7 days of growth, and slowly growing mycobacteria were extracted after 14 to 21 days.[90] The MALDI-TOF MS results were compared with results obtained from DNA sequencing of the 16S rRNA, *rpoB*, and/or *hsp65* genes. A total of 198 clinical strains, representing only 18 *Mycobacterium* species, were correctly identified to the species level 94.9% of the time using an extraction developed by the investigators, and compared with an augmented database. Both the Bruker MALDI Biotyper (Bruker, Fremont, CA) and the bioMerieux Vitek MS system (bioMerieux, Durham, NC) resulted in correct species-level identifications for 94.4% of these strains. The investigators noted that neither misidentification was clinically relevant. Furthermore, their data suggest that the age of the colonies used for testing should closely match the age of those colonies used for database creation.

GENOTYPING

Genotyping methods have been successfully applied to assess strain relatedness and recognize nosocomial outbreaks, pseudo-outbreaks, mixed infections, or laboratory contamination also with NTM.[2] A recent review by Jagielski and colleagues[91] provides a thorough overview on current methods of molecular typing of mycobacteria. The choice of molecular typing method highly depends on the species, the sample, the setting under investigation, and the expected outcome. The most commonly used methods are pulsed-field gel electrophoresis, insertion sequence (IS)-based typing, methods based on minisatellite sequences (eg, variable number of tandem repeat, major polymorphic tandem repeat), repetitive sequence-based PCR, random amplified polymorphic DNA analysis, amplified fragment length polymorphism analysis, or multilocus sequence typing.[91] With the advance of genotyping technologies, extensive intraspecies genetic divergence could be revealed in NTM, such as the *M avium* complex, *M kansasii,* or the *M abscessus* complex. These findings also suggested that particular subgroups of an NTM species may be associated with different degree of pathogenicity in humans, distinct clinical manifestation, disease progression, and susceptibility to certain antibiotics.[6,92–95] More recently, a whole-genome sequencing–based study, which provides higher resolution than more conventional typing methods, has identified less diversity of *M abscessus* subsp *massiliense* in clustered patients with cystic fibrosis than that observed within serial isolates from a single individual. This finding strongly indicates transmission between patients during an outbreak investigation. In addition the clusters of *M abscessus* subsp *massiliense* also showed evidence of transmission from a patient with mutations associated with macrolide and amikacin resistance to other patients.[7] Newer molecular typing methods, such as whole-genome sequencing, will likely be able to help identify more reliable and meaningful markers associated with the adaption of particular NTM in specific hosts and environmental habitats, or the evolutionary development of clinically significant NTM and their clinically significant subtypes. This new information also should help to better understand why certain species or certain intraspecies subtypes become clinically more significant while others rarely do. In addition, it is also important to collect genetic typing information on patients with different NTM infections so that we not only can understand what is the link between NTM infections and associated diseases (such as cystic fibrosis, different stages of chronic obstructive bronchitis, or bronchiectasis), but can better identify individuals at risk for these infections or determine differences in prognosis.

ANTIMICROBIAL SUSCEPTIBILITY TESTING

The presently accepted recommendations and guidelines for *in vitro* AST of clinically significant NTM isolates are summarized in the recent recommendation of the American Thoracic Society (ATS) and Infectious Disease Society of America (IDSA) from 2007 and the revised guidelines of the Clinical and Laboratory Standards Institute (CLSI) from 2011.[1,96] A more recent review by Brown-Elliott and colleagues[8] provides additional important recommendations and updates.

The role and relevance of *in vitro* AST of NTM to guide the treatment and clinical management of patients with NTM disease is under continuous debate. The basis of this debate is that in contrast to *M tuberculosis*, clinical response to antituberculosis drugs or antibiotics has been shown to correlate only with some compounds and only in some NTM (eg, *M avium* complex and macrolides or *M kansasii*, *M marinum*, or *M fortuitum*), whereas similar correlation for several other clinically significant NTM (eg, *M abscessus*) were not or could not be established. On the other hand, in contrast to *M tuberculosis*, most clinically significant initial NTM isolates already show natural resistance or high *in vitro* breakpoints for several antibiotics and, therefore, AST on NTM seems to be logical, and also to accumulate evidence on their *in vitro* AST patterns. However, it is important to keep in mind that performing AST on clinically nonsignificant NTM isolates is a waste of time and resources, and results may generate confusion in patient management. Because most NTM are ubiquitous in soil and water, determination of the clinical significance of an isolate is warranted before initiating any AST. A further problem is that determination of AST in NTM can be method and species dependent.[96]

Therefore, establishing valid, representative and reproducible AST breakpoints for therapeutic compounds is an important first step to reliably distinguish susceptible and resistant populations and to derive epidemiologic cut-offs (ECOFFs), as it was also indicated by a recent study by Hombach and colleagues[97] on slowly growing NTM. Determining such ECOFFs on a meaningful number of clinically significant isolates using wild-type drug susceptibility distributions, comparing these ECOFFs with pharmacokinetics and pharmadynamics data and subsequent selection of clinical antibiotic susceptibility breakpoints (CBP) in clinical studies has been suggested to determine the clinical value of *in vitro* AST findings and setting of CBPs.[98]

The gold standard method for AST of rapidly growing NTM is a broth microdilution assay.[1,8,96] AST testing of rapidly growing NTM should be guarded by quality control by using CLSI-recommended reference strains to ensure not only quality testing but also reproducibility of minimal inhibitory concentration (MICs) within the recommended and acceptable ranges of antimicrobials tested.[1,8,96] It is noteworthy that incubation due to acidification of broth pH in CO_2 should be avoided, as this can negatively influence testing for macrolides. In addition, MIC results for imipenem and meropenem, and tetracycline, may be invalid after more than 5 days of incubation because of stability-related problems. Isolates that are susceptible to clarithromycin should be further incubated for 14 days to rule out inducible macrolide resistance, which is a common phenomenon due to the presence of an rRNA methylase *erm* gene present in most clinically significant rapidly growing NTM.[99,100] To decrease turnaround time and save resources on prolonged incubation, routine DNA sequencing of particular *erm*, such as *erm* (41) in *M abscessus*, may facilitate both rapid macrolide inducibility detection and species identification within the *M abscessus* complex.[99,100] Additional methods, such as the agar disk diffusion method and Etest (bioMerieux), have not been standardized by CLSI regarding validation of end points or showed problems with reproducibility and therefore are not recommended for AST of rapidly growing NTM at this point.[1,8,96]

For slowly growing NTM, no single AST method is recommended. Both broth (microdilution or macrodilution) and solid AST (eg, agar disk elution for *M haemophilum* that requires more prolonged incubation) methods may be used following proper species-specific intralaboratory validation, and under adequate quality control measures.[1,8,96] Recommendations of the ATS, IDSA, and CLSI for slowly growing NTM AST are summarized in **Box 3**.[1,96]

Macrolides are playing a central role in treatment of *M avium* complex diseases, and *in vitro* AST for clarithromycin and clinical response has shown a good correlation.

Box 3
Recommendations of the American Thoracic Society and Infectious Disease Society of America for drug susceptibility testing of slowly growing mycobacteria

1. Clarithromycin susceptibility testing is recommended for new and previously untreated *M avium* complex isolates. No other drugs are recommended for susceptibility testing of new and previously untreated *M avium* complex isolates. There is no recognized value for testing of first-line antituberculosis agents with *M avium* complex.

2. Clarithromycin susceptibility testing should be performed for *M avium* complex isolates from patients who fail macrolide therapy or prophylaxis.

3. Previously untreated *M kansasii* isolates should be tested *in vitro* only to rifampin. Isolates of *M kansasii* that show susceptibility to rifampin will also be susceptible to rifabutin.

4. *M kansasii* isolates resistant to rifampin should be tested against a panel of secondary agents, including rifabutin, ethambutol, isoniazid, clarithromycin, fluoroquinolones, amikacin, sulfonamides, and linezolid.

5. *M marinum* isolates do not require susceptibility testing unless patient fails treatment after several months.

6. There are no current recommendations for one specific method of *in vitro* susceptibility testing for fastidious NTM species and some less commonly isolated NTM species.

7. Validation and quality control should be in place for susceptibility testing of antimicrobial agents with all species of NTM.

Reprinted with permission of the American Thoracic Society. Copyright © 2014 American Thoracic Society. Griffith DE, Aksamit T, Brown-Elliott BA, et al. An official ATS/IDSA statement: diagnosis, treatment, and prevention of nontuberculous mycobacterial diseases. Am J Respir Crit Care Med 2007;175:367–416. Official Journal of the American Thoracic Society.

Therefore, rapid molecular detection, predicting macrolide resistance in clinically significant isolates, may be beneficial to shorten turnaround times to identify patients with macrolide resistance and potential treatment failure. Previous studies have found that mutations in 80% to 100% of high-level macrolide-resistant *M avium* complex isolates could be detected at nucleotides 2058 and 2059 in the peptidyl transferase loop of the 23S rRNA gene.[1,101,102] However, the same mutations could be detected only between 10% and 20% of *M avium* complex strains with lower level of macrolide resistance. Recently, Maurer and colleagues[103] investigated the role of clarithromycin resistance–associated mutations in the 23S rRNA (*rrl*) gene in patients with chronic *M abscessus* infection undergoing clarithromycin therapy. Follow-up isolates demonstrated acquisition of resistance mutations in the *rrl* gene in addition to the presence of an inducible Erm methylase, indicating that routine 23S rRNA sequencing in *M abscessus* can be a valuable aid to rapidly detect high-level macrolide resistance in these patients.

IDENTIFIED FOCUS AREAS IN NTM RESEARCH

In a recent editorial, Daley and Glassroth[104] described difficulties finding answers to important NTM questions: (1) Robust multicenter trials, although more costly to conduct, would provide the patient numbers needed to conduct rigorous and adequately powered clinical trials in patients with NTM infections. (2) Studies that analyze trial results stratified by factors that are known to affect outcomes are important, as treatment outcomes are worse in patients who have acid-fast bacilli smear-positive disease and those with cavitary disease. (3) Patients with NTM have differing extent of disease, different clinical presentations, and various comorbidities. With limited resources, focus must be put on clinically relevant species, such as *M avium* complex and *M abscessus*, as there are more than 160 species of NTM, and the treatment of these infections varies. Precise speciation is very important because outcomes of treatment may vary by species and even subspecies. (4) *M avium* complex organisms are typically considered similar in the clinical response to therapy and clinical presentations, there are worse outcomes with treatment of *M intracellulare* compared with *M avium*; similarly, patients with *M abscessus* subsp *massiliense* have better treatment outcomes than those with *M abscessus* subsp *abscessus*. (5) Determination of the best measure of treatment success is still to be determined. Long-term follow-up is lacking, and the rate of reoccurrence needs to be evaluated versus reinfection.

REFERENCES

1. Griffith DE, Aksamit T, Brown-Elliott BA, et al. An official ATS/IDSA statement: diagnosis, treatment, and prevention of nontuberculous mycobacterial diseases. Am J Respir Crit Care Med 2007;175(4):367–416.
2. Somoskovi A, Mester J, Hale YM, et al. Laboratory diagnosis of nontuberculous mycobacteria. Clin Chest Med 2002;23(3):585–97.
3. Tortoli E. Impact of genotypic studies on mycobacterial taxonomy: the new mycobacteria of the 1990s. Clin Microbiol Rev 2003;16(2):319–54.
4. Tortoli E. The new mycobacteria: an update. FEMS Immunol Med Microbiol 2006;48(2):159–78.
5. Tortoli E. Phylogeny of the genus *Mycobacterium*: many doubts, few certainties. Infect Genet Evol 2012;12(4):827–31.
6. Aitken ML, Limaye A, Pottinger P, et al. Respiratory outbreak of *Mycobacterium abscessus* subspecies *massiliense* in a lung transplant and cystic fibrosis center. Am J Respir Crit Care Med 2012;185(2):231–2.
7. Bryant JM, Grogono DM, Greaves D, et al. Whole-genome sequencing to identify transmission of *Mycobacterium abscessus* between patients with cystic fibrosis: a retrospective cohort study. Lancet 2013;381(9877):1551–60.
8. Brown-Elliott BA, Nash KA, Wallace RJ Jr. Antimicrobial susceptibility testing, drug resistance mechanisms, and therapy of infections with nontuberculous mycobacteria. Clin Microbiol Rev 2012;25(3):545–82.
9. Prevots DR, Shaw PA, Strickland D, et al. Nontuberculous mycobacterial lung disease prevalence at four integrated health care delivery systems. Am J Respir Crit Care Med 2010;182(7):970–6.
10. Marras TK, Chedore P, Ying AM, et al. Isolation prevalence of pulmonary nontuberculous mycobacteria in Ontario, 1997 2003. Thorax 2007;62(8):661–6.
11. Marras TK, Mendelson D, Marchand-Austin A, et al. Pulmonary nontuberculous mycobacterial disease, Ontario, Canada, 1998-2010. Emerg Infect Dis 2013; 19(11):1889–91.
12. Billinger ME, Olivier KN, Viboud C, et al. Nontuberculous mycobacteria-associated lung disease in hospitalized persons, United States, 1998-2005. Emerg Infect Dis 2009;15(10):1562–9.
13. Adjemian J, Olivier KN, Seitz AE, et al. Prevalence of nontuberculous mycobacterial lung disease in U.S. Medicare beneficiaries. Am J Respir Crit Care Med 2012;185(8):881–6.
14. Gubler JG, Salfinger M, von Graevenitz A. Pseudoepidemic of nontuberculous mycobacteria due to a contaminated bronchoscope cleaning machine. Report of an outbreak and review of the literature. Chest 1992;101(5):1245–9.

15. Honeybourne D, Neumann CS. An audit of bronchoscopy practice in the United Kingdom: a survey of adherence to national guidelines. Thorax 1997;52(8):709–13.
16. Kaul K, Luke S, McGurn C, et al. Amplification of residual DNA sequences in sterile bronchoscopes leading to false-positive PCR results. J Clin Microbiol 1996;34(8):1949–51.
17. Mehta AC, Prakash UB, Garland R, et al. American College of Chest Physicians and American Association for Bronchology [corrected] consensus statement: prevention of flexible bronchoscopy-associated infection. Chest 2005;128(3): 1742–55.
18. Kent PT, Kubica GP. Public health mycobacteriology. A guide for a level III laboratory. Atlanta (GA): Center for Disease Control and Prevention; 1985.
19. Tang YW, Procop GW, Zheng X, et al. Histologic parameters predictive of mycobacterial infection. Am J Clin Pathol 1998;109(3):331–4.
20. Pfyffer GE, Palicova F. Mycobacterium: general characteristics, laboratory detection, and staining procedures. In: Versalovic J, Carroll KC, Jorgensen JH, et al, editors. Manual of clinical microbiology. 10th edition. Washington, DC: American Society for Microbiology; 2011. p. 472–502.
21. Whittier S, Olivier K, Gilligan P, et al. Proficiency testing of clinical microbiology laboratories using modified decontamination procedures for detection of nontuberculous mycobacteria in sputum samples from cystic fibrosis patients. The Nontuberculous Mycobacteria in Cystic Fibrosis Study Group. J Clin Microbiol 1997;35(10):2706–8.
22. De Bel A, De Geyter D, De Schutter I, et al. Sampling and decontamination method for culture of nontuberculous mycobacteria in respiratory samples of cystic fibrosis patients. J Clin Microbiol 2013;51(12):4204–6.
23. Somoskovi A, Hotaling JE, Fitzgerald M, et al. Lessons from a proficiency testing event for acid-fast microscopy. Chest 2001;120(1):250–7.
24. Ebersole LL. Acid-fast staining procedures. In: Isenberg HD, editor. Clinical microbiology procedures handbook, vol. 1. Washington, DC: American Society for Microbiology; 1992. p. 3.5.1–3.5.11.
25. Salfinger M, Pfyffer GE. The new diagnostic mycobacteriology laboratory. Eur J Clin Microbiol Infect Dis 1994;13(11):961–79.
26. Gruft H. Evaluation of mycobacteriology laboratories: the acid-fast smear. Health Lab Sci 1978;15(4):215–20.
27. Lipsky BA, Gates J, Tenover FC, et al. Factors affecting the clinical value of microscopy for acid-fast bacilli. Rev Infect Dis 1984;6(2):214–22.
28. Van Deun A, Maug AK, Hossain A, et al. Fluorescein diacetate vital staining allows earlier diagnosis of rifampicin-resistant tuberculosis. Int J Tuberc Lung Dis 2012;16(9):1174–9.
29. Fennelly KP, Morais CG, Hadad DJ, et al. The small membrane filter method of microscopy to diagnose pulmonary tuberculosis. J Clin Microbiol 2012;50(6): 2096–9.
30. Quinco P, Buhrer-Sekula S, Brandao W, et al. Increased sensitivity in diagnosis of tuberculosis in HIV-positive patients through the small-membrane-filter method of microscopy. J Clin Microbiol 2013;51(9):2921–5.
31. Bernard C, Wichlacz C, Rigoreau M, et al. Evaluation of the Fluo-RAL module for detection of tuberculous and nontuberculous acid-fast bacilli by fluorescence microscopy. J Clin Microbiol 2013;51(10):3469–70.
32. Minion J, Pai M, Ramsay A, et al. Comparison of LED and conventional fluorescence microscopy for detection of acid fast bacilli in a low-incidence setting. PLoS One 2011;6(7):e22495.

33. CLSI. Laboratory detection and identification of *Mycobacteria*. CLSI document M48-A. Approved Guideline. Wayne (PA): Clinical and Laboratory Standards Institute; 2008.
34. Centers for Disease Control and Prevention (CDC). Update: nucleic acid amplification tests for tuberculosis. MMWR Morb Mortal Wkly Rep 2000;49(26): 593–4.
35. Omar SV, Roth A, Ismail NA, et al. Analytical performance of the Roche LightCycler(R) Mycobacterium Detection Kit for the diagnosis of clinically important mycobacterial species. PLoS One 2011;6(9):e24789.
36. Franco-Alvarez de Luna F, Ruiz P, Gutierrez J, et al. Evaluation of the GenoType Mycobacteria Direct assay for detection of *Mycobacterium tuberculosis* complex and four atypical mycobacterial species in clinical samples. J Clin Microbiol 2006;44(8):3025–7.
37. Syre H, Myneedu VP, Arora VK, et al. Direct detection of mycobacterial species in pulmonary specimens by two rapid amplification tests, the gen-probe amplified mycobacterium tuberculosis direct test and the genotype mycobacteria direct test. J Clin Microbiol 2009;47(11):3635–9.
38. Mitarai S, Kato S, Ogata H, et al. Comprehensive multicenter evaluation of a new line probe assay kit for identification of *Mycobacterium* species and detection of drug-resistant *Mycobacterium tuberculosis*. J Clin Microbiol 2012;50(3): 884–90.
39. Styrt BA, Shinnick TM, Ridderhof JC, et al. Turnaround times for mycobacterial cultures. J Clin Microbiol 1997;35(4):1041–2.
40. Benjamin WH Jr, Waites KB, Beverly A, et al. Comparison of the MB/BacT system with a revised antibiotic supplement kit to the BACTEC 460 system for detection of mycobacteria in clinical specimens. J Clin Microbiol 1998;36(11):3234–8.
41. Hanna BA, Ebrahimzadeh A, Elliott LB, et al. Multicenter evaluation of the BACTEC MGIT 960 system for recovery of mycobacteria. J Clin Microbiol 1999; 37(3):748–52.
42. Pfyffer GE, Cieslak C, Welscher HM, et al. Rapid detection of mycobacteria in clinical specimens by using the automated BACTEC 9000 MB system and comparison with radiometric and solid-culture systems. J Clin Microbiol 1997;35(9): 2229–34.
43. Somoskovi A, Magyar P. Comparison of the mycobacteria growth indicator tube with MB Redox, Lowenstein-Jensen, and Middlebrook 7H11 media for recovery of mycobacteria in clinical specimens. J Clin Microbiol 1999;37(5):1366–9.
44. Tortoli E, Cichero P, Chirillo MG, et al. Multicenter comparison of ESP Culture System II with BACTEC 460TB and with Lowenstein-Jensen medium for recovery of mycobacteria from different clinical specimens, including blood. J Clin Microbiol 1998;36(5):1378–81.
45. Stockman L. Blood culture for mycobacteria: isolator method. In: Isenberg HD, editor. Clinical microbiology procedures handbook. Washington, DC: American Society for Microbiology; 1992. p. 3.9.1–3.9.5.
46. Brittle W, Marais BJ, Hesseling AC, et al. Improvement in mycobacterial yield and reduced time to detection in pediatric samples by use of a nutrient broth growth supplement. J Clin Microbiol 2009;47(5):1287–9.
47. White DA, Kiehn TE, Bondoc AY, et al. Pulmonary nodule due to *Mycobacterium haemophilum* in an immunocompetent host. Am J Respir Crit Care Med 1999; 160(4):1366–8.
48. Whittington RJ, Whittington AM, Waldron A, et al. Development and validation of a liquid medium (M7H9C) for routine culture of *Mycobacterium avium* subsp.

paratuberculosis to replace modified Bactec 12B medium. J Clin Microbiol 2013;51(12):3993–4000.

49. Thomsen VO, Dragsted UB, Bauer J, et al. Disseminated infection with *Mycobacterium genavense*: a challenge to physicians and mycobacteriologists. J Clin Microbiol 1999;37(12):3901–5.

50. Portaels F, Pattyn SR. Growth of mycobacteria in relation to the pH of the medium. Ann Microbiol (Paris) 1982;133(2):213–21.

51. Somoskovi A, Hotaling JE, Fitzgerald M, et al. False-positive results for *Mycobacterium celatum* with the AccuProbe *Mycobacterium tuberculosis* complex assay. J Clin Microbiol 2000;38(7):2743–5.

52. Cloud JL, Neal H, Rosenberry R, et al. Identification of *Mycobacterium* spp. by using a commercial 16S ribosomal DNA sequencing kit and additional sequencing libraries. J Clin Microbiol 2002;40(2):400–6.

53. Richter E, Niemann S, Rusch-Gerdes S, et al. Identification of *Mycobacterium kansasii* by using a DNA probe (AccuProbe) and molecular techniques. J Clin Microbiol 1999;37(4):964–70.

54. Zheng X, Pang M, Engler HD, et al. Rapid detection of *Mycobacterium tuberculosis* in contaminated BACTEC 12B broth cultures by testing with Amplified Mycobacterium Tuberculosis Direct Test. J Clin Microbiol 2001; 39(10):3718–20.

55. Wallace RJ Jr, Iakhiaeva E, Williams MD, et al. Absence of *Mycobacterium intracellulare* and presence of *Mycobacterium chimaera* in household water and biofilm samples of patients in the United States with *Mycobacterium avium* complex respiratory disease. J Clin Microbiol 2013;51(6):1747–52.

56. Ichimura S, Nagano M, Ito N, et al. Evaluation of the invader assay with the BACTEC MGIT 960 system for prompt isolation and identification of mycobacterial species from clinical specimens. J Clin Microbiol 2007;45(10):3316–22.

57. Taylor TB, Patterson C, Hale Y, et al. Routine use of PCR-restriction fragment length polymorphism analysis for identification of mycobacteria growing in liquid media. J Clin Microbiol 1997;35(1):79–85.

58. Telenti A, Marchesi F, Balz M, et al. Rapid identification of mycobacteria to the species level by polymerase chain reaction and restriction enzyme analysis. J Clin Microbiol 1993;31(2):175–8.

59. Brunello F, Ligozzi M, Cristelli E, et al. Identification of 54 mycobacterial species by PCR-restriction fragment length polymorphism analysis of the *hsp65* gene. J Clin Microbiol 2001;39(8):2799–806.

60. Sajduda A, Martin A, Portaels F, et al. *hsp65* PCR-restriction analysis (PRA) with capillary electrophoresis for species identification and differentiation of *Mycobacterium kansasii* and *Mycobacterium chelonae-Mycobacterium abscessus* group. Int J Infect Dis 2012;16(3):e193–7.

61. Kim BJ, Lee KH, Park BN, et al. Differentiation of mycobacterial species by PCR-restriction analysis of DNA (342 base pairs) of the RNA polymerase gene (*rpoB*). J Clin Microbiol 2001;39(6):2102–9.

62. Roth A, Reischl U, Streubel A, et al. Novel diagnostic algorithm for identification of mycobacteria using genus-specific amplification of the 16S-23S rRNA gene spacer and restriction endonucleases. J Clin Microbiol 2000;38(3): 1094–104.

63. Takewaki S, Okuzumi K, Manabe I, et al. Nucleotide sequence comparison of the mycobacterial *dnaJ* gene and PCR-restriction fragment length polymorphism analysis for identification of mycobacterial species. Int J Syst Bacteriol 1994;44(1):159–66.

64. Makinen J, Marjamaki M, Marttila H, et al. Evaluation of a novel strip test, Geno-Type Mycobacterium CM/AS, for species identification of mycobacterial cultures. Clin Microbiol Infect 2006;12(5):481–3.

65. Makinen J, Sarkola A, Marjamaki M, et al. Evaluation of genotype and LiPA MYCOBACTERIA assays for identification of Finnish mycobacterial isolates. J Clin Microbiol 2002;40(9):3478–81.

66. Russo C, Tortoli E, Menichella D. Evaluation of the new GenoType Mycobacterium assay for identification of mycobacterial species. J Clin Microbiol 2006; 44(2):334–9.

67. Tortoli E. Identification of mycobacteria by using INNO LiPA. J Clin Microbiol 2002;40(8):3111.

68. Tortoli E, Mariottini A, Mazzarelli G. Evaluation of INNO-LiPA MYCOBACTERIA v2: improved reverse hybridization multiple DNA probe assay for mycobacterial identification. J Clin Microbiol 2003;41(9):4418–20.

69. Perandin F, Pinsi G, Signorini C, et al. Evaluation of INNO-LiPA assay for direct detection of mycobacteria in pulmonary and extrapulmonary specimens. New Microbiol 2006;29(2):133–8.

70. Quezel-Guerraz NM, Arriaza MM, Avila JA, et al. Evaluation of the Speed-oligo(R) Mycobacteria assay for identification of *Mycobacterium* spp. from fresh liquid and solid cultures of human clinical samples. Diagn Microbiol Infect Dis 2010;68(2):123–31.

71. Kirschner P, Bottger EC. Species identification of mycobacteria using rDNA sequencing. Methods Mol Biol 1998;101:349–61.

72. Kirschner P, Rosenau J, Springer B, et al. Diagnosis of mycobacterial infections by nucleic acid amplification: 18-month prospective study. J Clin Microbiol 1996;34(2):304–12.

73. Kirschner P, Springer B, Vogel U, et al. Genotypic identification of mycobacteria by nucleic acid sequence determination: report of a 2-year experience in a clinical laboratory. J Clin Microbiol 1993;31(11):2882–9.

74. Kasai H, Ezaki T, Harayama S. Differentiation of phylogenetically related slowly growing mycobacteria by their gyrB sequences. J Clin Microbiol 2000;38(1): 301–8.

75. Kim BJ, Lee SH, Lyu MA, et al. Identification of mycobacterial species by comparative sequence analysis of the RNA polymerase gene (*rpoB*). J Clin Microbiol 1999;37(6):1714–20.

76. Macheras E, Roux AL, Ripoll F, et al. Inaccuracy of single-target sequencing for discriminating species of the *Mycobacterium abscessus* group. J Clin Microbiol 2009;47(8):2596–600.

77. Olsen RJ, Cernoch PA, Austin CM, et al. Validation of the MycoAlign system for *Mycobacterium* spp. identification. Diagn Microbiol Infect Dis 2007;59(1): 105–8.

78. Ringuet H, Akoua-Koffi C, Honore S, et al. hsp65 sequencing for identification of rapidly growing mycobacteria. J Clin Microbiol 1999;37(3):852–7.

79. Roth A, Fischer M, Hamid ME, et al. Differentiation of phylogenetically related slowly growing mycobacteria based on 16S-23S rRNA gene internal transcribed spacer sequences. J Clin Microbiol 1998;36(1):139–47.

80. Sassi M, Ben Kahla I, Drancourt M. *Mycobacterium abscessus* multispacer sequence typing. BMC Microbiol 2013;13:3.

81. Soini H, Bottger EC, Viljanen MK. Identification of mycobacteria by PCR-based sequence determination of the 32-kilodalton protein gene. J Clin Microbiol 1994; 32(12):2944–7.

82. Yamada-Noda M, Ohkusu K, Hata H, et al. *Mycobacterium* species identification—a new approach via *dnaJ* gene sequencing. Syst Appl Microbiol 2007; 30(6):453–62.

83. Turenne CY, Tschetter L, Wolfe J, et al. Necessity of quality-controlled 16S rRNA gene sequence databases: identifying nontuberculous *Mycobacterium* species. J Clin Microbiol 2001;39(10):3637–48.

84. Koh WJ, Jeon K, Lee NY, et al. Clinical significance of differentiation of *Mycobacterium massiliense* from *Mycobacterium abscessus*. Am J Respir Crit Care Med 2011;183(3):405–10.

85. Koh WJ, Jeong BH, Jeon K, et al. Clinical significance of the differentiation between *Mycobacterium avium* and *Mycobacterium intracellulare* in *M avium* complex lung disease. Chest 2012;142(6):1482–8.

86. Leao SC, Tortoli E, Euzeby JP, et al. Proposal that *Mycobacterium massiliense* and *Mycobacterium bolletii* be united and reclassified as *Mycobacterium abscessus* subsp. *bolletii* comb. nov., designation of *Mycobacterium abscessus* subsp. *abscessus* subsp. nov. and emended description of *Mycobacterium abscessus*. Int J Syst Evol Microbiol 2011;61(Pt 9):2311–3.

87. Macheras E, Konjek J, Roux AL, et al. Multilocus sequence typing scheme for the *Mycobacterium abscessus* complex. Res Microbiol 2014;165(2):82–90. http://dx.doi.org/10.1016/j.resmic.2013.12.003.

88. Shallom SJ, Gardina PJ, Myers TG, et al. New rapid scheme for distinguishing the subspecies of the *Mycobacterium abscessus* group and identifying *Mycobacterium massiliense* isolates with inducible clarithromycin resistance. J Clin Microbiol 2013;51(9):2943–9.

89. Simmon KE, Kommedal O, Saebo O, et al. Simultaneous sequence analysis of the 16S rRNA and *rpoB* genes by use of RipSeq software to identify *Mycobacterium* species. J Clin Microbiol 2010;48(9):3231–5.

90. Mather CA, Rivera SF, Butler-Wu SM. Comparison of the Bruker Biotyper and Vitek MS matrix-assisted laser desorption ionization-time of flight mass spectrometry systems for identification of mycobacteria using simplified protein extraction protocols. J Clin Microbiol 2014;52(1):130–8.

91. Jagielski T, Van Ingen J, Rastogi N, et al. Current methods in the molecular typing of *Mycobacterium tuberculosis* and other mycobacteria. BioMed Res Int 2014;2014:645802.

92. Kikuchi T, Watanabe A, Gomi K, et al. Association between mycobacterial genotypes and disease progression in *Mycobacterium avium* pulmonary infection. Thorax 2009;64(10):901–7.

93. Kim SY, Lee ST, Jeong BH, et al. Clinical significance of mycobacterial genotyping in *Mycobacterium avium* lung disease in Korea. Int J Tuberc Lung Dis 2012; 16(10):1393–9.

94. Shin SJ, Choi GE, Cho SN, et al. Mycobacterial genotypes are associated with clinical manifestation and progression of lung disease caused by *Mycobacterium abscessus* and *Mycobacterium massiliense*. Clin Infect Dis 2013;57(1): 32–9.

95. Tatano Y, Sano C, Yasumoto K, et al. Correlation between variable-number tandem-repeat-based genotypes and drug susceptibility in *Mycobacterium avium* isolates. Eur J Clin Microbiol Infect Dis 2012;31(4):445–54.

96. CLSI. Susceptibility testing of mycobacteria, norcardiae and other aerobic actinomycetes. CLSI Document M24–A2. Approved Standard-Second edition. Wayne (PA): Clinical and Laboratory Standards Institute; 2011.

97. Hombach M, Somoskovi A, Homke R, et al. Drug susceptibility distributions in slowly growing non-tuberculous mycobacteria using MGIT 960 TB eXiST. Int J Med Microbiol 2013;303(5):270–6.
98. Turnidge J, Paterson DL. Setting and revising antibacterial susceptibility breakpoints. Clin Microbiol Rev 2007;20(3):391–408 [table of contents].
99. Choi GE, Shin SJ, Won CJ, et al. Macrolide treatment for *Mycobacterium abscessus* and *Mycobacterium massiliense* infection and inducible resistance. Am J Respir Crit Care Med 2012;186(9):917–25.
100. Maurer FP, Castelberg C, Quiblier C, et al. Erm(41)-dependent inducible resistance to azithromycin and clarithromycin in clinical isolates of *Mycobacterium abscessus*. J Antimicrob Chemother 2014. [Epub ahead of print].
101. Christianson S, Grierson W, Wolfe J, et al. Rapid molecular detection of macrolide resistance in the *Mycobacterium avium* complex: are we there yet? J Clin Microbiol 2013;51(7):2425–6.
102. Meier A, Kirschner P, Springer B, et al. Identification of mutations in 23S rRNA gene of clarithromycin-resistant *Mycobacterium intracellulare*. Antimicrobial Agents Chemother 1994;38(2):381–4.
103. Maurer FP, Ruegger V, Ritter C, et al. Acquisition of clarithromycin resistance mutations in the 23S rRNA gene of *Mycobacterium abscessus* in the presence of inducible erm(41). J Antimicrob Chemother 2012;67(11):2606–11.
104. Daley CL, Glassroth J. Treatment of pulmonary nontuberculous mycobacterial infections: many questions remain. Ann Am Thorac Soc 2014;11(1):96–7.

Molecular Diagnosis of Tuberculosis and Drug Resistance

Shou-Yean Grace Lin, MS, Edward P. Desmond, PhD*

KEYWORDS

- Tuberculosis • Molecular detection • Drug resistance • GeneXpert • Line probes
- Pyrosequencing • Sequencing • Tuberculosis diagnostics

KEY POINTS

- Molecular drug susceptibility testing (MDST) provides rapid diagnosis of tuberculosis (TB) and drug-resistance detection with commendable sensitivity and specificity.
- In exceeding the performance of smear microscopy, MDST enables accurate diagnosis of TB, and improved patient management and TB control; MDST reduces unnecessary isolation or treatment, when a negative result for TB is obtained.
- The GeneXpert MTB/RIF assay provides rapid detection of multidrug-resistant TB. Because of the possibility of false detection of rifampin resistance, confirmation by sequencing is recommended, especially in regions where prevalence of resistance is low.
- Revealing mutation identity by sequencing offers opportunities to study drug minimum inhibitory concentrations for each mutation. Such information enables prediction of resistance levels, and may be helpful in formulating optimal regimens.
- Owing to false susceptibility and false resistance with MDST, culture-based drug susceptibility testing should follow. When resistance is detected, an expanded drug panel should be tested.

INTRODUCTION

A new era in tuberculosis (TB) control is beginning in the United States. In 2012, reported TB cases in this country were less than 10,000 for the first time since national reporting of TB began.[1] However, the global picture is different. TB continues to be the principal killer among infectious diseases. Multidrug-resistant TB (MDR TB) cases have almost reached a half million (450,000), 9.6% of which are extensively drug-resistant TB (XDR TB).[2,3] Rapid TB diagnosis and drug-resistance detection remains a sizable challenge in reducing TB-related morbidity and mortality, especially in

Neither author has affiliations with the companies whose products are discussed in this article.
California Department of Public Health, Richmond, CA, USA
* Corresponding author. Microbial Diseases Laboratory, California Department of Public Health, 850 Marina Bay Parkway, E164, Richmond, CA 94804.
E-mail address: Ed.Desmond@cdph.ca.gov

regions where coinfection with TB and human immunodeficiency virus (HIV) is prevalent. In combating TB, diagnosis of TB alone is inadequate; improving drug-resistance detection is an essential component for effective TB control and TB patient management.[2–7]

With the availability of molecular diagnostic tools, rapid diagnosis of TB and detection of drug resistance have made significant improvement in recent years.[8–10] The Centers for Disease Control and Prevention (CDC) guidelines published in 2009 recommended the use of nucleic acid amplification testing (NAAT) as standard practice for aiding in establishing TB diagnosis in persons with suspected TB.[11] Molecular assays that exceed the performance of acid-fast smear microscopy enable rapid diagnosis of TB and/or detection of drug resistance even for smear-negative patients.[8,12] As commercial products are now available at reduced prices in TB-endemic regions, molecular testing has become cost-effective and technically easy to implement worldwide.[5–7,13–15] While rapid identification of MDR TB is being realized, rapid detection of resistance to second-line drugs, and timely and effective treatment of patients with MDR/XDR TB, still present tremendous challenges.[2,16]

MICROBIOLOGY

Mycobacterium tuberculosis complex (MTBC) includes *Mycobacterium tuberculosis*, *Mycobacterium bovis*, *Mycobacterium africanum*, *Mycobacterium canettii*, *Mycobacterium caprae*, *Mycobacterium microti*, and *Mycobacterium pinnipedii*. Approximately 98% of human TB cases are caused by *M tuberculosis*. MTBC has a complex cell wall containing mycolic acids, and resists decolorization by acid alcohol when stained with carbol fuchsin or auramine (a fluorescent stain). Hence they are called acid-fast bacilli. *M tuberculosis* grows slowly in culture, requiring an average of 2 to 3 weeks of incubation before growth can be detected. Colonies on solid media are off-white or buff in color, with a rough appearance. The cellular morphology of TB bacilli grown in culture demonstrates cording or ropy clumps. The *M tuberculosis* genome contains 4,411,529 base pairs with high GC content (>65%).[17,18] *M bovis* causes 1% to 2% of human TB. *M bovis* differs from *M tuberculosis* by being niacin and nitrate negative, and inherently pyrazinamide resistant.

EPIDEMIOLOGY

Approximately one-third third of the human population can be demonstrated to have immunologic evidence of current or past infection with *M tuberculosis*. In 2012, it was estimated that there were approximately 8.6 million human cases worldwide with 1.3 million deaths.[3] The average global incidence rate was 122 new cases per 100,000 population per year. By contrast, in the United States, the TB incidence rate was 3.2 new cases per 100,000 population in 2012.[1] Serious concerns remain for the United States, however, because 63% of TB cases and 88% of MDR TB cases were foreign-born from countries where TB prevalence and drug-resistance rates are high.

CLINICAL PRESENTATION

Pulmonary TB, the most common form of the disease, is chronic and slowly progressive. Patients commonly experience cough, weight loss, night sweats, fever, and occasionally chest pain and dyspnea.[18] Early in the course of the disease, cough may be nonproductive; as inflammation and tissue necrosis ensue, sputum is usually produced. Pulmonary infiltrates and cavitary lesions may often be observed on chest radiographs. Dyspnea with parenchymal lung involvement is less common but may manifest in extensive disease.[19] Extrapulmonary tuberculosis also occurs frequently, and can involve nearly any organ system of the body including the lymphatic system, heart, joints, bones, central nervous system, and internal organs. In patients coinfected with HIV, or in patients infected with *M bovis*, extrapulmonary disease is more common.

PATHOGENESIS OF PULMONARY TUBERCULOSIS

TB infection involves dynamic interaction between the host immune system and TB bacilli. Within the lungs, the inhaled TB bacilli may be eliminated by alveolar macrophages, or multiply and progress to form small caseous lesions. Once these lesions have developed, in patients with normal cell-mediated immunity activated macrophages may exert microbicidal activity. Small caseous lesions may heal, stabilize, or progress to larger caseous lesions. Within the infected lung, each lesion is independent and may be engaged in various phases of immunologic battles. Thus different types of lesions may exist, including encapsulated lesions, proliferative lesions, and cavities.[20] TB bacilli within these lesions may be either intracellular (especially within macrophages) or extracellular, and may be either actively replicating or dormant. The variety of lesions and the metabolic states of the TB bacilli have important implications for the design of effective treatment regimens. Different drugs may be required to treat different populations of TB bacilli.[21] In approximately 90% of patients, the disease is controlled as latent TB infection; TB bacilli may remain viable within dormant lesions over many years and can be reactivated when the host immune system weakens.

MOLECULAR DIAGNOSIS

Among the first US Food and Drug Administration (FDA)-approved nucleic acid amplification tests was the *M tuberculosis* direct test (MTD) (Hologic Gen-Probe, San Diego, CA) for detection of MTBC from *N*-acetyl-L-cysteine–NaOH (NALC-NaOH) concentrated specimens, either smear-positive or smear-negative. The test marked a successful beginning of the molecular era in the United States for TB diagnosis with high sensitivity and specificity, and remarkably shortened the turnaround time with cost savings.[12] Another significant breakthrough was the molecular detection of drug resistance, without which drug-resistant TB can only be suspected until proved by culture-based drug susceptibility testing (CDST) results obtained typically 4 weeks or longer after specimen collection.

Genes Associated with Drug Resistance

In 1992, Zhang and colleagues[22] provided the first evidence that mutations in *katG* encoding catalase-peroxidase were associated with isoniazid (INH) resistance. Since then, many studies have been devoted to molecular understanding of drug resistance. Molecular drug susceptibility testing (MDST) assays capable of being performed directly on clinical specimens without the requirement for growth in culture have brought significant impact on improved turnaround time for drug-resistance detection. **Table 1** provides a brief summary of genes associated with drug resistance and the most predominant mutations found in clinical isolates. Although major genes associated with drug resistance have been identified, the understanding of drug resistance at the genetic level remains incomplete. Therefore, 100% sensitivity for detecting all drug resistance is not achievable at present. Furthermore, there are mutations that do not confer resistance or are associated with unpredictable susceptibility by CDST.[23–26] Thus specificity for resistance detection by molecular methods for certain drugs is not 100%. To deliver accurate drug susceptibility results to physicians, CDST still

Table 1
Genes and mutations associated with drug resistance in *Mycobacterium tuberculosis*

Drug	Gene	Mutations	Comments
Isoniazid (INH)	*katG*	AGC315ACC	Most frequent mutation, associated with high-level INH resistance
			Some other mutations in codon 315: ACA, AAC, ATC, ACT, GGC
	inhA promoter	-15C/T	Often associated with low-level INH resistance and ethionamide resistance
			Some other mutations: -8T/C, -8T/A, -8T/G, -9G/T, -16A/G, -17G/T
	ahpC promoter	-12G/A	Compensatory to *katG* mutations; found in isolates with high-level INH resistance
			Some other mutations: -6C/T, -9C/T, -10G/A, -10G/T
Rifampin (RIF)	*rpoB*	TCG531TTG	Most frequent mutation in MDR TB
			Associated with RIF and RFB resistance
			Detectable by HAIN[a], specified
			Detectable by Probe E of GeneXpert[b], not specified
		CAC526TAC	Associated with RIF and RFB resistance
		CAC526GAC	Detectable by HAIN[a], specified
			Detectable by Probe D of GeneXpert[b], not specified
		GAC516GTC	Often are associated with RIF resistance but RFB susceptibility
			Detectable by HAIN[a], specified
			Detectable by Probe B of GeneXpert[b], not specified
		Silent mutation: TTC514TTT	Most frequent silent mutation. Not associated with RIF or RFB resistance. Falsely interpreted as RIF-resistance by probe methods.
			Detectable by HAIN[a], missing WT3, not specified
			Detectable by Probe B of GeneXpert[b], not specified
			• Incorrectly reported as "RIF resistance detected"
Ethambutol (EMB)	*embB*	ATG306GTG	Most frequent mutation associated with EMB resistance
			Some other mutations in codon 306: CTG, ATA, ACG, ATT, TTG
			Not all mutations in *embB* are associated with EMB resistance
Pyrazinamide (PZA)	*pncA*	No predominant mutations	Widely distributed throughout the gene and the promoter
			Not all mutations are associated with PZA resistance

(continued on next page)

Table 1
(continued)

Drug	Gene	Mutations	Comments
Quinolones	*gyrA*	GAC94GGC	Most frequent mutation, usually MOX MIC >1 µg/mL. MOX may still have clinical efficacy if MIC ≤2 µg/mL[49]; may need to increase dosage Some other mutations in codon 94: TAC, CAC, GCC, AAC Some other mutations: TCG91CCG; GGC88GCC, GGC88TGC
		GCG90GTG	A frequent mutation. Usually MOX MIC ≤1 µg/mL. MOX may still have clinical efficacy
Amikacin (AMK)	*rrs*	1401A/G	Most common mutation; associated with AMK resistance
		1402C/T	Usually not associated with AMK resistance
		1484G/T	Associated with AMK resistance
Capreomycin (CAP)	*rrs*	1401A/G	Most common mutation; usually associated with CAP resistance Some other mutations: 1402C/T, 1484G/T
	tlyA	No predominant mutations	Mutations are widely distributed throughout the gene Some mutations are highly associated with CAP resistance: GGG196GAG, GC insertion at nucleotide 202, GT insertion at nucleotide 755
Kanamycin (KAN)	*rrs*	1401A/G	Most common mutation. Associated with KAN resistance Some other mutations: 1402C/T, 1484G/T
	eis promoter	-10G/A	Highly associated with KAN resistance Some other mutations: -14C/T, -37G/T
Bedaquiline (BDQ)	*atpE*		Mutations in C ring of the adenosine triphosphate (ATP) synthase may be associated with BDQ resistance

Abbreviations: MOX, moxifloxacin; RFB, rifabutin.
[a] HAIN refers to GenoTypeMTBDR*plus* assay.
[b] GeneXpert refers to MTB/RIF assay.

plays an integral role in confirming MDST results and testing drugs for which MDST is not yet available.

Isoniazid

Genetic understanding of the resistance mechanisms of INH is still evolving. Mutations in *katG* and the promoters of *inhA* and *ahpC* are associated with INH resistance,[27,28] and account for 85% to 90% of INH-resistant isolates detected in the United States, with specificity approaching 100%.[22,23,29–32] Although there are INH-resistant isolates lacking mutations in these loci, with the INH resistance rate at 10% or lower throughout most of the United States, the predictive values for INH susceptibility in the absence of a detected mutation in *katG* or the *inhA* promoter are 98% or higher. This finding provides commendably high confidence for using MDST to detect INH resistance. It is noteworthy that the prevalence of mutations in those genes found in INH-resistant strains is often geographically dependent. In certain countries such as Russia, the *katG* 315ACC mutation is highly prevalent, and may account for 94% of INH-resistant strains.[33] Assays capable of detecting this mutation would yield higher sensitivity for INH resistance detection in those countries than in the United States. Mutations in the *inhA* promoter are often associated with low-level INH resistance and concurrent ethionamide resistance.[34] Mutations in other genes, such as *ndh*,[35] may also be associated with INH resistance, but have not been widely investigated.

Rifampin and rifabutin

Using MDST to evaluate mutations present in the RIF-resistance–determining region (RRDR) of *rpoB* for detection of resistance to rifampin (RIF) has high sensitivity and specificity. Greater than 95% of RIF-resistant strains have mutations in the RRDR, but not all mutations found there are equivalent.[23,36] The level of RIF resistance may vary with a variety of mutations.[37] The most common mutations found in MDR TB are TCG531TTG, CAC526GAC, and CAC526TAC, which are associated with high-level RIF resistance and rifabutin (RFB) resistance,[38] whereas other mutations, such as GAC516 GTC or CAC526 CTC, may be associated with resistance to RIF but susceptibility to RFB.[38] There is another group of mutations, such as CTG511CCG, GAC516TAC, CAC526AAC, and CTG533CCG, associated with highly discordant RIF results generated from various CDST methods.[25,26] Furthermore, silent mutations such as TTC514TTT, GGC507GGT, and others are not associated with phenotypic RIF or RFB resistance.[23,24] These findings affect the specificity of RIF-resistance detection by probe-based MDST assays that do not provide the mutation identity; therefore, users are unable to use available knowledge to evaluate whether a mutation confers resistance.

Recent publications have described relapsed TB cases carrying strains with certain *rpoB* mutations that tested RIF-susceptible phenotypically.[25,39,40] This finding calls for a review of the current RIF critical concentration, and raises a concern of clinical relevancy of RIF resistance caused by these "disputed" mutations. The validity of using CDST as a standard for characterizing MDST performance is also challenged. However, causes leading to treatment failures are multifaceted. Intensity of TB disease, presence of underlying diseases (diabetes, HIV, or other conditions), nutritional status, drug-absorbance efficacy from the gastrointestinal tract, patient adherence to treatment, quality of TB medications, extent of drug resistance, and other factors should also be evaluated when investigating treatment failures. A study aimed at documenting the prevalence and prognostic value of *rpoB* mutations with unclear phenotypic RIF resistance was conducted by van Deun and colleagues.[39] Among 345 first-line retreatment cases whose isolates had *rpoB* mutations, 63% of those experienced failure or relapse with equal occurrence between patients carrying a strain with disputed versus common mutations. Because these were retreatment cases, a higher rate of failure than initial treatment is to be expected. Therefore, the presence of a disputed mutation may not be a good indicator for evaluating the clinical relevancy of RIF resistance. In addition, this study did not report retreatment outcomes for the 80% of retreatment cases that did not have *rpoB* mutations. This group could have served as a comparison group to assess the impact of factors other than *rpoB* mutations. Nevertheless, this is a critical issue involving several aspects of MDST and CDST, and more studies should be conducted. Whether the disputed mutations are associated with clinically relevant resistance requires further investigation.

Ethambutol

Ethambutol (EMB) resistance is not fully understood at the genetic level. Studies have indicated that mutations in *embB* are often associated with EMB resistance[41,42]; those in codons 306, 319, 354, and 406 are most commonly found in EMB-resistant isolates.[29] Among those, the most predominant mutation is the ATG306GTG mutation. Other mutations in *embB* may also confer EMB resistance, but they are spread over more than 100 codons and are difficult to detect cost-effectively using probe-based methods or short-segment sequencing. The sensitivity for detection of EMB resistance in *embB* is in the range of 60% to 80%, the specificity being 93% to 100%.[29,32] Although mono-EMB resistance is rare, likelihood of EMB resistance increases when an isolate is resistant to other drugs. Therefore, molecular detection of EMB resistance should be considered as a reflex test in cases where resistance mutations to other drugs are detected. Under this circumstance, the molecular result of *embB* may greatly influence clinical decisions on whether EMB should be retained in the regimen.

Pyrazinamide

Mutations in *pncA* are often associated with pyrazinamide (PZA) resistance.[29,43] These mutations are widespread within the gene and the promoter region,[43,44] and detection by probe-based methods or short-segment sequencing is difficult and not cost-effective. Sanger sequencing or next-generation sequencing (NGS) capable of sequencing long segments is more suitable. Revealing mutation identity by these sequence-based methods is critical for proper interpretation of *pncA* results, because some mutations do not confer PZA resistance, and minimum inhibitory concentration (MIC) varies significantly with a variety of mutations.[43] A study conducted at the CDC showed that the sensitivity for detection of PZA resistance by sequencing *pncA* gene and the promoter region was 84.6% (55 of 65), with specificity of 85.8% (109 of 127).[29] Mono-PZA resistance in *M tuberculosis* is rare; molecular detection for PZA resistance becomes critical and should be considered as a reflex test when resistance mutations to other drugs are detected. *M bovis* is intrinsically resistant to PZA. If *M bovis* is suspected, a rapid identification of *M bovis* by molecular testing is clinically relevant for excluding PZA from treatment. Furthermore, because of problems with false resistance by CDST,[45,46] *pncA* sequencing along with pyrazinamidase testing may sometimes be recommended to confirm phenotypic PZA resistance.[47,48]

Fluoroquinolones

Fluoroquinolones (fQs), such as ofloxacin, levofloxacin, moxifloxacin (MOX), and others, have been used as second-line drugs to treat TB. Mutations detected in the quinolone resistance–determining region (QRDR) of *gyrA* are often associated with fQ resistance. The most common mutations are GAC94GGC and GCG90GTG. Mutations in the QRDR may confer different levels of resistance.[49] Isolates with the GAC94GGC mutation usually yield higher MICs than those with the GCG90GTG mutation. MOX is more potent than other older-generation fQs. Even in the presence of mutations in QRDR, if the MIC is 2 μg/mL or less, MOX may still have clinical efficacy and can be beneficial for treating XDR TB.[49,50] Establishing MIC ranges for each mutation will help in predicting the level of resistance; such information may be helpful to physicians in formulating optimal regimens in the face of resistance. The sensitivity of fQ-resistance detection by line-probe assay (HAIN), pyrosequencing, or Sanger sequencing is in the mid-80% range, and the specificity is close to 100%.[23,29,51] Mutations in *gyrB* may also be associated with fQ resistance, but the frequency of finding mutations in *gyrB* is much lower than in *gyrA*.[52]

Injectable drugs

Mutations in *rrs* are often associated with resistance to the injectable drugs, amikacin (AMK), capreomycin (CAP), and kanamycin (KAN).[53] The most common mutation is the 1401 A/G mutation. The association of this mutation with AMK and KAN resistance is near 100%, whereas association with CAP resistance is variable.[23,29,51,54] The sensitivity of *rrs* sequencing for detection of resistance to these drugs is in the mid-80% range. Mutations in *eis* promoter account for 20% to 30% of KAN resistance with specificity close to 100%.[29,55] A systematic review found that only 1% to 3% of CAP-resistant strains possessed mutations in *tlyA*, and no mutations in *tlyA* were detected in CAP-susceptible isolates.[55] This finding makes *tlyA* a highly specific target for detection of CAP resistance. However, another study found *tlyA* mutations accounted for 10% of CAP resistance with 98.8% specificity.[29]

MOLECULAR ASSAYS

Current molecular methods (**Table 2**) for the identification of MTBC and the detection of drug resistance can be divided into 2 major categories, probe-based methods and sequence-based methods (**Box 1**). The major advantage of the sequence-based methods is their ability to provide sequence information and reveal the identity of the mutation. Because mutations are not always associated with resistance, availability of mutation identity enables proper interpretation of MDST results. When a new mutation is detected whose association with resistance is unknown, the interpretation should be deferred to CDST results, and the risk of reporting false resistance can be avoided. In addition, the level of drug resistance may vary with different mutations. The availability of mutation identity offers an opportunity to study drug MIC for each specific mutation. The accumulation of this knowledge enables prediction of drug-resistance levels for each mutation. However, this will not be possible if the mutation identity is not provided.

Molecular Beacon Assays

The molecular beacon (MB) assay uses a real-time polymerase chain reaction (PCR) platform and MB probes to detect mutations. MB probes have a loop-and-stem structure with a fluorophore attached to one arm of the stem and a quencher to the other.[56,57] For effectiveness of detecting various mutations, the loop contains the wild-type sequences rather than a specific mutant sequence. When the test organism has wild-type sequences, the MB will change its loop-and-stem form to linear form and hybridize to the amplicon. This conformational change forces the fluorophore away from the quencher and permits the fluorophore to emit light. If the organism contains a mutation within the detectable range of the MB probe, the mutation prevents hybridization and no fluorescent signals will be generated. Absence of fluorescent signals is interpreted as presence of a mutation.

The GeneXpert MTB/RIF assay (Cepheid, Sunnyvale, CA) uses nested real-time PCR for qualitative detection of MTBC and RIF resistance. The assay amplifies an MTBC-specific sequence of the *rpoB* gene and uses 5 MB probes to detect mutations in the RRDR. Studies have shown that GeneXpert is more sensitive and specific than smear microscopy for detecting MTBC, and its excellent performance in detecting RIF resistance has yielded a positive impact on rapid detection of MDR TB in developing countries.[8,13,58]

This assay has been cleared by the US FDA for diagnostic testing of raw sputa or concentrated sediments prepared from induced or expectorated sputa. It does not include a specific probe to identify MTBC; rather, the identification of MTBC is

Table 2
Current molecular methods for detection of drug resistance in *Mycobacterium tuberculosis*

	Cepheid GeneXpert MTB/RIF	HAIN MTBDR*plus* & MTBDR*sl*	Pyrosequencing[a] (Laboratory-Developed, Noncommercial Tests)	Sanger Sequencing[a] (Laboratory-Developed, Noncommercial Tests)
Methodology	Real-time PCR Molecular beacon probes	PCR Line probes	PCR pyrosequencing	PCR Sanger sequencing
Specimen types	1. Direct specimen 2. Concentrated specimen[b]	1. Smear-positive, concentrated pulmonary specimen 2. Culture	1. Concentrated specimen[b] 2. Culture	1. Concentrated specimen[b] 2. Culture
Testing time	2 h	6–7 h	5–6 h	1–2 d
Drug-testing availability	RIF	INH, RIF, EMB, fQs, AMK, CAP, KAN	INH, RIF, EMB, fQs, AMK, CAP, KAN Other drugs	INH, RIF, EMB, fQs, AMK, CAP, KAN, PZA Other drugs
Results	1. Mutation detected or not detected 2. No sequences provided	1. Mutation detected or not detected 2. Sequences of few frequent mutations are provided	Sequences provided	Sequences provided
Methodology Limitations	1. Difficult to detect mixed population 2. Silent mutations and mutations not conferring resistance lead to false resistance interpretation	1. Difficult to detect mixed population 2. Silent mutations and mutations not conferring resistance lead to false resistance interpretation	1. Mixed population may not be detected if the minor population is <30% 2. Not suitable for detecting widely distributed mutations	1. Mixed population may not be detected if the minor population is <30%
Advantages	1. Little hands-on time 2. Easy to perform 3. Easy to implement 4. Point-of-care capability	Low cost of equipment	1. Users may evaluate association of a mutation with resistance 2. Fairly wide applicability 3. Possible to detect mixed population	1. Users may evaluate association of a mutation with resistance 2. Wide applicability 3. Possible to detect mixed population

a Assays using pyrosequencing or Sanger sequencing technologies are laboratory-developed tests. The performance characteristics may vary. Laboratories may validate their own assays for testing specimens from various sources not restricted to respiratory specimens.
b Clinical specimens concentrated by NALC-NaOH are suitable. Smear-negative specimens may be tested, but the sensitivity is lower than that for smear-positive specimens.

Box 1
Molecular drug susceptibility testing methods

1. Probe-based methods
   - Molecular beacon probe assay
     ○ GeneXpert MTB/RIF assay detects MTBC and resistance to RIF
   - Line-probe assay
     ○ HAIN MTBDR*plus* assay detects MTBC and resistance to INH and RIF
     ○ HAIN MTBDR*sl* assay detects MTBC and resistance to quinolones, injectable drugs, and EMB. Can be used as a reflex test when INH and/or RIF resistance is detected
     ○ INNO LIPA assay detects MTBC and resistance to RIF
2. Sequence-based methods: capable of detecting MDR and XDR TB, and beyond
   - Sanger sequencing
   - Pyrosequencing
   - Next-generation sequencing

---

established when at least 2 probes generate positive signals within the valid cycle threshold (Ct). RIF-resistance detection is determined when the "maximum delta Ct" (ΔCtmax) is greater than a cutoff value set by the manufacturer, indicating the presence of a mutation (or mutations) in the RRDR. Presence of a mutation, theoretically, prevents the probe from hybridizing to the DNA template and allows no production of fluorescent signals. However, factors such as probe design, location of a mutation within the functional part of a probe, and the DNA template's secondary/tertiary structure may tolerate the presence of a mutation to a certain extent, allowing some production of fluorescent signals. In addition, a mixed population may affect the Ct value and the end-point fluorescence level. Thus signal production is not an effect of "all or none". The GeneXpert software standardizes the interpretation by applying a ΔCtmax cutoff and several rules to Ct. Owing to the complexity of results generated from multiple probes, users should take extra precautions to evaluate the interpretation provided by GeneXpert, especially when Ct values are very high or the ΔCtmax is very close to the cutoff. Under these situations, evaluation of end-point fluorescence values and the graph of the fluorescence production of each probe besides Ct and ΔCt values may provide additional information. If the accuracy of an interpretation is in doubt, retesting or confirmation by a sequence-based method is warranted.

The MB technology has a limitation in its inability to reveal specific mutant sequences when mutations are detected. Although presence of mutations in the RRDR is highly associated with RIF resistance, false RIF resistance detected by GeneXpert has been reported.[24,59,60] RIF is the cornerstone of the standard regimen, and reporting of false RIF resistance may have adverse effects on the management of TB patients. In the United States or Western Europe where RIF-resistance prevalence is low, the effect of false resistance greatly affects the positive predictive value. Following the FDA clearance, the package insert of the GeneXpert MTB/RIF assay states that detection of RIF resistance must have results confirmed by a reference laboratory, and specimens should also be tested for the presence of mutations associated with resistance to other drugs. The CDC have also provided recommendations for GeneXpert MTB/RIF users, including the laboratory-reporting language and infection-control decisions.[61]

Line-Probe Assays

Line-probe (LP) assays include 3 major steps. The target sequence is amplified by PCR with one of the primers biotinylated. Reverse hybridization captures amplicons whose sequences are complementary to that of the probes immobilized on a strip. Colorimetric detection allows visualization of the bands where hybridization has occurred. Both GenoType MTBDR*plus* and MTBDR*sl* strips (HAIN Lifescience, Nehren, Germany) and INNO-LIPA RIF.TB strips (Fujirebio Europe N.V., Ghent, Belgium) contain a specific probe for identification of MTBC, several probes with wild-type sequences, and several probes with the most prevalent mutations associated with drug resistance for each locus. These LP assays can be performed on culture isolates or smear-positive pulmonary specimens. Interpretation of LP assays is outlined in **Box 2**. The performance of these LP assays[32,51,62,63] for drug-resistance detection is similar to that of other MDST assays.

Box 2
Interpretation of results of line-probe assays

- All wild-type bands are present with absence of all mutant bands:
  - No mutations are present within the targeted DNA segment; this suggests susceptibility to the drug.
- Missing at least 1 wild-type band and presence of one of the mutant bands:
  - A specific mutation is present and its sequence is provided. Drug resistance is predicted.
- Missing at least 1 wild-type band but none of the mutant bands are present:
  - A mutation is present but not one of those frequent mutations; the identity of the mutation is not given.
  - It is likely to be associated with drug resistance, but one cannot rule out mutations with unpredictable drug susceptibility or not conferring resistance.
- All wild-type bands are present and one of the mutant bands is also present:
  - Possible a mixed population, or a mixed infection with 2 different strains, a wild-type strain, and a drug-resistant strain.
  - The variable intensity of the band may add difficulties in interpretation for this scenario. It is advisable to confirm by a sequence-based method, or to defer the interpretation to culture-based drug susceptibility testing results.

Sanger Sequencing

Sanger sequencing using the dye-terminator methodology has been the gold standard of sequencing. As long as the gene and mutations associated with drug resistance have been identified, it is possible for laboratories to design primers and use this method to detect resistance to any drug. However, the procedure is somewhat lengthy and requires more hands-on time. At CDC, a service using this method for molecular detection of drug resistance (http://www.cdc.gov/tb/topic/laboratory/MDDRUsersGuide.pdf) is available for testing isolates grown in solid or liquid media, and NALC-NaOH concentrated, smear-positive specimens from known or suspected MDR TB patients. Sanger sequencing has been shown to correlate well with CDST by the conventional agar proportion method for drugs defining XDR TB, in addition to EMB and PZA.[29]

Pyrosequencing

There are several instrument platforms for pyrosequencing (PSQ). The PSQ platform discussed here, PyroMark (Qiagen, Hilden, Germany), sequences short segments

(<100 bp) of genomic DNA and is suitable for rapid detection of mutations with simple data handling. Assays using the PyroMark sequencer have been developed for detection of drug resistance in *M tuberculosis* from culture isolates or directly from clinical specimens.[30,31,64–70] A PSQ assay consists of 3 essential steps: PCR amplification of target sequences, capture of single-stranded DNA, and real-time sequencing by the PSQ technology[71] at a speed of 1 nucleotide per minute. The user defines the deoxyribonucleotide triphosphate (dNTP) dispensation order. When the dNTP being dispensed is complementary to the first available base in the DNA template, hybridization occurs and pyrophosphate is generated. The pyrophosphate triggers a cascade of chemical reactions involving enzymes (adenosine triphosphate sulfurylase and luciferase) and substrates (adenosine 5′-phosphosulfate and luciferine) with an end result of the emission of light. The light generated is proportional to the dNTP incorporated. The identity of dNTP incorporated represents the base(s) sequenced.

PSQ results provide sequence identities, wild-type or mutant, with high reproducibility and accuracy comparable with that of Sanger sequencing. A recent study performed on both culture isolates and clinical specimens for detection of XDR TB demonstrated a correlation between PSQ and CDST in the range of 94% to 99% (94.3% for INH, 98.7% for RIF, 97.6% for fQs, 99.2% for AMK and CAP, and 96.4% for KAN).[23]

Next-Generation Sequencing

Next-generation sequencing (NGS) platforms perform high-throughput automated sequencing using a parallelized sequencing process to generate thousands to millions of sequences concurrently.[72,73] Sophisticated software to analyze an enormous volume of data sets is required. A recent study used NGS for culture identification, drug-resistance screening to 39 antibiotics, and strain typing simultaneously with the MiSeq platform (Illumina, San Diego, CA). Sequencing was performed on a culture that turned positive within 3 days of incubation in a liquid culture system.[74] This finding demonstrates the potential of using NGS as a rapid tool for TB diagnosis, drug-resistance testing, and strain typing. However, at present NGS requires a relatively high DNA concentration (1 ng to 1 μg) for adequate sensitivity; therefore, it is necessary to use growth from positive cultures for DNA extraction. As many cultures require 1 to 3 weeks of incubation to demonstrate growth, this delays the turnaround time of NGS. Nevertheless, advances in sequencing technology are likely to overcome this problem in the foreseeable future, and offer better and quicker systems to serve the need for TB diagnosis, drug-resistance detection, and epidemiologic surveillance, all at the same time.

PRACTICAL USE OF MOLECULAR DIAGNOSTIC ASSAYS

The CDC published guidelines in 2009 on the use of NAATs for the diagnosis of TB[11] and recommended that NAATs be performed on at least one respiratory specimen from each patient suspected of having pulmonary TB for whom the NAAT results would alter case management or TB-control activities. These guidelines may apply to MDST assays that can concurrently detect MTBC and drug-resistance mutations. Suggestions for cost-effective and meaningful utilization of MDST assays in regions with low prevalence of drug resistance are shown in **Box 3**.

IMPACT ON PATIENT MANAGEMENT, TB CONTROL, AND INFECTION CONTROL

MDST enables early diagnosis of TB, and early initiation of treatment, contact investigation, and infection control in health care settings. It also increases case detection for pan-susceptible TB and drug-resistant TB, which may result in increased cost to a

---

Box 3
Suggestions for use of molecular testing in regions with low drug resistance

Molecular Detection of Drug Resistance is Indicated

- Drug resistance is suspected
  - Patients are immigrants whose original countries have a high prevalence of drug resistance
  - Patients have been exposed to drug-resistant TB cases
  - Patients are not responding to the current regimen
  - Patients were treated previously and have relapsed
- Patients have wide contacts, such as inmates, rest home residents, health care workers, or students, and may carry wider epidemiologic implications
- Patients are vulnerable individuals with debilitating health conditions or immunocompromised status
- Patients are in a household with vulnerable individuals, infants, or immunocompromised
- Laboratory issues
  - Cultures are mixed with other bacteria; CDST could not be performed
  - Smear positive but culture negative

Method Selection and Reflex Testing

- If sequence-based method is available, it is the method of choice
- If GeneXpert is readily available, it can be used for detection of MTBC and RIF resistance. When a mutation is detected, confirmation by a sequence-based method is recommended
- If INH resistance is suspected, use a method which can at least detect mutations in *katG* and *inhA*
- If RIF resistance is detected, the specimen should be tested for mutations associated with resistance to other drugs

---

TB-control program.[14] However, these costs would be offset by downstream savings from reduced transmission and better treatment outcome. A study evaluating the clinical impact of an MB assay on management of MDR TB patients demonstrated that the average initiation of MDR TB regimens was 41 days sooner and the average culture conversion was 27 days sooner for the group in which MDST was performed.[10]

SUMMARY

MDST has raised expectations for improved TB diagnosis and detection of drug resistance. With its excellent turnaround time, MDST has had a significant impact on the management of TB patients, TB control, and infection control.

With the realization that mutations do not always confer drug resistance, detection of the presence of a mutation alone may bear risks of reporting false resistance. Therefore, determining the mutation identity by a sequence-based method is recommended.

Various mutations may confer different levels of resistance. Establishment of a library containing reliable MIC ranges for each mutation will enable prediction of a drug-resistance level, especially for RIF, RFB, and fQs. When the treatment arsenal is limited, such information may be helpful to physicians for making dosage adjustments if indicated.

MDST has limitations. Both sensitivity and specificity are less than 100%, and MDST is not available for all drugs. Culturing TB organisms for CDST may still be required. With availability of rapid MDST results for key drugs, when resistance mutations are detected, CDST should be performed on expanded drug panels as soon as adequate growth is available. This approach will shorten the turnaround time in obtaining complete CDST results.

Borderline susceptibility or resistance associated with certain mutations has created a problem for current CDST, which uses the binary classification of either susceptible or resistant. Reporting MIC results for strains with those mutations may be more objective and truthful, and more useful to physicians.

Ever-evolving technologies are leading to a new era when diagnosis, drug-resistance detection, and genotyping of MTBC can be obtained within days of specimen collection. The impact on early diagnosis, patient management, contact investigation, and surveillance will be greater than what is currently achievable.

REFERENCES

1. CDC. Reported tuberculosis in the United States, 2012. Atlanta (GA): Center for the Diseases Control and Prevention; 2013.
2. Hoffner S. Unexpected high levels of multidrug-resistant tuberculosis present new challenges for tuberculosis control. Lancet 2012;380(9851):1367–9.
3. WHO. Global tuberculosis report. 2013. Geneva (Switzerland): World Health Organization. Available at: http://wh1libdoc.who.int/publications/2013/97892415 64656_eng.pdf. WHO/HTM/TB/2013.11.
4. WHO. Multidrug and extensively drug-resistant TB (M/XDR-TB): 2010 global report in surveillance and response. Geneva (Switzerland): World Health Organization; 2011. March, 6, 2011.
5. WHO. Molecular line probe assays for rapid screening of patients at risk of multidrug-resistant tuberculosis (MDR-TB). Policy statement. Geneva (Switzerland): World Health Organization; 2008.
6. WHO. Roadmap for rolling out Xpert MTB/RIF for rapid diagnosis of TB and MDR-TB. Geneva (Switzerland): World Health Organization; 2010.
7. WHO. Policy statement: Automated real-time nucleic acid amplification technology for rapid and simultaneous detection of tuberculosis and rifampin resistance: Xpert MTB/RIF system. Geneva (Switzerland): World Health Organization. Available at: http://whlibdoc.who.int/publications/2011/978924 1501545. WHO/HTM/TB/2011.4. 2011.
8. Boehme CC, Nabeta P, Hillemann D, et al. Rapid molecular detection of tuberculosis and rifampin resistance. N Engl J Med 2010;363(11):1005–15.
9. Drobniewski F, Nikolayevskyy V, Maxeiner H, et al. Rapid diagnostics of tuberculosis and drug resistance in the industrialized world: clinical and public health benefits and barriers to implementation. BMC Med 2013;11:190.
10. Banerjee R, Allen J, Lin SY, et al. Rapid drug susceptibility testing with a molecular beacon assay is associated with earlier diagnosis and treatment of multidrug-resistant tuberculosis in California. J Clin Microbiol 2010;48(10):3779–81.
11. CDC. Updated guidelines for the use of nucleic acid amplification tests in the diagnosis of tuberculosis. MMWR Morb Mortal Wkly Rep 2009;58(1):7–10.
12. Marks SM, Cronin W, Venkatappa T, et al. The health-system benefits and cost-effectiveness of using *Mycobacterium tuberculosis* direct nucleic acid amplification testing to diagnose tuberculosis disease in the United States. Clin Infect Dis 2013;57(4):532–42.
13. Boehme CC, Nicol MP, Nabeta P, et al. Feasibility, diagnostic accuracy, and effectiveness of decentralised use of the Xpert MTB/RIF test for diagnosis of

tuberculosis and multidrug resistance: a multicentre implementation study. Lancet 2011;377(9776):1495–505.

14. Meyer-Rath G, Schnippel K, Long L, et al. The impact and cost of scaling up GeneXpert MTB/RIF in South Africa. PLoS One 2012;7(5):e36966.

15. de Lange C. Diagnosis: waiting for results. Nature 2013;502(7470):S10–2.

16. WHO. Global tuberculosis report 2012. Geneva (Switzerland): World Health Organization; 2012.

17. Cole S, Brosch R, Parkhill J, et al. Deciphering the biology of *Mycobacterium tuberculosis* from the complete genome sequence. Nature 1998;393:537–44.

18. Pfyffer GE, Palicova F. *Mycobacterium*: general characteristics, laboratory detection and staining procedures. In: Versalovic J, Carroll K, Funke G, et al, editors. Manual of clinical microbiology. 10th edition. Washington, DC: ASM Press; 2011. p. 472–502.

19. Hopewell P. Overview of clinical tuberculosis. In: Bloom B, editor. Tuberculosis, pathogenesis, protection and control. Washington, DC: ASM Press; 1994. p. 25–46.

20. Dannenberg AJ, Rook G. Pathogenesis of pulmonary tuberculosis: an interplay of tissue-damaging and macrophage-activating immune responses–dual mechanisms that control bacillary multiplication. In: Bloom B, editor. Tuberculosis. Washington, DC: ASM Press; 1994. p. 459–81.

21. Burman W. The value of in vitro drug activity and pharmacokinetics in predicting the effectiveness of antimicrobial therapy: a critical review. Am J Med Sci 1997; 313(6):355–63.

22. Zhang Y, Heym B, Allen B, et al. The catalase-peroxidase gene and isoniazid resistance of *Mycobacterium tuberculosis*. Nature 1992;358:591–3.

23. Lin SY, Rodwell TC, Victor T, et al. Pyrosequencing for rapid detection of extensively drug-resistant *Mycobacterium tuberculosis* in clinical isolates and clinical specimens. J Clin Microbiol 2014;52:475–82.

24. Alonso M, Palacios JJ, Herranz M, et al. Isolation of *Mycobacterium tuberculosis* strains with a silent mutation in rpoB leading to potential misassignment of resistance category. J Clin Microbiol 2011;49(7):2688–90.

25. Rigouts L, Gumusboga M, de Rijk WB, et al. Rifampin resistance missed in automated liquid culture system for *Mycobacterium tuberculosis* isolates with specific rpoB mutations. J Clin Microbiol 2013;51(8):2641–5.

26. van Deun A, Barrera L, Bastian I, et al. *Mycobacterium tuberculosis* strains with highly discordant rifampin susceptibility test results. J Clin Microbiol 2009; 47(11):3501–6.

27. Hazbon MH, Brimacombe M, Bobadilla del Valle M, et al. Population genetics study of isoniazid resistance mutations and evolution of multidrug-resistant *Mycobacterium tuberculosis*. Antimicrob Agents Chemother 2006;50(8):2640–9.

28. Wilson TM, Collins DM. ahpC, a gene involved in isoniazid resistance of the *Mycobacterium tuberculosis* complex. Mol Microbiol 1996;19:1025–34.

29. Campbell PJ, Morlock GP, Sikes RD, et al. Molecular detection of mutations associated with first- and second-line drug resistance compared with conventional drug susceptibility testing of *Mycobacterium tuberculosis*. Antimicrob Agents Chemother 2011;55(5):2032–41.

30. Engström A, Morcillo N, Imperiale B, et al. Detection of first- and second-line drug resistance in *Mycobacterium tuberculosis* clinical isolates by pyrosequencing. J Clin Microbiol 2012;50(6):2026–33.

31. García-Sierra N, Lacoma A, Prat C, et al. Pyrosequencing for rapid molecular detection of rifampin and isoniazid resistance in *Mycobacterium tuberculosis* strains and clinical specimens. J Clin Microbiol 2011;49(10):3683–6.

32. Huang W-L, Chen H-Y, Kuo Y-M, et al. Performance assessment of the Geno-Type MTBDRplus test and DNA sequencing in detection of multidrug-resistant *Mycobacterium tuberculosis*. J Clin Microbiol 2009;47(8):2520–4.

33. Mokrousov I, Otten T, Filipenko M, et al. Detection of isoniazid-resistant *Mycobacterium tuberculosis* strains by a multiplex allele-specific PCR assay targeting katG Codon 315 variation. J Clin Microbiol 2002;40(7):2509–12.

34. Lee H, Cho SN, Bang HE, et al. Exclusive mutations related to isoniazid and ethionamide resistance among *Mycobacterium tuberculosis* isolates from Korea. Int J Tuberc Lung Dis 2000;4(5):441–7.

35. Lee AS, Teo AS, Wong S-Y. Novel mutations in ndh in isoniazid-resistant *Mycobacterium tuberculosis* isolates. Antimicrob Agents Chemother 2001;45(7):2157–9.

36. Williams DL, Spring L, Collins L, et al. Contribution of rpoB mutations to development of rifamycin cross-resistance in *Mycobacterium tuberculosis*. Antimicrob Agents Chemother 1998;42(7):1853–7.

37. Ohno H, Koga H, Kohno S, et al. Relationship between rifampin MICs for and rpoB mutations of *Mycobacterium tuberculosis* strains isolated in Japan. Antimicrob Agents Chemother 1996;40(4):1053–6.

38. Tan Y, Hu Z, Zhao Y, et al. The beginning of the rpoB gene in addition to the rifampin resistance determination region might be needed for identifying rifampin/rifabutin cross-resistance in multidrug-resistant *Mycobacterium tuberculosis* isolates from Southern China. J Clin Microbiol 2012;50(1):81–5.

39. van Deun A, Aung KJ, Bola V, et al. Rifampin drug resistance tests for tuberculosis: challenging the gold standard. J Clin Microbiol 2013;51(8):2633–40.

40. Williamson DA, Roberts SA, Bower JE, et al. Clinical failures associated with rpoB mutations in phenotypically occult multidrug-resistant *Mycobacterium tuberculosis*. Int J Tuberc Lung Dis 2012;16(2):216–20.

41. Plinke C, Rusch-Gerdes S, Niemann S. Significance of mutations in embB Codon 306 for prediction of ethambutol resistance in clinical *Mycobacterium tuberculosis* isolates. Antimicrob Agents Chemother 2006;50(5):1900–2.

42. Ahmad S, Jaber AA, Mokaddas E. Frequency of embB codon 306 mutations in ethambutol-susceptible and -resistant clinical *Mycobacterium tuberculosis* isolates in Kuwait. Tuberculosis 2007;87(2):123–9.

43. Morlock GP, Crawford JT, Butler WR, et al. Phenotypic characterization of pncA mutants of *Mycobacterium tuberculosis*. Antimicrob Agents Chemother 2000;44(9):2291–5.

44. Kim HJ, Kwak HK, Lee J, et al. Patterns of pncA mutations in drug-resistant *Mycobacterium tuberculosis* isolated from patients in South Korea. Int J Tuberc Lung Dis 2012;16(1):98–103.

45. Piersimoni C, Mustazzolu A, Giannoni F, et al. Prevention of false resistance results obtained in testing the susceptibility of *Mycobacterium tuberculosis* to pyrazinamide with the Bactec MGIT 960 system using a reduced inoculum. J Clin Microbiol 2013;51(1):291–4.

46. Chedore P, Bertucci L, Wolfe J, et al. Potential for erroneous results indicating resistance when using the Bactec MGIT 960 system for testing susceptibility of *Mycobacterium tuberculosis* to pyrazinamide. J Clin Microbiol 2010;48(1):300–1.

47. Werngren J, Sturegard E, Jureen P, et al. Reevaluation of the critical concentration for drug susceptibility testing of *Mycobacterium tuberculosis* against pyrazinamide using wild-type MIC distributions and pncA gene sequencing. Antimicrob Agents Chemother 2012;56(3):1253–7.

48. Simons SO, van Ingen J, van der Laan T, et al. Validation of pncA gene sequencing in combination with the mycobacterial growth indicator tube method to test susceptibility of *Mycobacterium tuberculosis* to pyrazinamide. J Clin Microbiol 2012;50(2):428–34.

49. Sirgel FA, Warren RM, Streicher EM, et al. gyrA mutations and phenotypic susceptibility levels to ofloxacin and moxifloxacin in clinical isolates of *Mycobacterium tuberculosis*. J Antimicrob Chemother 2012;67(5):1088–93.

50. Poissy J, Aubry A, Fernandez C, et al. Should moxifloxacin be used for the treatment of extensively drug-resistant tuberculosis? An answer from a murine model. Antimicrob Agents Chemother 2010;54(11):4765–71.

51. Huang W-L, Chi T-L, Wu M-H, et al. Performance assessment of the GenoType MTBDRsl test and DNA sequencing for detection of second-line and ethambutol drug resistance among patients infected with multidrug-resistant *Mycobacterium tuberculosis*. J Clin Microbiol 2011;49(7):2502–8.

52. Maruri F, Sterling TR, Kaiga AW, et al. A systematic review of gyrase mutations associated with fluoroquinolone-resistant *Mycobacterium tuberculosis* and a proposed gyrase numbering system. J Antimicrob Chemother 2012;67(4): 819–31.

53. Maus CE, Plikaytis BB, Shinnick TM. Molecular analysis of cross-resistance to capreomycin, kanamycin, amikacin, and viomycin in *Mycobacterium tuberculosis*. Antimicrob Agents Chemother 2005;49(8):3192–7.

54. Brossier F, Veziris N, Aubry A, et al. Detection by GenoType MTBDRsl test of complex mechanisms of resistance to second-line drugs and ethambutol in multidrug-resistant *Mycobacterium tuberculosis* complex isolates. J Clin Microbiol 2010;48(5):1683–9.

55. Georghiou SB, Magana M, Garfein RS, et al. Evaluation of genetic mutations associated with *Mycobacterium tuberculosis* resistance to amikacin, kanamycin and capreomycin: a systematic review. PLoS One 2012;7(3):e33275.

56. Piatek AS, Tyagi S, Pol AC, et al. Molecular beacon sequence analysis for detecting drug resistance in *Mycobacterium tuberculosis*. Nat Biotechnol 1998; 16(4):359–63.

57. Tyagi S, Kramer FR. Molecular beacons: probes that fluoresce upon hybridization. Nat Biotechnol 1996;14:303–8.

58. Lawn SD, Mwaba P, Bates M, et al. Advances in tuberculosis diagnostics: the Xpert MTB/RIF assay and future prospects for a point-of-care test. Lancet Infect Dis 2013;13(4):349–61.

59. Marlowe EM, Novak-Weekley SM, Cumpio J, et al. Evaluation of the cepheid Xpert MTB/RIF assay for direct detection of *Mycobacterium tuberculosis* complex in respiratory specimens. J Clin Microbiol 2011;49(4):1621–3.

60. van Rie A, Mellet K, John MA, et al. False-positive rifampicin resistance on Xpert(R) MTB/RIF: case report and clinical implications. Int J Tuberc Lung Dis 2012;16(2):206–8.

61. CDC. Availability of an assay for detecting *Mycobacterium tuberculosis*, including refiampin-resistant strains, and consideration for its use-United States, 2013. MMWR Morb Mortal Wkly Rep 2013;62(41):821–7.

62. Ferro BE, García PK, Nieto LM, et al. Predictive value of molecular drug resistance testing of *Mycobacterium tuberculosis* isolates in Valle del Cauca, Colombia. J Clin Microbiol 2013;51(7):2220–4.

63. Said HM, Kock MM, Ismail NA, et al. Evaluation of the GenoType(R) MTBDRsl assay for susceptibility testing of second-line anti-tuberculosis drugs. Int J Tuberc Lung Dis 2012;16(1):104–9.

64. Bravo LT, Tuohy MJ, Ang C, et al. Pyrosequencing for rapid detection of *Myco-bacterium tuberculosis* resistance to rifampin, isoniazid, and fluoroquinolones. J Clin Microbiol 2009;47(12):3985–90.

65. Garza-Gonzalez E, Gonzalez GM, Renteria A, et al. A pyrosequencing method for molecular monitoring of regions in the inhA, ahpC and rpoB genes of *Myco-bacterium tuberculosis*. Clin Microbiol Infect 2010;16(6):607–12.

66. Guo Q, Zheng RJ, Zhu CT, et al. Pyrosequencing for the rapid detection of rifam-picin resistance in *Mycobacterium tuberculosis*: a meta-analysis [review article]. Int J Tuberc Lung Dis 2013;17(8):1008–13.

67. Halse TA, Edwards J, Cunningham PL, et al. Combined real-time PCR and rpoB gene pyrosequencing for rapid identification of *Mycobacterium tuberculosis* and determination of rifampin resistance directly in clinical specimens. J Clin Microbiol 2010;48(4):1182–8.

68. Jureen P, Engstrand L, Eriksson S, et al. Rapid detection of rifampin resistance in *Mycobacterium tuberculosis* by pyrosequencing technology. J Clin Microbiol 2006;44(6):1925–9.

69. Marttila HJ, Makinen J, Marjamaki M, et al. Prospective evaluation of pyrose-quencing for the rapid detection of isoniazid and rifampin resistance in clinical *Mycobacterium tuberculosis* isolates. Eur J Clin Microbiol Infect Dis 2009;28:33–8.

70. Zhao J-R, Bai Y-J, Wang Y, et al. Development of a pyrosequencing approach for rapid screening of rifampin, isoniazid and ethambutol-resistant *Mycobacte-rium tuberculosis*. Int J Tuberc Lung Dis 2005;9:328–32.

71. Diggle MA, Clarke SC. Pyrosequencing (TM)—sequencing typing at the speed of light. Mol Biotechnol 2004;28(2):129–38.

72. Daum LT, Rodriguez JD, Worthy SA, et al. Next-generation ion torrent sequencing of drug resistance mutations in *Mycobacterium tuberculosis* strains. J Clin Microbiol 2012;50(12):3831–7.

73. Quail MA, Smith M, Coupland P, et al. A tale of three next generation sequencing platforms: comparison of Ion Torrent, Pacific Biosciences and Illumina MiSeq sequencers. BMC Genomics 2012;13:341.

74. Köser CU, Bryant JM, Becq J, et al. Whole-genome sequencing for rapid sus-ceptibility testing of *M. tuberculosis*. N Engl J Med 2013;369(3):290–2.

Nonmolecular Methods for the Diagnosis of Respiratory Fungal Infections

Frédéric Lamoth, MD[a,b,c,*], Barbara D. Alexander, MD, MHS[a,b,*]

KEYWORDS

- Galactomannan • β-glucan • *Cryptococcus* antigen test • Invasive aspergillosis
- Pulmonary cryptococcosis • *Pneumocystis jirovecii* pneumonia • Mucormycosis

KEY POINTS

- Nonmolecular fungal biomarkers are part of the diagnostic workup of invasive fungal pneumonia in conjunction with other clinical, radiologic, and microbiological criteria.
- Good evidence supports the use of the galactomannan (GM) test in serum or bronchoalveolar lavage fluid for the diagnosis and follow-up of invasive aspergillosis in patients who have hematologic cancer.
- The 1,3-β-D-glucan (BG) test in serum can detect a broad spectrum of invasive fungal pathogens, including *Pneumocystis jirovecii*.
- GM and BG testing cannot be recommended in patients who do not have cancer, because of their modest performance in this population; their inability to detect mucormycosis is another limitation.
- Detection of the cryptococcal antigen in serum is a cornerstone of the diagnosis of disseminated cryptococcosis, but its sensitivity is lower in patients who do not have human immunodeficiency virus, with disease limited to the lung.

INTRODUCTION

Fungal pneumonias are an important cause of mortality among an increasing diversity of immunosuppressed populations, such as patients who have hematologic cancer, transplant recipients, patients with human immunodeficiency virus (HIV) or individuals with chronic pulmonary or autoimmune diseases. Their diagnosis is difficult and often only presumptive, relying on a combination of clinical, radiologic, and microbiological

Disclosure Statement: All authors report no potential conflict of interests.
[a] Division of Infectious Diseases, Department of Medicine, Duke University Medical Center, Box 102359, Durham, NC 27710, USA; [b] Clinical Microbiology Laboratory, Department of Pathology, Duke University Medical Center, 108 Carl building, Durham, NC 27710, USA; [c] Infectious Diseases Service and Institute of Microbiology, Lausanne University Hospital, Rue du Bugnon 46, 1011 Lausanne, Switzerland
* Corresponding authors.
E-mail addresses: frederic.lamoth@dm.duke.edu; alexa011@mc.duke.edu

factors. Nonmolecular fungal markers in serum or other biological samples represent a noninvasive diagnostic tool, which can help in therapeutic decisions. The performance of nonmolecular fungal diagnostic tests for each type of fungal pneumonia is discussed in this article. This review provides the reader with a general overview of the performance and limitations of these tests, as well as some recommendations for their use in specific contexts (summarized in **Table 1**).

MICROBIOLOGY/EPIDEMIOLOGY

Pneumonia is the leading infectious cause of death in developed countries.[1] Among the broad variety of respiratory pathogens, fungi account for only a small proportion of community-acquired and nosocomial pneumonias.[2,3] However, fungal respiratory infections are of particular concern in the expanding population of immunosuppressed patients, and the spectrum of opportunistic fungi causing infections in predisposed individuals is constantly increasing, as shown in **Table 2**. *Aspergillus* represents the leading cause of invasive pulmonary fungal infection (IFI) and death in patients who have cancer, especially those with hematologic malignancies, and in transplant recipients.[4,5] Members of the subphylum Mucormycotina (previously referred to as the Zygomycetes and responsible for mucormycosis) and other emerging non-*Aspergillus* molds account

Table 1		
Nonmolecular diagnostic tests for the diagnosis of fungal pulmonary infections		
Disease	**Available Tests**	**Comments**
Invasive aspergillosis	Galactomannan (serum)	Good evidence supports use in patients with hematologic malignancies Caveat: negative test does not exclude disease (relatively low sensitivity) Not routinely recommended in other populations at risk of IFI
	Galactomannan (BAL)	Good evidence supports use in patients with hematologic malignancies as well as in other populations at risk of IFI Caveat: cannot differentiate *Aspergillus* pulmonary colonization from IA
	BG (serum)	Good evidence supports use in patients with hematologic malignancies Caveat: negative test does not exclude disease (low sensitivity) Not routinely recommended in other populations at risk of IFI
Other mold pulmonary infections	BG (serum)	Not routinely recommended. Does not detect agents of mucormycosis
Pneumocystis jirovecii pneumonia	BG (serum)	Good evidence supports use in patients with HIV and patients who do not have HIV
Pulmonary cryptococcosis	Cryptococcal antigen (serum)	Good evidence supports use in patients with HIV and patients who do not have HIV Caveat: lower sensitivity in patients who do not have HIV and in nondisseminated disease

Abbreviations: BAL, bronchoalveolar lavage fluid; BG, 1,3-β-D-glucan; IA, invasive aspergillosis; IFI, invasive fungal infection.

Table 2
Opportunistic fungi causing respiratory infections in different patient populations

Disease	Causal Agent (%)	Underlying Conditions at Risk
Invasive pulmonary fungal infection	*Aspergillus fumigatus* (50–90)[a] Other *Aspergillus* species[b] (5–40) Zygomycetes[c] (1–10) Other molds[d] (1–10)	High[e] HSCT or hematologic cancer, SOT Low/moderate[e] Solid tumor, ICU, chronic pulmonary diseases, systemic autoimmune disease
Chronic pulmonary aspergillosis	*Aspergillus* species (most cases) Other molds (rare cases)	Cavitary tuberculosis or other chronic pulmonary diseases
Pneumocystis jirovecii pneumonia	*Pneumocystis jirovecii*	High HIV, HSCT, or hematologic cancer Low/Moderate SOT, solid tumor, chronic pulmonary diseases, systemic autoimmune disease
Cryptococcosis	*Cryptococcus neoformans* *Cryptococcus gattii*	High HIV, SOT Low/Moderate General population, HSCT

Abbreviations: HIV, human immunodeficiency virus; HSCT, hematopoietic stem cell transplantation; ICU, intensive care unit; SOT, solid-organ transplantation.
[a] Values in brackets are estimated proportions (in percent) and may vary according to the epidemiologic context.
[b] Most frequent pathogens include: *Aspergillus flavus, A niger, A terreus.*
[c] Most frequent pathogens include: *Rhizopus* spp, *Mucor* spp, *Rhizomucor* spp, *Absidia (Lichtheimia)* spp.
[d] Most frequent pathogens include: *Fusarium* spp, *Scedosporium* spp, *Paecilomyces* spp, *Scopulariopsis* spp.
[e] High and low/moderate risks refer to an estimated 1-year cumulative incidence of 1%–10% and <1%, respectively.

for an increasing proportion of cases and are associated with a particularly bad prognosis.[6,7] Among patients with HIV, *Cryptococcus neoformans* and *Pneumocystis jirovecii* are the most frequent causes of fungal pneumonia. *Aspergillus* spp are also the cause of chronic pulmonary aspergillosis or aspergilloma, an insidious noninvasive form of pulmonary infection affecting nonimmunosuppressed individuals with preexisting cavitary lung lesions.[8] Endemic mycoses caused by dimorphic molds (eg, *Histoplasma capsulatum, Coccidioides immitis*) and affecting previously healthy individuals are not discussed in this article, because they represent a distinct group of diseases.

CLINICAL PRESENTATION

Signs and symptoms of fungal pneumonia are not specific and are indistinguishable from those associated with respiratory infections of other origins. Fever is often the only sign of infection in neutropenic patients, who are not able to mount an effective immune response. Albeit not specific, pulmonary nodules are present in most cases of fungal pneumonia. A ground-glass opacity surrounding a macronodule is referred to as the halo sign and is present in about 60% of cases of invasive aspergillosis (IA). The halo sign is present early in the course of IA and is associated with a better prognosis if promptly recognized and treated.[9] Tracheobronchial aspergillosis represents a rare and severe subset of IA, in which the disease is limited to the tracheobronchial tree, and which can be missed by conventional thoracic computed tomography imaging.[10] The typical underlying immunosuppression of hosts who develop fungal pneumonias provides the opportunity for these infections to disseminate from the lungs. Clinical manifestations of extrapulmonary invasive fungal disease may include sinusitis, brain or epidural abscesses, vertebral osteomyelitis, cutaneous lesions, endocarditis, or fungemia.[11] Rhinocerebral and cutaneous mucormycosis are the most common presentation of this particular fungal disease in diabetic and immunocompetent patients.[12]

PATHOGENESIS

Fungi may simply colonize body sites without overt disease or they may invade, producing a variety of clinical syndromes. Development of disease is based on the susceptibility of the host and virulence of the pathogen. For example, *Aspergillus fumigatus* conidia are continuously inhaled by humans but rarely result in disease, because they are eliminated efficiently by the innate immune response. Pulmonary alveolar macrophages ingest inhaled *A fumigatus* conidia and inhibit germination. If macrophages are unable to clear the organism, the conidia germinate into hyphae. The host must then rely on polymorphonuclear leukocytes to defend against continued fungal growth. Despite similar degrees of exogenous immunosuppression impairing the innate immune clearance of *Aspergillus* conidia, only a subset of immunosuppressed patients develop IA. There is growing evidence that genetic polymorphisms in host defenses may alter the balance toward establishment of IA.[13]

In patients who develop invasive disease, the spectrum of host reaction varies based on underlying type and degree of immunosuppression. Nonneutropenic patients still capable of an immune response tend to limit angioinvasion, resulting in disease confined to the initial site of infection, compared with neutropenic patients, for whom dissemination is more common. This situation in turn influences the probability of antigenic markers leaking into body fluids, the development of antibodies, and the performance of diagnostic tests based on their detection.

DIAGNOSIS

The mortality of fungal respiratory infections has remained high despite the advent of new antifungal therapies.[14,15] The lack of specific signs of infection and the low sensitivity of conventional culture-based methods for diagnosis of fungal diseases result in delayed initiation of antifungal therapy. The early recognition and treatment of these infections are crucial for optimal outcome and represent a major challenge for the clinicians. A consensus group of the European Organization for Research and Treatment of Cancer (EORTC) and the Mycoses Study Group (MSG) have established definitions for IFIs for clinical and epidemiologic research.[16,17] These definitions are based on host factors and clinical and microbiological criteria and allow the classification of IFI according to the level of probability (proven, probable, possible, or no IFI). When the EORTC/MSG diagnostic criteria were revised in 2008, a major change consisted in the implementation of non–culture-based diagnostic tests as microbiological criteria.[17] These tests detect the presence of specific cell wall fungal antigens and include the Platelia *Aspergillus* enzyme immunoassay (EIA) (Bio-Rad Laboratories, Marne-La-Coquette, France) for the detection of galactomannan (GM) in serum or bronchoalveolar lavage fluid (BAL) and various commercially available tests for the detection of the 1,3-β-D-glucan (BG) in serum (Fungitell, Associates of Cape Cod, East Falmouth, MA, USA; Fungitec-G, Seikagaku, Tokyo, Japan; Wako, Wako Pure Chemicals Industries, Tokyo, Japan; Maruha, Maruha-Nichiro Foods, Tokyo, Japan).

Although the GM test is specifically designed for the detection of *Aspergillus* spp, the BG assay can detect a broader range of pathogenic fungi. For *Cryptococcus neoformans*, EIAs, latex agglutination (LA) tests, and a lateral-flow assay for the detection of a capsular antigen in serum and cerebrospinal fluid (CSF) are available. These serologic markers of IFI (summarized in **Table 3**) are referred to as nonmolecular diagnostic tests in opposition to molecular tests (eg, fungal-specific or multiplex polymerase chain reaction [PCR] assays), which despite their promising diagnostic usefulness,[18] have not yet been included in the EORTC/MSG definitions of IFI, because of their lack of standardization and the lack of commercially available tests.[17] For the same reasons, the expert panel of the 3rd European Conference on Infections in Leukemia has published a recommendation grading the use of GM, BG, and the cryptococcal antigen tests, but not molecular tests.[19]

Invasive Aspergillosis (IA)

IA affects oncohematologic patients with a cumulative incidence of 1% to 10% per year.[4] The overall 1-year cumulative incidence of IA among solid-organ transplant recipients is 0.65% but varies considerably based on the organ transplanted.[5] IA is also increasingly recognized among nontraditionally immunosuppressed patients, such as those receiving intensive care support, and EORTC/MSG host criteria for IFI may be missing in this at-risk patient group.[20,21]

GM assay

Detection of circulating immunogenic polysaccharides of the cell wall of *Aspergillus* as a diagnostic tool of IA has been investigated for about 30 years.[22–24] An LA test (Pastorex *Aspergillus*, Sanofi Diagnostic, Pasteur) was first developed for GM detection in serum, but showed low sensitivity for the diagnosis of IA.[25–27] The current double-direct sandwich enzyme-linked immunosorbent assay (ELISA) (Platelia *Aspergillus*, Bio-Rad Laboratories) uses the same antibody as the LA test (galactofuranose-specific rat monoclonal antibody EB-A2) for both capture and detection of GM, resulting in a lower threshold of detection.[28] The result is expressed as a ratio dividing the optical density (OD) of the patient's sample by that of a control sample containing a defined concentration of GM.

The cutoff defining a positive result has been debated. Although the threshold of positivity was initially set at an OD index 1.5 or greater by the manufacturer, receiver operating characteristic (ROC) curve analyses support the choice of 0.5 or greater as the optimal cutoff to define a positive test in serum.[29–31] The requirement of 2 consecutive positive tests (index $\geq$0.5) results in the best diagnostic accuracy.[29,30] The lower cutoffs are also associated with an earlier detection of disease[29,30,32] and better sensitivity in patients under treatment with mold-active antifungal drugs.[33]

Various causes of false-positive results have been reported, concomitant administration of piperacillin-tazobactam being the most famous.[34] However, this problem seems to be minimized, with new commercialized preparations of the drug containing only residual GM.[35] Other β-lactam antibiotics,[36] blood transfusions, or blood-derived products,[37] sodium gluconate (contained in Plasma-Lyte solution and some food products)[38–40] or other food additives[41–43] and cross-reactivity with other fungi[44–52] are also causes of false-positive results (see **Table 3**).

In 2003, the US Food and Drug Administration (FDA) cleared the Platelia *Aspergillus* EIA GM test with a cutoff value of 0.5 or greater as an aid in the diagnosis of IA when used in conjunction with other diagnostic procedures such as microbiological culture, histologic examination of biopsy samples, and radiographic evidence. The performance of the GM test in serum for the diagnosis of IA has been assessed in many

Table 3
Currently available nonmolecular fungal diagnostic tests

Fungal Biomarker	Commercial Test	Biological Fluid	Positive Cutoff[a]	Detected Fungi[b]	Causes of False-Positive Results
Galactomannan	Platelia Aspergillus EIA (Bio-Rad Laboratories)	Serum BAL CSF	0.5 (optical density index)	Aspergillus spp	Fungal contaminants[c] β-lactam antibiotics Blood transfusions and blood-derived products Food additives (sodium gluconate)
BG	Fungitell (Associates of Cape Cod) Fungitec-G (Seikagaku) Wako (Wako Pure Chemicals Industries) Maruha (Maruha-Nichiro Foods)	Serum	60–80 pg/mL (Fungitell) 20 pg/mL (Fungitec-G) 11 pg/mL (Wako/Maruha)	Aspergillus spp, Candida spp, Pneumocystis jiroveci[d]	Blood transfusions and blood-derived products Renal replacement therapy β-lactam antibiotics Immunoglobulins Cellulose containing dressings Bacterial infections
Cryptococcal antigen	Premier EIA (Meridian Biosciences) CALAS (Meridian Biosciences) Murex Cryptococcus (Remel) Crypto-LA (Wampole Laboratories) Cryptococcal antigen lateral-flow assay (Immuno-Mycologics)	Serum CSF	Any positive titer	Cryptococcus spp	Trichosporon spp Starch Disinfectants Soap Transport devices

[a] As recommended by the manufacturer.

[b] Fungi for which the test can be recommended for diagnostic use from currently available data.

[c] Cross-reactivity was described for various non-Aspergillus fungi including: Penicillium spp, Paecilomyces spp, Blastomyces dermatitidis, Histoplasma capsulatum, Paracoccidioidomyces brasiliensis, Fusarium spp, Geotrichum capitatum, Trichosporon dermatis, Cryptococcus spp, Bifidobacterium spp, Cladosporium spp, Acremonium spp, Alternaria spp, Wangiella dermatitidis, Rhodotorula rubra, Nigrospora oryzae, Trichothecium roseum, Prototheca spp.

[d] BG tests can detect most fungal species with the exception of all Mucormycotina (zygomycetes) and Cryptococcus spp.

studies over the years. Two meta-analyses including approximately 30 studies reported pooled sensitivity of 79% and specificity of 82% to 86% for the diagnosis of proven/probable IFI based on an index of 0.5 or greater as the positive test cutoff (**Table 4**).[53,54] Large heterogeneity of results related to the differences in patient populations and study designs was reported among these studies. Test performance was acceptable among patients with hematologic malignancies, but it appeared to be lower in the few studies reporting data from solid-organ transplant recipients (see **Table 4**). Data on the pediatric population are scarce, with lower specificity reported among children in some studies,[54,55] although the test also gained FDA clearance for use in this setting[56,57] (Package insert: Platelia *Aspergillus* EIA, Bio-Rad, Redmond, WA, 6/2003). Because *A fumigatus* was the major cause of IA in these studies, the

Table 4
Performance of nonmolecular diagnostic tests for the diagnosis of fungal infections in meta-analyses

Reference	Cutoff	Population	Pooled Sensitivity (%) (95% CI)	Pooled Specificity (%) (95% CI)
GM in Serum for IA (Proven/Probable)				
Pfeiffer et al,[54] 2006	ODI 0.5–1.5	All	61 (59–63)	93 (92–94)
	ODI 0.5–1.5	HM	58 (52–64)	95 (94–96)
	ODI 0.5–1.5	SOT	41 (21–64)	85 (80–89)
Leeflang et al,[53] 2008	ODI ≥0.5	All	78 (61–89)	81 (72–88)
	ODI ≥1	All	75 (59–86)	91 (84–95)
GM in BAL for IA (Proven/Probable)				
Guo et al,[59] 2010	ODI ≥0.5	All	86 (70–94)	89 (85–92)
	ODI ≥1	All	85 (72–93)	94 (89–97)
Zou et al,[60] 2012	ODI ≥0.5	All	87 (79–92)	89 (85–92)
	ODI ≥1	All	86 (76–92)	95 (91–97)
BG in Serum for Invasive Fungal Infections (Proven/Probable)[a]				
Karageorgopoulos et al,[72] 2011	Variable[b]	All	77 (67–84)	85 (80–90)
Lamoth et al,[71] 2012	Recommended[c] Single test	HM	62 (48–73)	91 (83–95)
	Recommended[c] Two consecutive tests	HM	50 (34–65)	99 (97–100)
Onishi et al,[73] 2012	Variable[b]	All	80 (77–82)	82 (81–83)
Lu et al,[139] 2011	Variable[b]	All	76 (67–83)	85 (73–92)
BG in Serum for *Pneumocystis jirovecii* Pneumonia				
Karageorgopoulos et al,[103] 2013	Variable[b]	All	95 (91–97)	86 (82–90)
Onishi et al,[73] 2012	Variable[b]	All	96 (92–98)	84 (83–86)

Abbreviations: HM, hematologic malignancies; ODI, optical density index; SOT, solid-organ transplant recipients.
   [a] Values are reported for all invasive fungal infections (consisting mainly of IA and candidiasis), *Pneumocystis jirovecii* infections and cryptococcosis being excluded. No significant differences were found in separate analyses of IA and candidiasis.
   [b] BG cutoffs associated with the optimal diagnostic accuracy for each individual study were reported (including cutoffs different from those recommended by the manufacturer).
   [c] Recommended BG cutoffs (according to the manufacturers): 60–80 pg/mL (Fungitell), 11 pg/mL (Wako and Maruha), and 20 pg/mL (Fungitec-G).

performance of the test for *Aspergillus* spp other than *A fumigatus* is not known, and some reports have suggested that reactivity might differ between species.[44,58]

Overall, serum GM testing can be recommended in adult and pediatric patients undergoing intensive myeloablative chemotherapy or allogeneic hematopoietic stem cell transplantation (HSCT) for hematologic malignancies. A screening strategy with GM monitoring in serum on a weekly or biweekly basis is supported by the potential of the GM test to detect IA early in these high-risk patients.[19] Diagnosis of IA based on GM detection in serum usually precedes diagnosis by radiologic criteria and start of antifungal therapy by several days.[29,30,32,33] The usefulness of the serum GM assay in other groups at risk (especially patients who do not have cancer or nonneutropenic patients) is controversial and cannot be supported as a routine test from the current data.

Recently, the use of the GM test in BAL fluid for the diagnosis of IA has raised considerable interest. Results of about 30 case control or cohort studies have been summarized in 2 meta-analyses and showed a good diagnostic accuracy with better sensitivity compared with serum GM testing among studies in which the tests were performed in parallel (see **Table 4**).[59,60] In BAL the test also showed a high sensitivity among patients who have nonhematologic cancer (solid-organ transplant recipients, chronic obstructive pulmonary disease, patients in the intensive care unit [ICU]),[61–66] whereas the sensitivity of the test in serum was particularly low in this subgroup. These differences may be explained by a lower degree of angioinvasion in these patients who are still capable of having a local inflammatory reaction confining the disease to the lung. However, a lower specificity was observed for the test in BAL of lung transplant recipients, who often have *Aspergillus* colonization of the respiratory tree, thereby limiting the usefulness of BAL GM testing in surveillance bronchoscopic examinations from these patients. The GM test was also compared with molecular methods (*Aspergillus*-specific PCR) in BAL in several studies and showed a similar performance.[60,67] Combining both PCR and GM testing in BAL resulted in a significant increase of sensitivity without loss of specificity (about 97% sensitivity and specificity for IA defined as either positive PCR or GM in BAL).[67] Some controversial results have been reported about the optimal cutoff of the GM test in BAL. Results of meta-analyses and most relevant individual studies suggest that a higher index cutoff (1 instead of 0.5) results in the best diagnostic accuracy.[60,67–69]

BG assay

The first assay for the detection of BG, a major component of the cell wall of many fungal species, was a chromogenic test developed in Japan, in which BG activated the coagulation cascade of the amebocyte lysate of the horseshoe crab *Tachypleus tridentatus* via factor G.[70] As mentioned earlier, there are 4 commercial tests for BG detection in serum, which differ in the method of detection (colorimetric or turbidimetric) or the reaction substrate (derived from 2 different species of horseshoe crabs, *Limulus polyphemus* and *Tachypleus tridentatus*), which result in different cutoffs of positivity. The overall performance of these tests seems to be similar.[71] The BG assay is not specific for the diagnosis of IA and can detect most pathogenic molds and yeasts, with the important exceptions of mucormycosis and cryptococcosis. The performance of the BG assay for the diagnosis of IFI in serum has been evaluated in numerous studies, which used different methodological approaches and patient populations. Although most studies included patients with both IA and invasive candidiasis, separate analyses provided a similar diagnostic accuracy for both diseases.[71–73] Two meta-analyses, including 16 to 31 studies, reported a moderate overall diagnostic accuracy, with a sensitivity of about 75% to 80% and a specificity of 80% to 85% (see **Table 4**).[72,73] Another meta-analysis restricted to cohort studies in patients with hematologic malignancies showed a lower sensitivity.[71] With the requirement of 2 consecutive positive tests, the specificity approached 100%, whereas sensitivity remained low (about 50%). However, a recent single-center study restricted to patients who have hematologic cancer and not included in this meta-analysis found a low specificity, even with 2 consecutive positive tests.[74]

The cutoff of positivity for the tests is also debated. ROC curve analyses suggest that the optimal cutoff values may be lower than those recommended by the manufacturers (5–7 pg/mL instead of 11 pg/mL for the Wako and Maruha assay, and 60 pg/mL instead of 80 pg/mL for the Fungitell test).[71]

Few studies have assessed the usefulness of the BG test in patients who do not have cancer. The specificity was found to be particularly low in lung transplant recipients; 92% (54/59) of patients not diagnosed with IFI had BG levels of 60 pg/mL or greater.[75] A low specificity of the BG assay for the diagnosis of IA was also reported among ICU patients.[76] Renal replacement therapy, blood transfusions or blood-derived products, concomitant bacterial infection, and β-lactam antibiotics have been implicated as possible causes of false-positive results (see **Table 3**).[74,75,77,78] The performance of the BG assay in samples other than serum (eg, BAL) has not been investigated. The effect of antifungal drug exposure at time of BG testing was assessed in 1 study and did not seem to affect the performance of the test.[79] Based on these data, the use of the BG test should be restricted to patients who have hematologic cancer, and, even in this setting, its role remains controversial, because of the relatively low sensitivity and contradictory results regarding the specificity.

Aspergillus lateral-flow devices

New technologies based on the incorporation of immune-chromatographic assays into lateral-flow devices (LFDs) have recently been used for the development of a specific and rapid test for detection of *Aspergillus* spp in serum and BAL.[80] This test uses a murine monoclonal antibody (JF5) binding to a glycoprotein antigen and is highly specific to *Aspergillus* spp, without cross-reaction with other fungal species. In animal models, this test showed good performance for the early detection of IA (3–7 days after infection) and good interlaboratory reproducibility.[81,82] There have been few studies reporting the clinical performance of the *Aspergillus* LFD test. In a study limited to HSCT recipients, the LFD had a performance comparable with GM, but sensitivity was low (40%) for both tests among the few IFI cases (1 proven and 9 probable IFI).[83] Promising results were also obtained in a small series of BAL testing.[84]

Another LFD immunochromatographic assay has been designed to detect GM in urine samples using an IgM monoclonal antibody (MAb476).[85] The convenience of these easy and rapid tests providing results in about 15 minutes deserves further investigation.

Anti-Aspergillus antibodies

Detection of specific anti-*Aspergillus* antibodies, identifying no more than one-third of cases, is not considered useful for the diagnosis of IA.[55,86] Historically, this situation was believed to be because IA usually occurs in patients who have hematologic cancer with profound leukopenia and are not able to mount an effective antibody response. However, the clinical spectrum of IA has changed over the last years, with an increasing proportion of nonneutropenic patients, including HSCT recipients in the immune reconstitution phase and patients who do not have cancer.[20,21] This situation has led to a renewed interest in antibody detection for the diagnosis of IA, with some results suggesting that detection of anti-*Aspergillus* antibodies before HSCT might be predictive of the development of IA during the postengraftment phase.[87,88] This approach needs further investigation and suffers from lack of standardization, as a result of different methods used for antibody detection (immunoelectrophoresis, immunodiffusion, complement fixation, hemagglutination, indirect immunofluorescence, radioimmunoassay, ELISA) and different in-house batches of antigens for detection.

Chronic Pulmonary Aspergillosis

This entity includes a large spectrum of pulmonary *Aspergillus* infections with various clinical presentations (aspergilloma, chronic necrotizing aspergillosis) occurring in otherwise immunocompetent patients with underlying pulmonary disease (eg, cavitary tuberculosis, chronic obstructive pulmonary disease, cystic fibrosis, pulmonary fibrosis).[8] The diagnosis of chronic pulmonary aspergillosis CPA is difficult and usually relies on the detection of precipitating antibody (IgG) against *Aspergillus*, along with consistent radiologic findings and clinical signs of chronic pulmonary infection.[89] Increased total and *Aspergillus*-specific IgE levels may be present.[89] Because of the physiopathology of the disease, which is localized to the lungs with no or minimal angioinvasion, detection of serum fungal markers is not helpful.[90,91] One study suggested that the GM test in BAL samples can be of some usefulness, with a sensitivity and specificity of 77%,[90] and deserves further investigation.

Pneumonia Caused by Non-Aspergillus Molds

Mucormycosis represents the second most common cause of fungal pneumonia, accounting for approximately 10% of all IFI in immunocompromised patients and resulting in significant morbidity and mortality.[4,92] Patients with hematologic malignancies have the highest risk of mucormycosis, but uncontrolled diabetes mellitus and iron overload (after therapy with iron chelators) are important predisposing factors defining additional populations at significant risk.[92] *Rhizopus* spp, *Mucor* spp, and *Absidia* (*Lichtheimia*) spp account for most cases, followed by *Rhizomucor* spp, *Cunninghamella* spp and *Apophysomyces* spp.[92] These molds, which are members of the subphylum Mucormycotina, do not contain GM or a significant amount of BG in their cell wall. Thus, neither the BG nor the GM assays are able to diagnose them.

Although the GM assay is specifically designed for the detection of *Aspergillus* spp, cross-reactivity with some non-*Aspergillus* molds such as *Fusarium* spp, the third most common cause of invasive pulmonary mold infections, has been reported.[44,51,93] However, detection of GM has not been systematically studied for the diagnosis of these non-*Aspergillus* invasive mold infections. Results of 1 small series and isolated cases from large cohort studies have suggested that the BG test may also be useful for the early detection of some of these less common molds.[94-96] Again, further study is required to confirm.

Pneumocystis jirovecii Pneumonia

Pneumocystis jirovecii pneumonia (PJP) is one of the most frequent opportunistic infections among patients with HIV, with a mortality of about 10% to 20%.[97] Although its incidence has decreased in this population with the use of highly active antiretroviral therapy and prophylaxis, an increasing number of cases are reported among patients who do not have HIV with other causes of immunosuppression, such as hematologic malignancies, solid-organ transplantation, solid tumors, connective tissue diseases, and underlying lung diseases.[98,99] Dry cough is a hallmark of the disease, and the diagnosis usually requires induced sputum or bronchoscopy for BAL fluid, which may not be feasible in patients with deep immunosuppression or severe underlying conditions. Detection of markers of the disease in serum thus represents an attractive alternative strategy.

In 2003, measurement of plasma S-adenosylmethionine concentrations was proposed as a diagnostic tool of PJP.[100] Because P jirovecii is not able to synthesize this essential metabolic intermediate, plasma S-adenosylmethionine from the host serves as an exogenous source for the pathogen and accordingly is depleted during PJP infection. Although this approach provided interesting results in patients with HIV,[100,101] it was not able to discriminate infected versus noninfected patients in populations who did not have HIV.[102]

Because BG is a major component of the cyst wall of P jirovecii, it has recently been investigated as a marker of the disease. The use of the BG assay for the diagnosis of PJP is supported by many studies, with pooled sensitivity and specificity of about 95% and 85%, respectively (see **Table 4**).[73,103] Performance seems similar between patients who have HIV and those who do not have HIV. The high sensitivity is an important result, because it implies that a negative BG test is sufficient to reasonably exclude PJP in patients with a low or moderate pretest probability. The interpretation of a positive test should be more cautious, considering the possible cause of false-positive results (as discussed earlier) and particularly, the possibility of a concomitant alternative IFI in these similarly at-risk populations.

Pulmonary Cryptococcosis

The encapsulated yeast, Cryptococcus neoformans, is the major cause of cryptococcosis, followed in some parts of the world by Cryptococcus gattii.[104] C neoformans is a leading opportunistic pathogen in patients with HIV and represents the third most common cause of IFIs in solid-organ transplant recipients.[5,104,105] Although meningitis is the most common presentation, the infection is primarily acquired by inhalation. Respiratory symptoms are often present and underdiagnosed and can be predominant in cases in which the infection is confined to the lungs, especially in patients who do not have HIV or patients with mild immunosuppression.[106,107] The outbreak of C gattii occurring over the last decade in North America is associated with predominantly pulmonary disease rather than meningitis and affects immunocompetent as well as immunocompromised individuals.[108]

The diagnosis of pulmonary cryptococcosis is particularly difficult, because of the paucity and nonspecificity of clinical signs and symptoms. Isolation of the fungus from respiratory specimens often requires invasive procedures and may provide false-negative results.[107,109] Serologic testing for antibodies against the polysaccharide capsule shows that asymptomatic or mild past cryptococcal infection is frequent (even during early childhood) and is thus not useful for diagnosis of acute cryptococcosis.[110]

Detection of the polysaccharide capsule antigen can be performed in serum and CSF by LA or EIA. Various kits are commercially available and showed similar performance, with high concordance values (>90%).[111,112] The performance of the cryptococcal antigen test was evaluated in various clinical subsets (disseminated cryptococcosis, cryptococcal meningitis, and pulmonary cryptococcosis) via a systematic review including 7 studies performed between 2001 and 2008.[19] Specificity is high (93%–100%), but rare false-positive reactions may occur in patients with malignancies or rheumatoid diseases, as well as cross-reactions with other yeasts (Trichosporon spp).[46,113,114] The sensitivity of the test in serum is higher among patients with HIV with disseminated disease compared with patients who do not have HIV, who are less likely to have disseminated infection (95% vs 77%); subgroup analysis restricted to patients with pulmonary disease showed a lower sensitivity (approximately 60%).[115] In another study, the overall sensitivity of the serum antigen test for the diagnosis of pulmonary cryptococcosis among solid-organ transplant recipients was 83%, but decreased to 73% in the absence of extrapulmonary infection.[116] Thus, a negative result in serum should be interpreted cautiously and does not exclude the disease, especially in patients with infection limited to the lungs. Cryptococcal antigen testing can be performed in BAL, but few data support its use in this setting, as a result of a lack of specificity because colonization of the lungs may occur.[117,118] A lateral-flow assay (LFA, Immuno-Mycologics, OK, USA) for the rapid detection of the cryptococcal antigen in serum, CSF, and urine was cleared by the FDA in 2011 and showed a high level of agreement with the EIA among patients with HIV in Thailand and Africa.[119,120] Similar performance was found among patients who do not have HIV.[121]

TREATMENT

Although the performance of nonmolecular fungal markers for the diagnosis of IFI has been evaluated in multiple analyses, few studies have focused on their role in triggering therapeutic decisions. Overall, it is estimated that the GM and BG test anticipate the diagnosis of IFI by approximately 1 week (2–10 days) compared with conventional clinical, radiologic, and microbiological criteria,[29,30,32,33,122] which supports their usefulness as screening tests for the early initiation of antifungal therapy in high-risk patients. Recent data have also suggested that GM or BG levels in serum may be predictive of IFI outcome and thus may be useful in assessing the response to therapy and guiding adjustments of antifungal treatment. Some single studies and 1 systematic review showed a strong correlation between the kinetics of GM indexes and survival outcomes of IA.[123–126] The initial value of GM at diagnosis was also found to be predictive of outcome.[123,124] Some studies have supported the use of the BG test as a surrogate marker for response to therapy in invasive candidiasis, but BG decline seems to become evident relatively late in the course of the disease (>7–14 days).[127–130] Data of the utility of BG in the follow-up of IA or PJP are scarce and not conclusive.[122,128] Monitoring the cryptococcal antigen titer is not useful in determining response to therapy in patients with HIV.[131–133] A small series[134] showed declining titers in patients who do not have HIV presenting mainly with pulmonary involvement, but the study did not allow definitive conclusions.

DISCUSSION/SUMMARY

Non–culture-based diagnostic tools represent an attractive alternative approach for the diagnosis of fungal pneumonia. Because these infections are life threatening and have a low prevalence, a valuable diagnostic test should be both highly sensitive and specific. Although the cryptococcal antigen has been admitted as a conventional test in the diagnostic workup of cryptococcosis, the role of the GM and BG tests for diagnosis of IFIs is still controversial. Many studies have reported data on sensitivity and specificity of these tests in various patient populations. Reviewing this abundant literature leads to the first conclusions that none of them has an optimal diagnostic accuracy and that heterogeneity of results is a hallmark of the systematic reviews and meta-analyses on this topic. These discrepancies can be easily related to important differences inherent to the study designs, including the type of analysis (retrospective case control vs prospective cohort studies), the type of population (neutropenic patients who have cancer vs nonneutropenic patients who have cancer), the reference standard of IFI (inclusion or not of possible and probable IFI cases according to EORTC-MSG criteria), the strategy of testing (serial monitoring vs punctual testing based on clinical suspicion), and the epidemiologic context (prevalence of fungal infections and distribution of their causative agents). Subanalyses of selected groups of patients show, not surprisingly, that antigen detection in serum is more sensitive in more immunosuppressed populations with a high risk of disseminated disease than in patients still capable of an effective immune response. This finding highlights the important fact that fungal infections are not a well-defined entity but a spectrum of diseases, in which the host immune status is a major determinant.

As outlined by the EORTC-MSG consensus group, the diagnosis of IFI still relies on a constellation of factors defining the presence of the disease on a scale of probability.[17] Serologic fungal markers are pieces of the puzzle and need to be interpreted in conjunction with other hints of the disease. Most of the studies have assessed the single value of these tests for the diagnosis of IFI, providing raw data of performance irrespective of these concomitant factors. Few analyses addressed the question of their usefulness when used in combination with radiologic or other microbiological tools in a defined algorithm for therapeutic decisions. Some studies compared a preemptive strategy based on GM detection and suggestive radiologic findings versus empirical antifungal therapy.[135–137] As expected, the use of antifungal drugs was decreased with a preemptive approach, but there was a concern about undetected IFI cases (especially non-*Aspergillus* IFI) and an increased incidence of IFI, although this had no impact on mortality. As discussed by Marr and colleagues[138] in an editorial comment, the prevalence of disease in a defined population and its pretest probability are crucial elements in the decision to start antifungal therapy, because these parameters define the positive and negative predictive values of a test with a given sensitivity and specificity. From this point of view, to decide which patients will be started on preemptive antifungal therapy, systematically monitoring for GM or BG antigenemia can be considered in the homogenous population of patients who have hematologic cancer in which the prevalence of disease is relatively high (about 10%) and the specificity of the test is high (especially for 2 consecutive tests). However, punctual testing driven by a clinical suspicion of IFI is less useful, because a negative result is not sufficient to exclude the disease (relatively low sensitivity for a high pretest probability) and should not affect the decision to treat the patient. Following the same argument, these tests have a limited value in patients who do not have cancer or solid-organ transplant patients, in whom the prevalence of IFI is lower and both sensitivity and specificity are not optimal. In this case, unless there is a high pretest probability of IFI based on clinical or radiologic findings, a positive test is more likely to result in useless antifungal treatment, whereas a negative test is not interpretable.

Increasing interest has been focused on the use of fungal markers in BAL instead of serum with the GM assay, showing a relatively high diagnostic accuracy in certain populations. However, testing in BAL still requires an invasive procedure, which is usually performed at the stage of relatively advanced disease, when the diagnosis of IA is already supported by radiologic findings of lung lesions. The test may be useful to confirm the diagnosis or to turn it toward other causes of pneumonia, but it cannot exclude a fungal infection caused by non-*Aspergillus* molds and it cannot differentiate *Aspergillus* colonization from invasive disease.

Several other issues or unsolved questions need to be addressed in the future. Nonmolecular fungal markers are particularly attractive as a noninvasive diagnostic tool with the ability to anticipate the diagnosis of IFI compared with other microbiological or radiologic criteria. From this perspective, the impact of BG or GM monitoring on the timing of diagnosis and the start of antifungal therapy has been rarely considered in previous performance analyses.[30,71] The cost-effectiveness of such monitoring strategies should be evaluated, because the tests are time consuming and labor intensive for the laboratory to perform.

Fungal pneumonias represent a large and heterogeneous group of diseases, with different pathogenic processes and clinical features. Characteristics of the fungal pathogen as well as of the host immunity contribute to defining them within a continuous spectrum of infection, ranging from transient colonization to invasive infection and from disease localized to lung to disseminated infection. It seems unreasonable to expect 1 single test to be sensitive and specific enough to define the spectrum. Future studies on this topic should include nonmolecular fungal markers as part of a global diagnostic approach and assessment of their impact on the timing of diagnosis and therapeutic decisions as well as on clinical outcomes in comparative interventional trials.

REFERENCES

1. Restrepo MI, Faverio P, Anzueto A. Long-term prognosis in community-acquired pneumonia. Curr Opin Infect Dis 2013;26(2):151–8.
2. American Thoracic Society, Infectious Diseases Society of America. Guidelines for the management of adults with hospital-acquired, ventilator-associated, and healthcare-associated pneumonia. Am J Respir Crit Care Med 2005;171(4):388–416.
3. Echols RM, Tillotson GS, Song JX, et al. Clinical trial design for mild-to-moderate community-acquired pneumonia–an industry perspective. Clin Infect Dis 2008;47(Suppl 3):S166–75.
4. Kontoyiannis DP, Marr KA, Park BJ, et al. Prospective surveillance for invasive fungal infections in hematopoietic stem cell transplant recipients, 2001-2006: overview of the Transplant-Associated Infection Surveillance Network (TRANSNET) Database. Clin Infect Dis 2010;50(8):1091–100.
5. Pappas PG, Alexander BD, Andes DR, et al. Invasive fungal infections among organ transplant recipients: results of the Transplant-Associated Infection Surveillance Network (TRANSNET). Clin Infect Dis 2010;50(8):1101–11.
6. Nucci M, Marr KA. Emerging fungal diseases. Clin Infect Dis 2005;41(4):521–6.
7. Park BJ, Pappas PG, Wannemuehler KA, et al. Invasive non-*Aspergillus* mold infections in transplant recipients, United States, 2001-2006. Emerg Infect Dis 2011;17(10):1855–64.
8. Denning DW. Chronic forms of pulmonary aspergillosis. Clin Microbiol Infect 2001;7(Suppl 2):25–31.
9. Greene RE, Schlamm HT, Oestmann JW, et al. Imaging findings in acute invasive pulmonary aspergillosis: clinical significance of the halo sign. Clin Infect Dis 2007;44(3):373–9.
10. Fernandez-Ruiz M, Silva JT, San-Juan R, et al. *Aspergillus* tracheobronchitis: report of 8 cases and review of the literature. Medicine (Baltimore) 2012;91(5):261–73.
11. Paterson DL. New clinical presentations of invasive aspergillosis in non-conventional hosts. Clin Microbiol Infect 2004;10(Suppl 1):24–30.
12. Roden MM, Zaoutis TE, Buchanan WL, et al. Epidemiology and outcome of zygomycosis: a review of 929 reported cases. Clin Infect Dis 2005;41(5):634–53.
13. Lamoth F, Rubino I, Bochud PY. Immunogenetics of invasive aspergillosis. Med Mycol 2011;49(Suppl 1):S125–36.
14. Neofytos D, Fishman JA, Horn D, et al. Epidemiology and outcome of invasive fungal infections in solid organ transplant recipients. Transpl Infect Dis 2010;12(3):220–9.

15. Neofytos D, Horn D, Anaissie E, et al. Epidemiology and outcome of invasive fungal infection in adult hematopoietic stem cell transplant recipients: analysis of Multicenter Prospective Antifungal Therapy (PATH) Alliance registry. Clin Infect Dis 2009;48(3):265–73.

16. Ascioglu S, Rex JH, de Pauw B, et al. Defining opportunistic invasive fungal infections in immunocompromised patients with cancer and hematopoietic stem cell transplants: an international consensus. Clin Infect Dis 2002;34(1):7–14.

17. De Pauw B, Walsh TJ, Donnelly JP, et al. Revised definitions of invasive fungal disease from the European Organization for Research and Treatment of Cancer/ Invasive Fungal Infections Cooperative Group and the National Institute of Allergy and Infectious Diseases Mycoses Study Group (EORTC/MSG) Consensus Group. Clin Infect Dis 2008;46(12):1813–21.

18. Mengoli C, Cruciani M, Barnes RA, et al. Use of PCR for diagnosis of invasive aspergillosis: systematic review and meta-analysis. Lancet Infect Dis 2009; 9(2):89–96.

19. Marchetti O, Lamoth F, Mikulska M, et al. ECIL recommendations for the use of biological markers for the diagnosis of invasive fungal diseases in leukemic patients and hematopoietic SCT recipients. Bone Marrow Transplant 2012;47(6): 846–54.

20. Cornillet A, Camus C, Nimubona S, et al. Comparison of epidemiological, clinical, and biological features of invasive aspergillosis in neutropenic and nonneutropenic patients: a 6-year survey. Clin Infect Dis 2006;43(5):577–84.

21. Meersseman W, Vandecasteele SJ, Wilmer A, et al. Invasive aspergillosis in critically ill patients without malignancy. Am J Respir Crit Care Med 2004;170(6): 621–5.

22. de Repentigny L, Boushira M, Ste-Marie L, et al. Detection of galactomannan antigenemia by enzyme immunoassay in experimental invasive aspergillosis. J Clin Microbiol 1987;25(5):863–7.

23. Dupont B, Huber M, Kim SJ, et al. Galactomannan antigenemia and antigenuria in aspergillosis: studies in patients and experimentally infected rabbits. J Infect Dis 1987;155(1):1–11.

24. Reiss E, Lehmann PF. Galactomannan antigenemia in invasive aspergillosis. Infect Immun 1979;25(1):357–65.

25. Machetti M, Feasi M, Mordini N, et al. Comparison of an enzyme immunoassay and a latex agglutination system for the diagnosis of invasive aspergillosis in bone marrow transplant recipients. Bone Marrow Transplant 1998; 21(9):917–21.

26. Stynen D, Sarfati J, Goris A, et al. Rat monoclonal antibodies against Aspergillus galactomannan. Infect Immun 1992;60(6):2237–45.

27. Verweij PE, Stynen D, Rijs AJ, et al. Sandwich enzyme-linked immunosorbent assay compared with Pastorex latex agglutination test for diagnosing invasive aspergillosis in immunocompromised patients. J Clin Microbiol 1995;33(7): 1912–4.

28. Stynen D, Goris A, Sarfati J, et al. A new sensitive sandwich enzyme-linked immunosorbent assay to detect galactofuran in patients with invasive aspergillosis. J Clin Microbiol 1995;33(2):497–500.

29. Kawazu M, Kanda Y, Nannya Y, et al. Prospective comparison of the diagnostic potential of real-time PCR, double-sandwich enzyme-linked immunosorbent assay for galactomannan, and a (1->3)-beta-D-glucan test in weekly screening for invasive aspergillosis in patients with hematological disorders. J Clin Microbiol 2004;42(6):2733–41.

30. Maertens JA, Klont R, Masson C, et al. Optimization of the cutoff value for the *Aspergillus* double-sandwich enzyme immunoassay. Clin Infect Dis 2007; 44(10):1329–36.

31. Marr KA, Balajee SA, McLaughlin L, et al. Detection of galactomannan antigenemia by enzyme immunoassay for the diagnosis of invasive aspergillosis: variables that affect performance. J Infect Dis 2004;190(3):641–9.

32. Maertens J, Theunissen K, Verbeken E, et al. Prospective clinical evaluation of lower cut-offs for galactomannan detection in adult neutropenic cancer patients and haematological stem cell transplant recipients. Br J Haematol 2004;126(6): 852–60.

33. Marr KA, Laverdiere M, Gugel A, et al. Antifungal therapy decreases sensitivity of the *Aspergillus* galactomannan enzyme immunoassay. Clin Infect Dis 2005; 40(12):1762–9.

34. Sulahian A, Touratier S, Ribaud P. False positive test for *Aspergillus* antigenemia related to concomitant administration of piperacillin and tazobactam. N Engl J Med 2003;349(24):2366–7.

35. Mikulska M, Furfaro E, Del Bono V, et al. Piperacillin/tazobactam (Tazocin) seems to be no longer responsible for false-positive results of the galactomannan assay. J Antimicrob Chemother 2012;67(7):1746–8.

36. Aubry A, Porcher R, Bottero J, et al. Occurrence and kinetics of false-positive *Aspergillus* galactomannan test results following treatment with beta-lactam antibiotics in patients with hematological disorders. J Clin Microbiol 2006;44(2): 389–94.

37. Martin-Rabadan P, Gijon P, Alonso Fernandez R, et al. False-positive *Aspergillus* antigenemia due to blood product conditioning fluids. Clin Infect Dis 2012;55(4): e22–7.

38. Guigue N, Menotti J, Ribaud P. False positive galactomannan test after ice-pop ingestion. N Engl J Med 2013;369(1):97–8.

39. Hage CA, Reynolds JM, Durkin M, et al. Plasmalyte as a cause of false-positive results for *Aspergillus* galactomannan in bronchoalveolar lavage fluid. J Clin Microbiol 2007;45(2):676–7.

40. Petraitiene R, Petraitis V, Witt JR 3rd, et al. Galactomannan antigenemia after infusion of gluconate-containing Plasma-Lyte. J Clin Microbiol 2011;49(12):4330–2.

41. Ansorg R, van den Boom R, Rath PM. Detection of *Aspergillus* galactomannan antigen in foods and antibiotics. Mycoses 1997;40(9–10):353–7.

42. Girmenia C, Santilli S, Ballaro D, et al. Enteral nutrition may cause false-positive results of *Aspergillus* galactomannan assay in absence of gastrointestinal diseases. Mycoses 2011;54(6):e883–4.

43. Murashige N, Kami M, Kishi Y, et al. False-positive results of *Aspergillus* enzyme-linked immunosorbent assays for a patient with gastrointestinal graft-versus-host disease taking a nutrient containing soybean protein. Clin Infect Dis 2005;40(2):333–4.

44. Cummings JR, Jamison GR, Boudreaux JW, et al. Cross-reactivity of non-*Aspergillus* fungal species in the *Aspergillus* galactomannan enzyme immunoassay. Diagn Microbiol Infect Dis 2007;59(1):113–5.

45. Dalle F, Charles PE, Blanc K, et al. *Cryptococcus neoformans* galactoxylomannan contains an epitope(s) that is cross-reactive with *Aspergillus* galactomannan. J Clin Microbiol 2005;43(6):2929–31.

46. Fekkar A, Brun S, D'Ussel M, et al. Serum cross-reactivity with *Aspergillus* galactomannan and cryptococcal antigen during fatal disseminated *Trichosporon dermatis* infection. Clin Infect Dis 2009;49(9):1457–8.

47. Giacchino M, Chiapello N, Bezzio S, et al. *Aspergillus* galactomannan enzyme-linked immunosorbent assay cross-reactivity caused by invasive *Geotrichum capitatum*. J Clin Microbiol 2006;44(9):3432–4.
48. Kappe R, Schulze-Berge A. New cause for false-positive results with the Pastorex *Aspergillus* antigen latex agglutination test. J Clin Microbiol 1993;31(9): 2489–90.
49. Mennink-Kersten MA, Ruegebrink D, Klont RR, et al. Bifidobacterial lipoglycan as a new cause for false-positive Platelia *Aspergillus* enzyme-linked immunosorbent assay reactivity. J Clin Microbiol 2005;43(8):3925–31.
50. Swanink CM, Meis JF, Rijs AJ, et al. Specificity of a sandwich enzyme-linked immunosorbent assay for detecting *Aspergillus* galactomannan. J Clin Microbiol 1997;35(1):257–60.
51. Tortorano AM, Esposto MC, Prigitano A, et al. Cross-reactivity of *Fusarium* spp. in the *Aspergillus* galactomannan enzyme-linked immunosorbent assay. J Clin Microbiol 2012;50(3):1051–3.
52. Wheat LJ, Hackett E, Durkin M, et al. Histoplasmosis-associated cross-reactivity in the BioRad Platelia *Aspergillus* enzyme immunoassay. Clin Vaccine Immunol 2007;14(5):638–40.
53. Leeflang MM, Debets-Ossenkopp YJ, Visser CE, et al. Galactomannan detection for invasive aspergillosis in immunocompromised patients. Cochrane Database Syst Rev 2008;(4):CD007394.
54. Pfeiffer CD, Fine JP, Safdar N. Diagnosis of invasive aspergillosis using a galactomannan assay: a meta-analysis. Clin Infect Dis 2006;42(10):1417–27.
55. Herbrecht R, Letscher-Bru V, Oprea C, et al. *Aspergillus* galactomannan detection in the diagnosis of invasive aspergillosis in cancer patients. J Clin Oncol 2002;20(7):1898–906.
56. Choi SH, Kang ES, Eo H, et al. *Aspergillus* galactomannan antigen assay and invasive aspergillosis in pediatric cancer patients and hematopoietic stem cell transplant recipients. Pediatr Blood Cancer 2013;60(2):316–22.
57. Steinbach WJ, Addison RM, McLaughlin L, et al. Prospective *Aspergillus* galactomannan antigen testing in pediatric hematopoietic stem cell transplant recipients. Pediatr Infect Dis J 2007;26(7):558–64.
58. Xavier MO, Araujo JS, Aquino VR, et al. Variability in Galactomannan detection by Platelia *Aspergillus* EIA according to the *Aspergillus* species. Rev Inst Med Trop Sao Paulo 2013;55(3). pii:S0036-46652013000300145.
59. Guo YL, Chen YQ, Wang K, et al. Accuracy of BAL galactomannan in diagnosing invasive aspergillosis: a bivariate metaanalysis and systematic review. Chest 2010;138(4):817–24.
60. Zou M, Tang L, Zhao S, et al. Systematic review and meta-analysis of detecting galactomannan in bronchoalveolar lavage fluid for diagnosing invasive aspergillosis. PLoS One 2012;7(8):e43347.
61. Clancy CJ, Jaber RA, Leather HL, et al. Bronchoalveolar lavage galactomannan in diagnosis of invasive pulmonary aspergillosis among solid-organ transplant recipients. J Clin Microbiol 2007;45(6):1759–65.
62. He H, Ding L, Sun B, et al. Role of galactomannan determinations in bronchoalveolar lavage fluid samples from critically ill patients with chronic obstructive pulmonary disease for the diagnosis of invasive pulmonary aspergillosis: a prospective study. Crit Care 2012;16(4):R138.
63. Luong ML, Clancy CJ, Vadnerkar A, et al. Comparison of an *Aspergillus* real-time polymerase chain reaction assay with galactomannan testing of bronchoalvelolar lavage fluid for the diagnosis of invasive pulmonary

aspergillosis in lung transplant recipients. Clin Infect Dis 2011;52(10): 1218–26.

64. Meersseman W, Lagrou K, Maertens J, et al. Galactomannan in bronchoalveolar lavage fluid: a tool for diagnosing aspergillosis in intensive care unit patients. Am J Respir Crit Care Med 2008;177(1):27–34.

65. Pasqualotto AC, Xavier MO, Sanchez LB, et al. Diagnosis of invasive aspergillosis in lung transplant recipients by detection of galactomannan in the bronchoalveolar lavage fluid. Transplantation 2010;90(3):306–11.

66. Zhang XB, Chen GP, Lin QC, et al. Bronchoalveolar lavage fluid galactomannan detection for diagnosis of invasive pulmonary aspergillosis in chronic obstructive pulmonary disease. Med Mycol 2013;51(7):688–95.

67. Avni T, Levy I, Sprecher H, et al. Diagnostic accuracy of PCR alone compared to galactomannan in bronchoalveolar lavage fluid for diagnosis of invasive pulmonary aspergillosis: a systematic review. J Clin Microbiol 2012;50(11):3652–8.

68. D'Haese J, Theunissen K, Vermeulen E, et al. Detection of galactomannan in bronchoalveolar lavage fluid samples of patients at risk for invasive pulmonary aspergillosis: analytical and clinical validity. J Clin Microbiol 2012;50(4): 1258–63.

69. Maertens J, Maertens V, Theunissen K, et al. Bronchoalveolar lavage fluid galactomannan for the diagnosis of invasive pulmonary aspergillosis in patients with hematologic diseases. Clin Infect Dis 2009;49(11):1688–93.

70. Obayashi T, Tamura H, Tanaka S, et al. A new chromogenic endotoxin-specific assay using recombind limulus coagulation enzymes and its clinical applications. Clin Chim Acta 1985;149(1):55–65.

71. Lamoth F, Cruciani M, Mengoli C, et al. β-Glucan antigenemia assay for the diagnosis of invasive fungal infections in patients with hematological malignancies: a systematic review and meta-analysis of cohort studies from the Third European Conference on Infections in Leukemia (ECIL-3). Clin Infect Dis 2012; 54(5):633–43.

72. Karageorgopoulos DE, Vouloumanou EK, Ntziora F, et al. β-D-glucan assay for the diagnosis of invasive fungal infections: a meta-analysis. Clin Infect Dis 2011; 52(6):750–70.

73. Onishi A, Sugiyama D, Kogata Y, et al. Diagnostic accuracy of serum 1,3-beta-D-glucan for Pneumocystis jiroveci pneumonia, invasive candidiasis, and invasive aspergillosis: systematic review and meta-analysis. J Clin Microbiol 2012; 50(1):7–15.

74. Racil Z, Kocmanova I, Lengerova M, et al. Difficulties in using 1,3-{beta}-D-glucan as the screening test for the early diagnosis of invasive fungal infections in patients with haematological malignancies–high frequency of false-positive results and their analysis. J Med Microbiol 2010;59(Pt 9):1016–22.

75. Alexander BD, Smith PB, Davis RD, et al. The (1,3){beta}-D-glucan test as an aid to early diagnosis of invasive fungal infections following lung transplantation. J Clin Microbiol 2010;48(11):4083–8.

76. Acosta J, Catalan M, del Palacio-Perez-Medel A, et al. A prospective comparison of galactomannan in bronchoalveolar lavage fluid for the diagnosis of pulmonary invasive aspergillosis in medical patients under intensive care: comparison with the diagnostic performance of galactomannan and of (1–> 3)-beta-d-glucan chromogenic assay in serum samples. Clin Microbiol Infect 2011; 17(7):1053–60.

77. Albert O, Toubas D, Strady C, et al. Reactivity of (1–>3)-beta-d-glucan assay in bacterial bloodstream infections. Eur J Clin Microbiol Infect Dis 2011;30(11):1453–60.

78. Mennink-Kersten MA, Warris A, Verweij PE. 1,3-beta-D-glucan in patients receiving intravenous amoxicillin-clavulanic acid. N Engl J Med 2006;354(26): 2834–5.
79. Koo S, Bryar JM, Page JH, et al. Diagnostic performance of the (1–>3)-beta-D-glucan assay for invasive fungal disease. Clin Infect Dis 2009;49(11): 1650–9.
80. Thornton CR. Development of an immunochromatographic lateral-flow device for rapid serodiagnosis of invasive aspergillosis. Clin Vaccine Immunol 2008; 15(7):1095–105.
81. Wiederhold NP, Najvar LK, Bocanegra R, et al. Interlaboratory and interstudy reproducibility of a novel lateral-flow device and influence of antifungal therapy on detection of invasive pulmonary aspergillosis. J Clin Microbiol 2013;51(2): 459–65.
82. Wiederhold NP, Thornton CR, Najvar LK, et al. Comparison of lateral flow technology and galactomannan and (1->3)-beta-D-glucan assays for detection of invasive pulmonary aspergillosis. Clin Vaccine Immunol 2009;16(12):1844–6.
83. Held J, Schmidt T, Thornton CR, et al. Comparison of a novel *Aspergillus* lateral-flow device and the Platelia galactomannan assay for the diagnosis of invasive aspergillosis following haematopoietic stem cell transplantation. Infection 2013; 41(6):1163–9.
84. Hoenigl M, Koidl C, Duettmann W, et al. Bronchoalveolar lavage lateral-flow device test for invasive pulmonary aspergillosis diagnosis in haematological malignancy and solid organ transplant patients. J Infect 2012;65(6):588–91.
85. Dufresne SF, Datta K, Li X, et al. Detection of urinary excreted fungal galactomannan-like antigens for diagnosis of invasive aspergillosis. PLoS One 2012;7(8):e42736.
86. Chan CM, Woo PC, Leung AS, et al. Detection of antibodies specific to an antigenic cell wall galactomannoprotein for serodiagnosis of *Aspergillus* fumigatus aspergillosis. J Clin Microbiol 2002;40(6):2041–5.
87. Du C, Wingard JR, Cheng S, et al. Serum IgG responses against *Aspergillus* proteins before hematopoietic stem cell transplantation or chemotherapy identify patients who develop invasive aspergillosis. Biol Blood Marrow Transplant 2012;18(12):1927–34.
88. Sarfati J, Monod M, Recco P, et al. Recombinant antigens as diagnostic markers for aspergillosis. Diagn Microbiol Infect Dis 2006;55(4):279–91.
89. Denning DW, Riniotis K, Dobrashian R, et al. Chronic cavitary and fibrosing pulmonary and pleural aspergillosis: case series, proposed nomenclature change, and review. Clin Infect Dis 2003;37(Suppl 3):S265–80.
90. Izumikawa K, Yamamoto Y, Mihara T, et al. Bronchoalveolar lavage galactomannan for the diagnosis of chronic pulmonary aspergillosis. Med Mycol 2012;50(8):811–7.
91. Kitasato Y, Tao Y, Hoshino T, et al. Comparison of *Aspergillus* galactomannan antigen testing with a new cut-off index and *Aspergillus* precipitating antibody testing for the diagnosis of chronic pulmonary aspergillosis. Respirology 2009;14(5):701–8.
92. Petrikkos G, Skiada A, Lortholary O, et al. Epidemiology and clinical manifestations of mucormycosis. Clin Infect Dis 2012;54(Suppl 1):S23–34.
93. Mikulska M, Furfaro E, Del Bono V, et al. Galactomannan testing might be useful for early diagnosis of fusariosis. Diagn Microbiol Infect Dis 2012;72(4):367–9.
94. Cuetara MS, Alhambra A, Moragues MD, et al. Detection of (1–>3)-beta-D-glucan as an adjunct to diagnosis in a mixed population with uncommon proven

invasive fungal diseases or with an unusual clinical presentation. Clin Vaccine Immunol 2009;16(3):423–6.

95. Odabasi Z, Mattiuzzi G, Estey E, et al. Beta-D-glucan as a diagnostic adjunct for invasive fungal infections: validation, cutoff development, and performance in patients with acute myelogenous leukemia and myelodysplastic syndrome. Clin Infect Dis 2004;39(2):199–205.

96. Ostrosky-Zeichner L, Alexander BD, Kett DH, et al. Multicenter clinical evaluation of the (1–>3) beta-D-glucan assay as an aid to diagnosis of fungal infections in humans. Clin Infect Dis 2005;41(5):654–9.

97. Thomas CF Jr, Limper AH. *Pneumocystis* pneumonia. N Engl J Med 2004; 350(24):2487–98.

98. Maini R, Henderson KL, Sheridan EA, et al. Increasing *Pneumocystis* pneumonia, England, UK, 2000-2010. Emerg Infect Dis 2013;19(3):386–92.

99. Reid AB, Chen SC, Worth LJ. *Pneumocystis jirovecii* pneumonia in non-HIV-infected patients: new risks and diagnostic tools. Curr Opin Infect Dis 2011; 24(6):534–44.

100. Skelly M, Hoffman J, Fabbri M, et al. S-adenosylmethionine concentrations in diagnosis of *Pneumocystis carinii* pneumonia. Lancet 2003;361(9365):1267–8.

101. Skelly MJ, Holzman RS, Merali S. S-adenosylmethionine levels in the diagnosis of *Pneumocystis carinii* pneumonia in patients with HIV infection. Clin Infect Dis 2008;46(3):467–71.

102. de Boer MG, Gelinck LB, van Zelst BD, et al. beta-D-glucan and S-adenosylmethionine serum levels for the diagnosis of *Pneumocystis* pneumonia in HIV-negative patients: a prospective study. J Infect 2011;62(1):93–100.

103. Karageorgopoulos DE, Qu JM, Korbila IP, et al. Accuracy of beta-D-glucan for the diagnosis of *Pneumocystis jirovecii* pneumonia: a meta-analysis. Clin Microbiol Infect 2013;19(1):39–49.

104. Chayakulkeeree M, Perfect JR. Cryptococcosis. Infect Dis Clin North Am 2006; 20(3):507–44, v–vi.

105. Singh N, Dromer F, Perfect JR, et al. Cryptococcosis in solid organ transplant recipients: current state of the science. Clin Infect Dis 2008;47(10):1321–7.

106. Shirley RM, Baddley JW. Cryptococcal lung disease. Curr Opin Pulm Med 2009; 15(3):254–60.

107. Vilchez RA, Irish W, Lacomis J, et al. The clinical epidemiology of pulmonary cryptococcosis in non-AIDS patients at a tertiary care medical center. Medicine (Baltimore) 2001;80(5):308–12.

108. Harris JR, Lockhart SR, Debess E, et al. *Cryptococcus gattii* in the United States: clinical aspects of infection with an emerging pathogen. Clin Infect Dis 2011;53(12):1188–95.

109. Meyohas MC, Roux P, Bollens D, et al. Pulmonary cryptococcosis: localized and disseminated infections in 27 patients with AIDS. Clin Infect Dis 1995;21(3):628–33.

110. Goldman DL, Khine H, Abadi J, et al. Serologic evidence for *Cryptococcus neoformans* infection in early childhood. Pediatrics 2001;107(5):E66.

111. Babady NE, Bestrom JE, Jespersen DJ, et al. Evaluation of three commercial latex agglutination kits and a commercial enzyme immunoassay for the detection of cryptococcal antigen. Med Mycol 2009;47(3):336–8.

112. Binnicker MJ, Jespersen DJ, Bestrom JE, et al. Comparison of four assays for the detection of cryptococcal antigen. Clin Vaccine Immunol 2012;19(12): 1988–90.

113. Campbell CK, Payne AL, Teall AJ, et al. Cryptococcal latex antigen test positive in patient with *Trichosporon beigelii* infection. Lancet 1985;2(8445):43–4.

114. McManus EJ, Jones JM. Detection of a *Trichosporon beigelii* antigen cross-reactive with *Cryptococcus neoformans* capsular polysaccharide in serum from a patient with disseminated *Trichosporon* infection. J Clin Microbiol 1985;21(5):681–5.

115. Pappas PG, Perfect JR, Cloud GA, et al. Cryptococcosis in human immunodeficiency virus-negative patients in the era of effective azole therapy. Clin Infect Dis 2001;33(5):690–9.

116. Singh N, Alexander BD, Lortholary O, et al. Pulmonary cryptococcosis in solid organ transplant recipients: clinical relevance of serum cryptococcal antigen. Clin Infect Dis 2008;46(2):e12–8.

117. Baughman RP, Rhodes JC, Dohn MN, et al. Detection of cryptococcal antigen in bronchoalveolar lavage fluid: a prospective study of diagnostic utility. Am Rev Respir Dis 1992;145(5):1226–9.

118. Kralovic SM, Rhodes JC. Utility of routine testing of bronchoalveolar lavage fluid for cryptococcal antigen. J Clin Microbiol 1998;36(10):3088–9.

119. Jarvis JN, Percival A, Bauman S, et al. Evaluation of a novel point-of-care cryptococcal antigen test on serum, plasma, and urine from patients with HIV-associated cryptococcal meningitis. Clin Infect Dis 2011;53(10):1019–23.

120. Lindsley MD, Mekha N, Baggett HC, et al. Evaluation of a newly developed lateral flow immunoassay for the diagnosis of cryptococcosis. Clin Infect Dis 2011;53(4):321–5.

121. McMullan BJ, Halliday C, Sorrell TC, et al. Clinical utility of the cryptococcal antigen lateral flow assay in a diagnostic mycology laboratory. PLoS One 2012; 7(11):e49541.

122. Senn L, Robinson JO, Schmidt S, et al. 1,3-Beta-D-glucan antigenemia for early diagnosis of invasive fungal infections in neutropenic patients with acute leukemia. Clin Infect Dis 2008;46(6):878–85.

123. Bergeron A, Porcher R, Menotti J, et al. Prospective evaluation of clinical and biological markers to predict the outcome of invasive pulmonary aspergillosis in hematological patients. J Clin Microbiol 2012;50(3):823–30.

124. Koo S, Bryar JM, Baden LR, et al. Prognostic features of galactomannan antigenemia in galactomannan-positive invasive aspergillosis. J Clin Microbiol 2010; 48(4):1255–60.

125. Miceli MH, Grazziutti ML, Woods G, et al. Strong correlation between serum *Aspergillus* galactomannan index and outcome of aspergillosis in patients with hematological cancer: clinical and research implications. Clin Infect Dis 2008;46(9):1412–22.

126. Woods G, Miceli MH, Grazziutti ML, et al. Serum *Aspergillus* galactomannan antigen values strongly correlate with outcome of invasive aspergillosis: a study of 56 patients with hematologic cancer. Cancer 2007;110(4):830–4.

127. Jaijakul S, Vazquez JA, Swanson RN, et al. (1,3)-beta-D-glucan as a prognostic marker of treatment response in invasive candidiasis. Clin Infect Dis 2012;55(4): 521–6.

128. Koo S, Baden LR, Marty FM. Post-diagnostic kinetics of the (1–> 3)-beta-D-glucan assay in invasive aspergillosis, invasive candidiasis and *Pneumocystis jirovecii* pneumonia. Clin Microbiol Infect 2012;18(5):E122–7.

129. Sims CR, Jaijakul S, Mohr J, et al. Correlation of clinical outcomes with beta-glucan levels in patients with invasive candidiasis. J Clin Microbiol 2012; 50(6):2104–6.

130. Tissot F, Lamoth F, Hauser PM, et al. Beta-glucan antigenemia anticipates diagnosis of blood culture-negative intra-abdominal candidiasis. Am J Respir Crit Care Med 2013;188(9):1100–9.

131. Aberg JA, Watson J, Segal M, et al. Clinical utility of monitoring serum crypto-coccal antigen (sCRAG) titers in patients with AIDS-related cryptococcal disease. HIV Clin Trials 2000;1(1):1–6.

132. Antinori S, Radice A, Galimberti L, et al. The role of cryptococcal antigen assay in diagnosis and monitoring of cryptococcal meningitis. J Clin Microbiol 2005; 43(11):5828–9.

133. Powderly WG, Cloud GA, Dismukes WE, et al. Measurement of cryptococcal antigen in serum and cerebrospinal fluid: value in the management of AIDS-associated cryptococcal meningitis. Clin Infect Dis 1994;18(5):789–92.

134. Lin TY, Yeh KM, Lin JC, et al. Cryptococcal disease in patients with or without human immunodeficiency virus: clinical presentation and monitoring of serum cryptococcal antigen titers. J Microbiol Immunol Infect 2009;42(3):220–6.

135. Cordonnier C, Pautas C, Maury S, et al. Empirical versus preemptive antifungal therapy for high-risk, febrile, neutropenic patients: a randomized, controlled trial. Clin Infect Dis 2009;48(8):1042–51.

136. Girmenia C, Micozzi A, Gentile G, et al. Clinically driven diagnostic antifungal approach in neutropenic patients: a prospective feasibility study. J Clin Oncol 2010;28(4):667–74.

137. Maertens J, Theunissen K, Verhoef G, et al. Galactomannan and computed tomography-based preemptive antifungal therapy in neutropenic patients at high risk for invasive fungal infection: a prospective feasibility study. Clin Infect Dis 2005;41(9):1242–50.

138. Marr KA, Leisenring W, Bow E. Empirical versus preemptive antifungal therapy for fever during neutropenia. Clin Infect Dis 2009;49(7):1138–9 [author reply 1139–40].

139. Lu Y, Chen YQ, Guo YL, et al. Diagnosis of invasive fungal disease using serum (1–>3)-beta-D-glucan: a bivariate meta-analysis. Intern Med 2011;50(22): 2783–91.

Interferon-Gamma Release Assays

Robert Belknap, MD[a],*, Charles L. Daley, MD[b]

KEYWORDS

- Latent tuberculosis infection • Interferon-gamma release assays • Tuberculosis
- Tuberculin skin test • QuantiFERON • T-SPOT

KEY POINTS

- Diagnosis of latent tuberculosis infection (LTBI) should be targeted toward individuals and groups with high risk of progression to active tuberculosis (TB). Low-risk populations should not be screened.
- Interferon-gamma release assays (IGRAs) perform as well or better than the tuberculin skin test (TST) in most targeted populations. IGRAs are preferred for bacille Calmette-Guérin (BCG)-vaccinated populations.
- A positive IGRA in a person at low risk for TB exposure should be confirmed with a repeat test or another method before recommending LTBI treatment.
- The choice of which IGRA to use is generally based on the costs and feasibility of performing the test.

INTRODUCTION

TB remains a major global health problem. Worldwide, there are an estimated 2 billion people infected with *Mycobacterium tuberculosis* and from this large reservoir approximately 8.6 million people develop TB each year.[1] A staggering 1.3 million people die from TB annually, including more than 300,000 with HIV infection. Although the rates of TB are declining at approximately 2% per year, HIV coinfection and the emergence of drug-resistant strains of *M tuberculosis* threaten to undermine global TB control.

Identification and treatment of LTBI can substantially reduce the risk of developing TB and is a major focus of TB control in the United States.[2] Identification of all persons with LTBI would require screening large numbers of low-risk individuals that would not be cost-effective and would result in many false-positive test results.[3] Instead, the Centers for Disease Control and Prevention (CDC) recommends targeted testing in order to identify persons with LTBI who are at greater risk of progressing to TB and who

[a] Denver Public Health Department, University of Colorado School of Medicine, 605 Bannock Street, Denver, CO 80204, USA; [b] National Jewish Health, University of Colorado School of Medicine, 1400 Jackson Street, Denver, CO 80206, USA
* Corresponding author.
E-mail address: robert.belknap@dhha.org

Clin Lab Med 34 (2014) 337–349
http://dx.doi.org/10.1016/j.cll.2014.02.007
0272-2712/14/$ – see front matter © 2014 Elsevier Inc. All rights reserved.

would benefit from treatment of LTBI.[2] Persons with increased risk for developing TB include those who have been recently infected with *M tuberculosis* and those who have medical conditions that are associated with an increased risk of developing TB.

For nearly a century, the TST has been used to identify persons with TB infection. The TST is performed by the intradermal injection of purified protein derivative (PPD) that contains more than 200 proteins.[4] With such a diverse collection of antigens, it is not surprising that the TST lacks sensitivity and specificity, resulting in false-positive and false-negative test results. The 2 most important causes of false-positive results are infection with nontuberculous mycobacteria (NTM) and prior BCG vaccination. IGRAs are in vitro blood tests that measure the production of interferon gamma after stimulation with more specific mycobacterial antigens.[5] Because these antigens are not contained within BCG strains or most NTM, they provide a more specific test than the TST. This review focuses on IGRAs and their strengths and limitations for screening for LTBI.

MICROBIOLOGY

The genus *Mycobacterium* consists of slow-growing organisms that are widely distributed throughout the world and range from organisms that cause no human disease to those like *M tuberculosis* and *M leprae* that cause enormous morbidity and mortality.[6] TB is caused by members of the *M tuberculosis* complex that includes the clinically relevant species *M tuberculosis*, *M bovis*, and *M africanum*. All members of the *M tuberculosis* complex, except BCG substrains, contain a region of the genome referred to as the deleted region 1 (RD1); this region distinguishes virulent strains of *M bovis* from all BCG strains and is thought to represent part of the original attenuation during 1908–1921.[7] Within RD1 are genes that encode for the antigens, early secreted antigenic target 6 (ESAT-6) and culture filtrate protein 10 (CFP-10); these antigens are more specific than PPD for *M tuberculosis* and are absent from all available strains of *M bovis* BCG.[8]

NTM refer to nonlepromatous organisms that are not members of the *M tuberculosis* complex.[6] NTM have been referred to as mycobacteria other than TB, atypical mycobacteria, and environmental mycobacteria. The latter designation refers to their widespread presence in the environment. NTM have several features that distinguish them from *M tuberculosis*. They have a wide range of pathogenicity, are not always associated with disease, and, unlike *M tuberculosis*, are not transmissible from human to human. Importantly, the incidence of NTM disease is increasing in many areas of the world, and the cause for this increase is unknown.[9] NTM share many antigens with *M tuberculosis* and thus can result in a false-positive TST result. Most strains of NTM, however, except *M marinum*, *M kansasii*, *M szulgai*, and *M flavescens*, do not encode for the antigens ESAT-6 and CFP-10, so they do not affect the results of IGRAs.[10]

EPIDEMIOLOGY

Understanding the epidemiology of TB is necessary to develop successful TB control interventions. As discussed previously, there were an estimated 8.6 million people who developed TB in 2012.[1] Twenty-two high-burden countries accounted for 81% of all estimated incident cases worldwide, with rates of approximately 150 to 300 cases per 100,000 population. In these high-burden countries, stopping transmission through TB case detection and treatment is the most important TB control intervention.

The prevalence of LTBI in the United States was estimated to be approximately 4.2% in 1999–2000; an estimated 11,213,000 individuals had LTBI.[11] Higher prevalence rates were noted in those who were foreign born (18.7%), non-Hispanic blacks (7.0%), Mexican Americans (9.4%), and individuals living in poverty (6.1%). This reservoir of infected persons was the source for most of the 9951 new TB cases in 2012, resulting in an incidence rate of 3.2 per 100,000 population[12]; this represents a 6.1% decline compared with 2011. Four states reported half of the total cases (California, Texas, New York, and Florida) but rates of TB were highest in Alaska (9.0/100,000) and Hawaii (8.4/100,000). In countries like the United States, where the number of active TB cases are relatively few, prevention of cases through identification and treatment of LTBI is paramount; developing effective targeted testing programs requires being able to identify individuals and populations with higher rates of disease.

One such population is those who are foreign born, who make up a disproportionate burden of TB cases in the United States. Foreign-born cases in the United States made up 63% of all cases with an incidence of 15.8 per 100,000 population.[12] In contrast, the rate of TB among US-born cases was only 1.4 per 100,000 population. More than half of the foreign-born cases originated from 5 countries: Mexico (20.9%), Philippines (8.5%), India (8.5%), Vietnam (7.2%), and China (5.6%).

Studies have shown that the risk of TB in those who are foreign born is substantially higher than that in US-born persons. This rate is highest in the first year likely due to prevalent TB at the time of immigration but remains elevated above the US-born rate for several years.[13,14] The highest rates are in immigrants and refugees from high-incidence countries (defined as ≥100 cases/100,000 population), students/exchange visitors and temporary workers from high-incidence countries, and immigrants and refugees from medium-incidence countries.[15] According to a recent study, the risk of reactivation among Filipino immigrants was 25 times higher than that of the 2012 TB rate among US-born persons and did not decline significantly over a 9-year period.[14] Molecular genotyping studies have documented that more than 80% of TB in those who are foreign born in the United States is due to reactivation of LTBI.[16] Therefore, targeted testing for LTBI among those who are foreign born is a major strategic component of TB control. The CDC currently recommends that foreign-born individuals from high-prevalence countries be tested for LTBI if they have been in the United States for less than 5 years. The studies, cited previously, however, as well as a cost-effective analysis argue for testing this population regardless of the amount of time in the United States.[17]

Persons who have been recently infected with *M tuberculosis* as well as certain medical conditions (**Table 1**) are at high risk of developing TB and, therefore, should be targeted for screening.[2] Recently infected persons, such as contacts to infectious TB cases and persons who have converted their TST (or IGRA) from negative to positive over the previous 2 years, have a high rate of progression to TB (discussed later). In a controlled clinical trial evaluating the efficacy of isoniazid treatment of LTBI among contacts to infectious cases, the rate of developing TB in the first year among converters in the placebo arm was 12.9 cases per 100,000 compared with 1.6 per 100,000 in the subsequent 7 years of the study.[18] More than half of the risk of developing TB is in the first 1 year after infection.[2]

CLINICAL PRESENTATION

TB represents a spectrum of disease ranging from LTBI, in which patients are asymptomatic, to active TB, where patients are symptomatic and infectious. LTBI is defined solely by evidence of sensitization to mycobacterial proteins in the absence of

Table 1
Medical conditions associated with high risk of progression to active TB

HIV infection	Injection drug use
Other immunosuppressive diseases	End-stage renal disease
Diabetes mellitus	Silicosis
Immunosuppressive drugs	Intestinal bypass
Hematologic/reticuloendothelial malignancies	Malabsorption
Postgastrectomy	<10% Below ideal body weight
Carcinomas of head and neck	Smoking (tobacco)

symptoms or signs of active TB.[19] In some instances, a chest radiograph may show the remnants of previous disease, such as calcified granulomas or apical pleural parenchymal fibrosis. By definition, however, there are no clinical symptoms or signs of TB disease and cultures, if obtained, are negative.

Once active TB develops, the clinical manifestations are protean and represent a balance between host defenses and bacterial virulence. Patterns of disease vary depending on whether the disease is primary or reactivation in nature, the host's immune status, and possibly the strain of M tuberculosis.[6] Most patients present with pulmonary disease. Primary infection may cause an inflammatory infiltrate in the lung that usually clears as cell-mediated immunity develops. If the parenchymal disease persists beyond the development of cell-mediated immunity, progressive primary disease occurs. During most initial infections with M tuberculosis, small numbers of organisms are disseminated hematogenously and some become seeded in the apices of the lung, which accounts for the characteristic radiographic location of reactivation disease in the apical or posterior segments of the upper lobes.[6] Fibrocaseous lesions may contain live mycobacteria for many years, and these are the lesions that may reactivate years later.

PATHOGENESIS

M tuberculosis is spread from person to person through the air by droplet nuclei—particles 1 to 5 μm in diameter that contain viable M tuberculosis.[6] Droplet nuclei are expelled into the air when patients with infectious TB create an aerosol by talking, coughing, or singing. The likelihood of transmitting the bacilli depends on the number of bacilli expelled into the air, the concentration of organisms in the air, and the length of time the contact breathes the infected air. Whether or not an inhaled tubercle bacillus establishes an infection in a contact's lung depends on both the bacterial virulence and the innate immune response of the host. If the bacillus survives the initial defenses, it can multiply within the alveolar macrophage and infection occurs.

Once cell-mediated immunity develops, collections of activated T cells and macrophages form granulomas that wall off the tubercle bacilli.[6,19,20] For most persons with normal immune function, infection with M tuberculosis is arrested once cell-mediated immunity develops, even though small numbers of viable bacilli remain within the granuloma. If cell-mediated immunity cannot contain infection, the person progresses to active disease. Untreated, approximately 10% of persons develop active TB, 5% within the first 1 to 2 years of infection and the rest over their lifetime.[6] Molecular epidemiology studies have shown that more than 80% of TB cases in the United States arise from reactivation of LTBI.[2,13] Persons who are coinfected with HIV have a 5% to 10% annual risk of developing active disease. Patients with low CD4 cell counts have increased susceptibility to TB and those with the lowest CD4 counts have the highest risk.[19] The CD4 T cell produces interferon-gamma, which is a key element in the adaptive immune response to TB. The measurement of this cytokine after stimulation of peripheral blood cells is also a key component of IGRAs.

Although the previous discussion dichotomizes TB into LTBI and active TB, in reality, there is likely a dynamic spectrum of disease in which there are several possible outcomes after exposure to an infectious patient[19,20]:

1. Infection may be eliminated through the innate immune system and without priming antigen-specific T cells.
2. Infection may be eliminated by T-cell priming through an acquired immune response.
3. Infection is controlled with some bacteria persisting in a nonreplicating quiescent state.
4. Bacterial replication occurs but at a subclinical level, as demonstrated during prevalence surveys.
5. Bacterial replication occurs and produces symptoms.

In setting 1, neither the TST nor the IGRA is positive and the person is not at risk of progressing to active TB. In setting 2, the TST and/or IGRA is positive but, again, the individual is not at risk of progressing to active TB. In the third setting, however, the TST and/or IGRA is positive and the person is at risk of developing active TB because viable bacteria are present. Ideally, a test would be able to distinguish persons in setting 2 from those in setting 3 because only the latter group would be at risk for developing TB. Unfortunately, neither the TST nor IGRAs are able to do so.

DIAGNOSIS

The TST had been the only test for diagnosing LTBI but has several well-described limitations. These include the need for 2 visits, subjective results, low sensitivity for active TB, and false-positive results due to prior BCG vaccination or NTM infection.[21] The IGRAs were developed to overcome many of these limitations. They require a single blood draw and assess the cell-mediated immune response by measuring interferon gamma produced after incubation with TB-specific antigens.

Interferon-Gamma Release Assays

Two commercially available tests are approved by the US Food and Drug Administration, QuantiFERON-TB Gold In-Tube (QFT-GIT) (Cellestis/Qiagen, Venlo, Limburg) and T-SPOT.*TB* (Oxford Immunotec, Abingdon, UK).[22,23] The antigens used for QFT-GIT and T-SPOT.*TB* have been selected from the RD1 portion of the TB genome, which is absent from BCG vaccine strains and most commonly occurring NTM, as discussed previously.

QFT-GIT and T-SPOT.*TB* have several similarities. Both assays use ESAT-6 and CFP-10 whereas QFT-GIT includes a third antigen, TB 7.7. Both IGRAs have internal controls, termed the nil and mitogen, in addition to the TB antigen stimulation. The nil determines the amount of interferon gamma detected after incubation without antigens. The result from the nil control is subtracted from the result after stimulation with the TB antigens to determine the interferon gamma that is attributable to TB. The mitogen control is used to confirm that an individual's cells are capable of responding to antigen stimulation and that the test was performed correctly. Phytohemagglutinin (PHA) is used as a nonspecific antigen stimulant and failure to respond appropriately suggests an inadequate number of functional effector T cells or an error in processing the blood or performing the test.

QFT-GIT and T-SPOT.*TB* differ in how the interferon-gamma response is measured. QFT-GIT uses an ELISA that measures interferon gamma produced in heparinized whole blood after stimulation. Blood is collected into 3 specialized tubes, approximately 1 mL in each of the nil, TB antigen, and mitogen tubes. The tubes must be shaken after collection to ensure the antigens dried on the inner surface of the TB and mitogen tubes are adequately mixed with the blood. They are then incubated for 16 to 24 hours at 37°C. After incubation, the tubes are centrifuged, plasma is extracted, and interferon gamma levels are measured using an ELISA. The results are measured in international units per milliliter and should be reported as both the quantitative values and qualitative interpretation of positive, negative, or indeterminate (**Table 2**).

T-SPOT.*TB* is based on an enzyme-linked immunospot (ELISPOT) method that determines the quantity of effector T cells responding to antigen stimulation. For most individuals, 8 mL of heparinized whole blood is adequate to supply enough cells. From the blood, peripheral blood mononuclear cells (PBMCs) are separated, washed, and counted. The PBMCs are then added into microtiter wells at a concentration of 250,000 ± 50,000 PBMCs per well. Each test uses 4 wells: a nil control, a mitogen-containing PHA, and 2 separate wells for ESAT-6 and CFP-10. The microtiter plates are then incubated at 37°C with 5% CO_2 for 16 to 20 hours. Interferon gamma secreted from the cells is captured by specific antibodies on the base of the wells. These appear as dark blue spots after the wells are washed and subjected to another conjugation step. The spot counts are used to determine if the test is positive, negative, borderline, or invalid (**Table 3**).

Test Performance of IGRAs

Precisely determining the sensitivity and specificity of the IGRAs is difficult due to lack of a gold standard for TB infection. As a result, the sensitivity has primarily been estimated using culture-proved TB as a surrogate for infection. Many studies have compared the IGRA results with the TST. In a meta-analysis of the commercially available IGRAs, the pooled sensitivity for active TB was 81% (95% CI, 0.78 to 0.83) for QFT-GIT and 88% (95% CI, 0.86 to 0.90) for T-SPOT.*TB* compared with 70% (95% CI, 0.67 to 0.72) for TST.[24] A separate analysis in low- and middle-income countries found similar results in HIV-uninfected individuals but a lower sensitivity for all 3 tests in HIV-infected persons.[25] The conclusion is that although the sensitivities are higher than the TST, they are not high enough to use the IGRAs to exclude active TB in someone with symptoms.

The specificity has been estimated using populations at low risk for TB exposure based on country of origin and epidemiologic history. These estimates have included

Table 2
Interpretation of QFT-GIT results

Nil (IU/mL)	TB Ag Minus Nil (IU/mL)	Mitogen Minus Nil (IU/mL)	Qualitative Result
≤8.0	<0.35	≥0.5	Negative
	≥0.35 and <25% of nil value	≥0.5	
	≥0.35 and ≥25% of nil value	Any	Positive
	<0.35	<0.5	Indeterminate
	≥0.35 and <25% of nil value	<0.5	
>8.0	Any	Any	

Abbreviation: Ag, antigen.

Table 3			
Interpretation of T-SPOT.*TB* results			
Nil (Spots)	TB Ag Minus Nil[a] (Spots)	Mitogen (Spots)	Qualitative Result
≤10	≤4	≥20	Negative
	5, 6, 7	Any	Borderline
	≥8	Any	Positive
	≤4	<20	Invalid
>10	Any	Any	

Abbreviation: Ag, antigen.

 [a] Highest spot count of (panel A—nil) or (panel B—nil).

BCG-vaccinated persons from countries with a low burden of TB. The manufacturers' estimated specificities from the package inserts are 99.1% for QFT-GIT and 97.1% for T-SPOT.*TB*.[22,23] These estimates were based on small numbers of people, 576 for QFT-GIT and 306 for T-SPOT.*TB*. Subsequent studies looking at serial testing in low-risk populations suggest the specificity for both tests is lower when used commercially.[26]

More important than sensitivity and specificity of the IGRAs is their ability to predict who will develop active TB if untreated. The estimated lifetime risk for active TB in a healthy person with a positive TST is 10%, 5% in the first few years after infection and 5% later.[3] The risk increases when other medical diagnoses or immunosuppressive medications are present. The data for QFT-GIT and T-SPOT.*TB* in predicting future active TB are limited. The short-term risk of developing active TB after a positive IGRA is low.[27–29] One meta-analysis found that the short-term risk of active TB after a positive IGRA or positive TST is similar.[30] Therefore, a risk assessment that evaluates the likelihood of recent infection and any medical risks for reactivation is still valuable to counsel patients about the risks and benefits of treating TB infection.

Some investigators have suggested that having a single dichotomous cutpoint for defining a positive IGRA, including conversions, may be inappropriate.[10] For TST, the cutpoint for a positive varies based on risk, and a conversion requires a quantitative increase of 10 mm in induration. Many studies have assessed alternative cutpoints for the IGRAs but none has proved consistently superior to the manufacturers' defined cutpoints thus far. A positive IGRA should be interpreted in the context of clinical and epidemiologic risk, and the manufacturers recommend repeating a positive test in people at low risk for TB exposure to avoid unnecessarily treating someone who does not have LTBI.

IGRAs in Targeted Populations

Clinically, IGRAs are primarily used to diagnose TB infection and guide prevention efforts. TB prevention is predicated on targeted testing of individuals at increased risk for TB infection, risk for progression to active TB, or both. Determining the performance of the IGRAs in these groups has been a priority. Because the risk of developing active TB is high in the first few years after infection, recent close contacts to active pulmonary TB patients are a high priority group for testing. Again, because there is not a gold standard diagnostic test for TB infection, surrogate markers based on exposure history have been used to stratify individual risk and assess IGRA performance. Two large prospective studies found that the IGRAs correlated with the surrogate marker for exposure whereas the TST correlated with older age and/or prior BCG vaccination.[31,32]

The patients at highest risk for developing active TB after infection are people coinfected with HIV.[3] The performance of the IGRAs in these patients depends on the degree of immune dysfunction and the risk for TB exposure. Indeterminate QFT-GIT results are more common in patients with lower CD4 counts presumably due to a lack of sufficient effector T-cells.[33] The T-SPOT.*TB* seems less affected as long as enough blood is drawn such that there are sufficient PBMCs to run the assay.[34] Some patients are still able to respond at low CD4 counts and the tests are considered valid if the nil and mitogen controls react appropriately. Indeterminate QFT-GITs or invalid T-SPOT.*TB*s in HIV-infected patients with low CD4 counts should be retested after antiretroviral therapy is started and CD4 recovery occurs. The best timing for retesting has not been established but a general recommendation is to wait for the CD4 to increase to greater than 200 cells/μL. In contrast, a failed TST looks the same as a negative result and anergy skin testing is unreliable to differentiate between the two.[35]

In HIV-infected patients at lower risk for TB exposure, the correlation between a positive TST, QFT-GIT, and T-SPOT.*TB* is decreased. One study of HIV-infected patients at low risk for TB exposure found that among 27 patients with a positive TST, QFT-GIT, or T-SPOT.*TB*, only 1 was positive by all 3 tests.[36] Another study found that in 41 US-born, HIV-infected patients with a positive QFT-GIT and no risk for TB exposure, 33 (80%) tested negative on a repeat QFT-GIT approximately 1 month later without TB treatment.[37]

Several published studies have evaluated the use of IGRAs in patients with non-HIV immune disorders.[38–41] Most of the studies have been small and in patients with varying risks for TB exposure or proportions with a history of BCG vaccination. As with studies in nonimmunocompromised patients, the IGRAs seem to perform better in BCG-vaccinated people. In others, the IGRAs are not clearly superior to the TST.

Children represent another important group that is targeted for TB prevention. Children have a higher risk of progressing to active TB early and developing severe, life-threatening TB compared with adults. Increasingly, studies have evaluated the performance of the IGRAs in children. These studies have again used either culture-proved active TB or an exposure gradient as a surrogate for TB infection. Test failure due to an insufficient blood volume or functional T cells is more common at younger ages.[42] As a result, there are few data published on the use of IGRAs in children less than 2 years old. Overall, the IGRAs and TST perform similarly in children ages 2 years or older.[43] The IGRAs may be slightly better than the TST for detecting active TB but still are not sufficient to confirm or exclude disease.

Health care workers are another large group that is routinely tested for TB infection. Due to the occupational risk for TB exposure and the risk of transmission to immunocompromised patients, most US health care workers undergo annual testing for TB. Historically, new infections defined by converting from negative to positive on TST have been rare.[44] The primary problem with the TST is the need for 2 visits within 2 to 3 days. The convenience of a single blood draw prompted some health care systems to adopt IGRAs for annual testing. After this, several observational studies reported higher than expected numbers of health care workers with a positive test.[45–49] Subsequently, a large prospective study compared the performance of the TST, QFT-GIT, and T-SPOT.*TB* for serially testing US health care workers.[26] That study found that unexpected conversions were more common with the IGRAs than the TST. Most of the IGRA conversions occurred as an isolated positive test and were negative on follow-up 6 months later consistent with a false-positive result.

Table 4
Treatment regimens for LTBI (adults)

Drugs	Dose	Interval	Duration	Comments
Isoniazid[a]	300 mg	Daily	9 mo	Standard regimen
Isoniazid[a]	900 mg	Twice weekly	9 mo	Use DOT
Rifampin	600 mg	Daily	4 mo	Well tolerated, improved adherence
Isoniazid[a] plus rifapentine	900 mg 900 mg	Once weekly	3 mo	As effective as isoniazid, less hepatotoxic, improved adherence; should use DOT

Abbreviation: DOT, directly observed therapy.
[a] Use pyridoxine 25–50 mg per day.

TREATMENT

Treating patients with LTBI to prevent future active TB has been a recommended strategy for TB control in the United States since 1965.[50] As discussed previously, early placebo-controlled trials showed that isoniazid effectively decreased the risk of future TB in people with a positive TST.[18] Because LTBI treatment has a proved benefit, similar controlled studies based on IGRA testing have not been conducted to date.

The recommended regimens for LTBI treatment are listed in **Table 4**. Isoniazid for 9 months remains a first-line option based on its established efficacy. Clinically significant toxicity, such as drug-induced hepatitis, is rare but treatment completion rates are low in clinical practice due to the duration of therapy and minor side effects, such as headache and fatigue.[51,52] Subsequent studies of shorter course treatments have demonstrated better completion rates.[53,54] A trial of once-weekly isoniazid and rifapentine given for 12 doses (3 months) was shown safe and effective compared with 9 months of isoniazid with a significantly higher completion rate.[54] The major limitation with this regimen is the recommendation to give it by directly observed therapy, as was done in the study. An ongoing trial is evaluating the adherence to once-weekly treatment when patients take it self-administered. Rifampin daily for 4 months is a second-line regimen for treating LTBI. Despite few data for its efficacy, this regimen has gained in popularity based on its tolerability and high completion rates compared with isoniazid.[51–53,55] A large trial evaluating the efficacy of rifampin is currently under way.

In addition to higher completion rates, the shorter course regimens have shown less hepatotoxicity compared with isoniazid.[53,54] A limiting factor for regimens that contain rifampin or rifapentine is the high potential for drug-drug interactions. Both medications are potent inducers of the cytochrome P450 enzyme system and require a careful review of any concomitant medications before being prescribed.

SUMMARY/DISCUSSION

Compared with the TST, the IGRAs perform as well or better in most targeted populations. Ongoing challenges include a low sensitivity for active TB, limited ability to predict future progression to disease, and poor specificity in groups at lower risk for TB exposure. The IGRAs have overcome several limitations of the TST by requiring a single visit, providing objective results that are retrievable electronically, and being more specific in BCG-vaccinated people.[56] Because BCG vaccine is used in countries with a higher burden of TB, the people at greatest risk for TB infection are often the ones who benefit most from screening with an IGRA. Comparing QFT-GIT and

T-SPOT.*TB*, neither has proved definitively better, so the choice is generally made based on the local cost and feasibility for each test.

REFERENCES

1. World Health Organization. Global Tuberculosis Report 2013. Geneva, Switzerland: World Health Organization; 2013.
2. Centers for Disease Control and Prevention, Targeted tuberculin testing and treatment of latent tuberculosis infection. Am J Respir Crit Care Med 2000; 161:S221–47.
3. Horsburgh CR Jr, Rubin EJ. Clinical practice. Latent tuberculosis infection in the United States. N Engl J Med 2011;364(15):1441–8.
4. Prasad TS, Verma R, Kumar S, et al. Proteomic analysis of purified protein derivative of Mycobacterium tuberculosis. Clin Proteomics 2013;10(1):8.
5. Mazurek M, Jereb J, Vernon A, et al. Updated guidelines for using interferon gamma release assays to detect Mycobacterium tuberculosis infection - United States, 2010. MMWR Recomm Rep 2010;59(RR-5):1–25.
6. Walter N, Daley CL. Tuberculosis and nontuberculous mycobacterial infection. In: Spiro SG, Silvestri GA, Agusti A, editors. Clinical Respiratory Medicine. Philadelphia: Elsevier Saunders; 2012. p. 385–408.
7. Behr MA. BCG–different strains, different vaccines? Lancet Infect Dis 2002;2(2): 86–92.
8. Andersen P, Munk ME, Pollock JM, et al. Specific immune-based diagnosis of tuberculosis. Lancet 2000;356(9235):1099–104.
9. Adjemian J, Olivier KN, Seitz AE, et al. Prevalence of nontuberculous mycobacterial lung disease in U.S. Medicare beneficiaries. Am J Respir Crit Care Med 2012;185(8):881–6.
10. Pai M, Denkinger CM, Kik SV, et al. Gamma interferon release assays for detection of mycobacterium tuberculosis infection. Clin Microbiol Rev 2014;27(1): 3–20.
11. Bennett DE, Courval JM, Onorato I, et al. Prevalence of tuberculosis infection in the United States population: the national health and nutrition examination survey, 1999-2000. Am J Respir Crit Care Med 2008;177(3):348–55.
12. Centers for Disease Control and Prevention (CDC). Trends in tuberculosis - United States, 2012. MMWR Morb Mortal Wkly Rep 2013;62:201–5.
13. Cain KP, Haley CA, Armstrong LR, et al. Tuberculosis among foreign-born persons in the United States: achieving tuberculosis elimination. Am J Respir Crit Care Med 2007;175(1):75–9.
14. Walter ND, Painter J, Parker M, et al. Persistent latent tuberculosis reactivation risk in United States immigrants. Am J Respir Crit Care Med 2014; 189(1):88–95.
15. Liu Y, Painter JA, Posey DL, et al. Estimating the impact of newly arrived foreign-born persons on tuberculosis in the United States. PLoS One 2012;7(2):e32158.
16. Ricks PM, Cain KP, Oeltmann JE, et al. Estimating the burden of tuberculosis among foreign-born persons acquired prior to entering the U.S., 2005-2009. PLoS One 2011;6(11):e27405.
17. Linas BP, Wong AY, Freedberg KA, et al. Priorities for screening and treatment of latent tuberculosis infection in the United States. Am J Respir Crit Care Med 2011;184(5):590–601.
18. Ferebee SH. Controlled chemoprophylaxis trials in tuberculosis. A general review. Bibl Tuberc 1970;26:28–106.

19. Barry CE 3rd, Boshoff HI, Dartois V, et al. The spectrum of latent tuberculosis: rethinking the biology and intervention strategies. Nat Rev Microbiol 2009; 7(12):845–55.
20. Modlin RL, Bloom BR. TB or not TB: that is no longer the question. Sci Transl Med 2013;5(213):213sr6.
21. Farhat M, Greenaway C, Pai M, et al. False-positive tuberculin skin tests: what is the absolute effect of BCG and non-tuberculous mycobacteria? Int J Tuberc Lung Dis 2006;10(11):1192–204.
22. Cellestis. QuantiFERON-TB Gold Package Insert. 2011. Available at: http://www.cellestis.com/IRM/Content/pdf/QuantiFeron%20US%20VerJ_JULY2011_ttf.pdf. Accessed January 28, 2014.
23. Oxford Immunotec. T-SPOT.TB Package Insert. 2013. Available at: http://www.tspot.com/wp-content/uploads/2012/01/PI-TB-US-v4.pdf. Accessed January 28, 2014.
24. Diel R, Loddenkemper R, Nienhaus A. Evidence-based comparison of commercial interferon-gamma release assays for detecting active TB: a metaanalysis. Chest 2010;137(4):952–68.
25. Metcalfe JZ, Everett CK, Steingart KR, et al. Interferon-gamma release assays for active pulmonary tuberculosis diagnosis in adults in low- and middle-income countries: systematic review and meta-analysis. J Infect Dis 2011; 204(Suppl 4):S1120–9.
26. Dorman SE, Belknap R, Graviss EA, et al. Interferon-gamma release assays and tuberculin skin testing for diagnosis of latent tuberculosis infection in Healthcare Workers in the United States. Am J Respir Crit Care Med 2014;189(1):77–87.
27. Kim YJ, Kim SI, Kim YR, et al. Predictive value of interferon-gamma ELISPOT assay in HIV 1-infected patients in an intermediate tuberculosis-endemic area. AIDS Res Hum Retroviruses 2012;28(9):1038–43.
28. Lange B, Vavra M, Kern WV, et al. Development of tuberculosis in immunocompromised patients with a positive tuberculosis-specific IGRA. Int J Tuberc Lung Dis 2012;16(4):492–5.
29. Machingaidze S, Verver S, Mulenga H, et al. Predictive value of recent QuantiFERON conversion for tuberculosis disease in adolescents. Am J Respir Crit Care Med 2012;186(10):1051–6.
30. Rangaka MX, Wilkinson KA, Glynn JR, et al. Predictive value of interferon-gamma release assays for incident active tuberculosis: a systematic review and meta-analysis. Lancet Infect Dis 2012;12(1):45–55.
31. Arend SM, Thijsen SF, Leyten EM, et al. Comparison of two interferon-gamma assays and tuberculin skin test for tracing tuberculosis contacts. Am J Respir Crit Care Med 2007;175(6):618–27.
32. Diel R, Loddenkemper R, Meywald-Walter K, et al. Comparative performance of tuberculin skin test, QuantiFERON-TB-Gold in Tube assay, and T-Spot.TB test in contact investigations for tuberculosis. Chest 2009;135(4):1010–8.
33. Aichelburg MC, Rieger A, Breitenecker F, et al. Detection and prediction of active tuberculosis disease by a whole-blood interferon-gamma release assay in HIV-1-infected individuals. Clin Infect Dis 2009;48(7):954–62.
34. Cattamanchi A, Smith R, Steingart KR, et al. Interferon-gamma release assays for the diagnosis of latent tuberculosis infection in HIV-infected individuals: a systematic review and meta-analysis. J Acquir Immune Defic Syndr 2011; 56(3):230–8.
35. Slovis BS, Plitman JD, Haas DW. The case against anergy testing as a routine adjunct to tuberculin skin testing. JAMA 2000;283(15):2003–7.

36. Talati NJ, Seybold U, Humphrey B, et al. Poor concordance between interferon-gamma release assays and tuberculin skin tests in diagnosis of latent tuberculosis infection among HIV-infected individuals. BMC Infect Dis 2009;9:15.

37. Gray J, Reves R, Johnson S, et al. Identification of false-positive QuantiFERON-TB Gold In-Tube assays by repeat testing in HIV-infected patients at low risk for tuberculosis. Clin Infect Dis 2012;54(3):e20–3.

38. Smith R, Cattamanchi A, Steingart KR, et al. Interferon-gamma release assays for diagnosis of latent tuberculosis infection: evidence in immune-mediated inflammatory disorders. Curr Opin Rheumatol 2011;23(4):377–84.

39. Chung WK, Zheng ZL, Sung JY, et al. Validity of interferon-gamma-release assays for the diagnosis of latent tuberculosis in haemodialysis patients. Clin Microbiol Infect 2010;16(7):960–5.

40. Leung CC, Yam WC, Yew WW, et al. T-Spot.TB outperforms tuberculin skin test in predicting tuberculosis disease. Am J Respir Crit Care Med 2010;182(6): 834–40.

41. Kim EY, Lim JE, Jung JY, et al. Performance of the tuberculin skin test and interferon-gamma release assay for detection of tuberculosis infection in immunocompromised patients in a BCG-vaccinated population. BMC Infect Dis 2009;9:207.

42. Haustein T, Ridout DA, Hartley JC, et al. The likelihood of an indeterminate test result from a whole-blood interferon-gamma release assay for the diagnosis of Mycobacterium tuberculosis infection in children correlates with age and immune status. Pediatr Infect Dis J 2009;28(8):669–73.

43. Mandalakas AM, Detjen AK, Hesseling AC, et al. Interferon-gamma release assays and childhood tuberculosis: systematic review and meta-analysis. Int J Tuberc Lung Dis 2011;15(8):1018–32.

44. Larsen NM, Biddle CL, Sotir MJ, et al. Risk of tuberculin skin test conversion among health care workers: occupational versus community exposure and infection. Clin Infect Dis 2002;35(7):796–801.

45. Gandra S, Scott WS, Somaraju V, et al. Questionable effectiveness of the QuantiFERON-TB Gold Test (Cellestis) as a screening tool in healthcare workers. Infect Control Hosp Epidemiol 2010;31(12):1279–85.

46. Ringshausen FC, Nienhaus A, Schablon A, et al. Predictors of persistently positive Mycobacterium-tuberculosis-specific interferon-gamma responses in the serial testing of health care workers. BMC Infect Dis 2010;10:220.

47. Ringshausen FC, Nienhaus A, Torres Costa J, et al. Within-subject variability of Mycobacterium tuberculosis-specific gamma interferon responses in German health care workers. Clin Vaccine Immunol 2011;18(7):1176–82.

48. Torres Costa J, Silva R, Ringshausen FC, et al. Screening for tuberculosis and prediction of disease in Portuguese healthcare workers. J Occup Med Toxicol 2011;6:19.

49. Slater ML, Welland G, Pai M, et al. Challenges with QuantiFERON-TB Gold assay for large-scale, routine screening of U.S. healthcare workers. Am J Respir Crit Care Med 2013;188(8):1005–10.

50. Runyon EH. Preventive treatment in tuberculosis: a statement by the Committee on Therapy, American Thoracic Society. Am Rev Respir Dis 1965;91: 297–8.

51. Lardizabal A, Passannante M, Kojakali F, et al. Enhancement of treatment completion for latent tuberculosis infection with 4 months of rifampin. Chest 2006;130(6):1712–7.

52. Page KR, Sifakis F, Montes de Oca R, et al. Improved adherence and less toxicity with rifampin vs isoniazid for treatment of latent tuberculosis: a retrospective study. Arch Intern Med 2006;166(17):1863–70.
53. Menzies D, Long R, Trajman A, et al. Adverse events with 4 months of rifampin therapy or 9 months of isoniazid therapy for latent tuberculosis infection: a randomized trial. Ann Intern Med 2008;149(10):689–97.
54. Sterling TR, Villarino ME, Borisov AS, et al. Three months of rifapentine and isoniazid for latent tuberculosis infection. N Engl J Med 2011;365(23):2155–66.
55. Hong Kong Chest Service/Tuberculosis Research Centre, M.B.M.R.C., A double-blind placebo-controlled clinical trial of three antituberculosis chemoprophylaxis regimens in patients with silicosis in Hong Kong. Am Rev Respir Dis 1992;145(1):36–41.
56. Diel R, Goletti D, Ferrara G, et al. Interferon-gamma release assays for the diagnosis of latent Mycobacterium tuberculosis infection: a systematic review and meta-analysis. Eur Respir J 2011;37(1):88–99.

Respiratory Fungal Infections

Molecular Diagnostic Tests

Kevin C. Hazen, PhD, D(ABMM)

KEYWORDS

- Assay • Fungal infection • PCR • Species

KEY POINTS

- A variety of polymerase chain reaction (PCR)-based assays have been developed for detection of *Aspergillus* spp. in respiratory specimens and in blood.
- Positive blood specimens suggest invasive infection and are less likely to be positive due to contamination.
- Ribosomal RNA gene is an effective target for the PCR assays and can be used to develop assays that distinguish species.
- At least 2 commercial assays are available outside of the United States. No assay has been approved by the Food and Drug Administration.
- Galactomannan detection is equally effective for diagnosis of aspergillosis.
- In general, the sensitivity and specificity of conventional PCR and real-time PCR assays for pneumocystis jirovecii pneumonia (PjP) are excellent.
- Real-time PCR allows quantification, which is potentially useful to distinguish PjP colonization from infection.
- Currently the decision of colonization versus infection based on molecular results must be driven by clinical information.

INTRODUCTION

Fungal infection of the respiratory tract can take several forms, the most common of which is pneumonia. Fungal infection can occur in the immunocompetent typically as a result of inhalation of a large inoculum of fungal elements (eg, histoplasmosis). However, the number of etiologic agents attacking immunocompetent individuals and causing significant infection is limited. A much larger menu of fungi is associated with respiratory disease in immunocompromised patients. The most common of these are *Aspergillus* species, *Pneumocystis jirovecii*, *Scedosporium* species, *Fusarium* species, *Candida* species, *Cryptococcus* species, and members of the *Mucorales* within the *Mucoromycotina*.[1]

Clinical Microbiology Laboratory, Department of Pathology, Duke University Health System, 2902 DUMC, 116 CARL Building, Durham, NC 27710, USA
E-mail address: kevin.hazen@duke.edu

Clin Lab Med 34 (2014) 351–364
http://dx.doi.org/10.1016/j.cll.2014.02.008
0272-2712/14/$ – see front matter © 2014 Elsevier Inc. All rights reserved.

Given the high level of attributable mortality associated with these fungi in immuno-compromised patients, the need for rapid diagnosis is self-evident. As reviewed in the previous article (by Lamoth and Alexander), traditional culture-based methods lack sensitivity and are generally too slow to provide useful information for therapeutic management. Nonculture-based methods, such as antigen testing, are helpful but lack specificity due to crossreactivity with various fungi and with nonfungal materials. To be useful, repeat testing may be required (eg, galactomannan). Nucleic acid–based diagnostics offer the potential for high sensitivity, high specificity, and rapid turn-around time. Despite such potential, there is currently no Food and Drug Administration (FDA)-approved nucleic acid–based test for diagnosis of fungal infection directly from a specimen. One assay that has received CE marking is the SeptiFast produced by Roche Diagnostics. This assay is LightCycler based and targets several *Candida* species and *Aspergillus fumigatus.* The performance of this assay in prospective clinical trials requires additional study. A second assay, MycAssay *Aspergillus* (Myconostica), is also CE-marked. This relatively new real-time PCR assay also awaits extensive prospective evaluation.

The most recent European Organization for Research and Treatment of Cancer/Invasive Fungal Infections Cooperative Group and the National Institute of Allergy and Infectious Diseases Mycoses Study Group (EORTC/MSG) consensus documents regarding diagnosis of invasive fungal infections do not include the use of molecular assays as an adjunct for diagnosis due to the lack of standardization.[2] Interest in trying to incorporate PCR assays into the guideline is high.

Laboratories are faced with several challenges when considering the development of a molecular assay for diagnosis of respiratory fungal infections. For example, should the test target single or multiple specific pathogens or be a single target with broad specificity (eg, ribosomal DNA)? The answer to this is, of course, driven by the frequency of infection by different fungi, the patient population intended for the assay, the resources of the laboratory, and other factors. Also at issue in design of a molecular test is consideration for targeting organisms that are either part of the host microbiota or are common contaminants of the respiratory tract. Although *Candida* species are considered part of the normal microbiota of the oropharynx, other organisms, such as *Cladosporium, Aspergillus,* and *Fusarium* may also be commensals in some individuals.[3] Additionally, these organisms may simply be acquired through consumption of foods and be transient colonizers.

Another challenge for design of a molecular test is choice of specimen. Sputum specimens, which are relatively easy to collect and do not require invasive procedures, have the risk of poor sensitivity and poor specificity if the target is a common contaminant or part of the commensal population or if the specimen is not well produced. Bronchoalveolar lavage (BAL) may be preferable from the viewpoint of minimizing contamination but has a higher risk to the patient than collection of sputum and may be insensitive. Blood specimens may be insufficient for organisms that do not invade or have not invaded into the pulmonary vasculature, and for those that do invade, whether whole blood or a blood fraction provides highest sensitivity must be determined. Furthermore, some fungi causing respiratory disease may enter the blood stream but will not result in a positive blood culture (eg, *Aspergillus* spp.), making assessment of a molecular assay's performance characteristics for blood specimens difficult.

The design of molecular assays for fungal respiratory pathogens that are common contaminants or members of the normal respiratory microbiota must also consider whether the intent of the assay is for screening or for diagnosis. Within the concept of screening is the issue of whether patient sampling is a one-time event or occurs at regular intervals. The type of sample, the sensitivity and specificity of the assay (and hence positive and negative likelihood values), and the limit of detection become variables of consideration. Optimally, a test with high sensitivity and high specificity in the face of low pretest probability is desired.

This article reviews developments in molecular testing for detection of *Aspergillus* species and *Pneumocystis jirovecii*, which represent (arguably) the most common fungal agents of respiratory infection. Not surprisingly, the molecular assays for these 2 agents have received the most effort to standardize. Laboratory-developed molecular assays have been described for specific detection of other fungal agents causing respiratory disease, such as members of the Mucorales (eg, *Mucor* spp., *Rhizopus* spp., *Rhizomucor* spp., *Absidia* spp., *Cunninghamella* spp.); *Candida* species (most effort in this case is not specifically for respiratory disease but rather systemic disease); *Scedosporium* spp.; and the systemic, thermally dimorphic fungi (ie, the endemic fungi such as *Histoplasma capsulatum, Blastomyces dermatitidis, Coccidioides* spp., *Paracoccidioides brasiliensis*).[4–15] However, further developmental progress is needed before these will attain general utility.

ASPERGILLOSIS

The microbiology, epidemiology, pathogenesis, and clinical presentation of *Aspergillus* species and aspergillosis have been described in a previous article in this issue (see Lamoth and Alexander).

Diagnosis

During recent years, molecular assay development for aspergillosis has received significant attention resulting in several excellent reviews being published (eg, see Refs.[16–21]). As is evident from these reviews, a wide range of assays have been developed targeting just genus-specific sequences, just *Aspergillus fumigatus*–specific sequences, or sequences allowing multiple species identification. In general, the most common target is the 18S rDNA gene. However, the ITS1-58S-ITS2 region or parts thereof, the 28S gene, cytochrome b gene, and repetitive sequences have also been targeted (eg, see references[22–34]). Other groups have targeted mitochondria DNA for similar readouts as those for nuclear DNA. Targets include mitochondrial rRNA genes and the mitochondrial cytochrome b gene.[35–39] An advantage of the cytochrome b gene is that it allows for quantification, which is difficult to achieve with multicopy gene targets. The CE marking of 2 different *Aspergillus* assays (MycAssay and SeptiFast) exemplifies the progress that has been achieved. Unlike some of the assays referenced earlier, the MycAssay reports the presence of *Aspergillus* species but not the specific species (15 species were targeted), whereas the SeptiFast reports only *Aspergillus fumigatus*. Of note with the MycAssay, a false-positive result can occur due to *Penicillium* species. As noted earlier, however, neither of these assays has obtained FDA approval for distribution in the United States.

In response, in part, to the desire to include molecular testing in the EORTC/MSG definitions for proven, probable, and possible aspergillosis,[2] several organizations, namely the European *Aspergillus* PCR Initiative (EAPCRI), United Kingdom Fungal Polymerase Chain Reaction Consensus Group (UKFPCRCG), and the *Aspergillus* Technology Consortium (AsTeC) have initiated efforts to help standardize laboratory-developed PCR tests.[40–44] In one such effort, calibrator material was evaluated for its reproducibility, robustness, and stability among 12 laboratories and thus its potential use for assay development and target quantification.[44] The calibrator material consisted of DNA isolated from conidia of *Aspergillus fumigatus* strain AF293.

Although the material appeared to provide satisfactory results and was stable to 10 freeze-thaw cycles, the investigators point out that all of the participating laboratories used PCR assays that target the rRNA gene. As there are multiple copies of this gene in the fungal genome, it is not possible to correlate the results to genome equivalents and consequently the material is not useful for assessing extraction methods for specific specimen types.

A second study was based on the results of an earlier investigation where the UKFPCRCG distributed specimen control panels to 6 laboratories.[45] These 6 laboratories represented 5 different laboratory-developed PCR tests for *Aspergillus* spp. The purpose of the study was to interrogate which method provided the best detection limits. Two methods were found to be superior (detection limit of 10^1 conidia). Ten laboratories were involved that allowed the investigators to assess specific amplification systems. The results showed that the amplification system used by each laboratory had little effect on the results, thus the main issue was the method of extraction. This observation was supported by a subsequent study performed under the auspices of the EAPCRI involving 24 testing centers.[41]

Other efforts by the EAPCRI, UKFPCRCG, and AsTeC include establishing a standard for PCR that is validated as a screening tool using an animal model for specimens and evaluation of PCR methods for testing serum and whole blood specimens.[40,42] In separate meta-analyses White and colleagues[42,43] concluded that serum is a satisfactory specimen type and requires less standardization, allowing detection of 10 genomes/ml. Additionally, serum can be used for the galactomannan assay (see later discussion). Thus, the laboratories that offer both PCR and galactomannan may prefer serum as a specimen. Otherwise whole blood is a good candidate for PCR assays because it may provide an earlier positive result and may be more sensitive.[46] The use of serum or blood as a specimen type rather than BAL comes from observations that BAL specimens may be contaminated with *Aspergillus* species conidia or may detect colonizing but not parasitic organisms (reviewed in Refs.[20,21]). Indeed, Cahill and colleagues[47] have reported that approximately 40% of lung transplant patients become colonized with *Aspergillus* spp. Positive serum, plasma, or blood specimens, on the other hand, would indicate invasive aspergillosis. As a screening tool, PCR assays using serum, blood, or plasma provide excellent sensitivity; hence a single negative result is sufficient to exclude the diagnosis of proven or probable invasive aspergillosis.[48] However, a single positive result has lower specificity than 2 positive results.[48]

Combination Testing

Although the incorporation of PCR assays into the diagnostic EORTC criteria for proven, probable, and possible aspergillosis awaits further studies, the question of whether PCR assays are necessary when there exist commercial assays for the *Aspergillus* species antigen, galactomannan. Several studies have compared laboratory-developed PCR assays with antigen testing, primarily galactomannan, for serum or whole blood specimens (eg, see Refs.[28,46,49]) and BAL specimens (eg, see Refs.[33,50]).

In a mixed retrospective and prospective specimen study but retrospective patient study in which proven and probable cases of invasive aspergillosis were compared with controls, Springer and colleagues[46] noted no significant differences in use of serum versus whole blood for PCR diagnosis but there were indications that whole blood could be more sensitive and could allow diagnosis earlier than serum (15 days vs 36 days). Noteworthy in the study was that galactomannan detection had the highest specificity and better sensitivity than serum PCR. However, these results may likely be biased because the galactomannan assay was used as an inclusion criterion by the EORTC/MSG for defining probable disease. The authors also noted that combination tests in which 2 different assays were used provided the highest specificity although lowered sensitivity. Using a serum PCR assay compared with galactomannan antigen, Lopes da Silva and colleagues[49] found no difference in the sensitivity and specificity between the 2 serum assays in neutropenic patients. No information regarding the time to positivity was provided. These investigators also observed that 2 consecutive positive results for both assays predicted invasive aspergillosis. In their study, the serum PCR assays were performed on a different group of patients than the galactomannan assays. Both of these studies did experience single test false-positive results with both the galactomannan and the PCR assays, which may explain why combining both tests provides better specificity.

In a limited but apparently prospective study, a real-time PCR assay was compared with galactomannan detection for diagnosis of invasive aspergillosis where the diagnosis of possible and probable disease was based on EORTC/MSG criteria.[33] The dynamic detection range of the PCR assay was 10 to 10^6 plasmid copies of an *Aspergillus* species conserved sequence (representing *A. fumigatus, A. flavus, A. glaucus, A. niger,* and *A. terreus*) within the 18S rRNA gene. Using this approach to estimate dynamic range, the number of genome equivalents is unclear. Of 20 patients diagnosed with probable or possible invasive aspergillosis, 18 were positive by real-time PCR and all were positive by galactomannan antigen assay. For this study, the results suggest possible superiority of galactomannan detection over the investigators' real-time PCR assay. The 2 patients in which the galactomannan was positive and the PCR assay was negative grew out *Candida albicans* on culture. Both patients were characterized as having probable invasive aspergillosis. *C. albicans* is not known to express galactomannans in its cell wall protein *N*-glycans.[51,52] A second study also looked as probable and possible invasive aspergillosis but included a third category, *Aspergillus* colonization, which was defined as growth from BAL of *Aspergillus* species but normal bronchoscopic and chest computed tomography findings. In the study, the investigators compared a PCR assay that was pan specific for *Aspergillus* species, a separate assay specific to *A. fumigates,* and a third assay specific to *A. terreus* developed in collaboration with Immunocompromised Host Section of the National Cancer Institute with galactomannan antigen detection. The sensitivity of the pan-specific PCR assay compared to galactomannan was 100% versus 93%, respectively, whereas the specificities were 88% and 89%. The galactomannan assay had a higher specificity than the pan-specific PCR assay for *Aspergillus* colonization specimens, whereas the specificity of the pan-specific PCR assay specificity was higher than antigen testing for negative control samples. The investigators also noted that positive results for both assays improved specificity to 97%.

A meta-analysis was performed to determine whether PCR could potentially serve as a criterion for diagnosis of probable or possible invasive aspergillosis.[53] Both prospective and retrospective cohort and case-control studies were included. Similar to the 2 studies mentioned earlier, the investigators concluded that PCR of BAL is comparable to galactomannan detection in BAL fluid and that using both tests optimizes sensitivity without compromising specificity. No attempt to determine if the methods differ in time to positivity was done.

The Need for Prospective Clinical Trials

The studies described earlier demonstrate that various PCR assays have the potential to be useful in assisting physicians in diagnosing invasive aspergillosis and for inclusion in EORTC/MSG definitions for proven, probable, or possible invasive aspergillosis. Unfortunately, the prospective studies used to assess the potential of PCR assays were based on specimens from patients who were classified as proven, probable, or possible aspergillosis using current non-PCR data. Before PCR assays can be included into the EORTC/MSG definitions, large prospective studies in which PCR is evaluated as an independent versus contributory indicator of disease must be done. The potential role of quantitative PCR as a possible adjunct to these PCR-based definitions still requires further investigation.

PNEUMOCYSTIS JIROVECII PNEUMONIA
Introduction

In 1909, Chagas discovered an organism, which he considered to be a trypanosome, in the lungs of guinea pigs. He named the organism *Schizotrypanum cruzi* and considered it related to *Trypanosoma cruzi*.[54] Later studies by others demonstrated the organism, now called *Pneumocystis carinii*, was a separate genus and species. Before the AIDS epidemic, disease caused by *P. jirovecii* (the human adapted species of *Pneumocystis*) was recognized as a cause of lung disesae in post–World War II infants who had been institutionalized and were debilitated. It was also seen in immunocompromised individuals starting in the early 1960s. Once effective therapy was developed, the disease's prevalence diminished until the beginning of the AIDS epidemic when the disease was commonly seen in patients with low CD4 counts. The frequency with which pneumocystosis was associated with AIDS patients resulted in it being listed as an AIDS defining illness. Diagnosis of the disease has progressed from radiographic and microscopic methods to molecular-based approaches.

Microbiology

The inability to cultivate *P. jirovecii* and other species of *Pneumocystis* impeded progress in assigning the organism to its appropriate Kingdom and phylum. Most studies based its taxonomy on its life cycle in the host where it produces trophic forms, which can undergo fission and can conjugate followed by meiosis and mitosis to form haploid spores. The spores are contained within a cyst (8 spores/cyst). Following excystment, the spores are released and the cycle begins again. Both the trophic forms and the cysts can be seen in clinical material, the trophic forms often clumping together. Further studies, primarily molecular, demonstrated that the organism is actually a fungus belonging to the phylum Ascomycota, subphylum *Taphrinomycotina*, class Pneumocystidomycetes, order Pneumocystidales.[55] The surface of *P. jirovecii* has several proteins. One of these, the major surface glycoprotein (MSG), has multiple isoforms. Antigenic variation of the *P. jirovecii* surface occurs as a result of expression of the different MSG isoforms and possibly also because a second surface protein, a protease encoded by the *PRT1* gene, may modify the MSG.

Epidemiology

Acquisition of *P. jirovecii* occurs early in life and has been thought to lead to asymptomatic colonization. However, recent studies suggest that *P. jirovecii* may cause or contribute to acute respiratory disease in immunocompetent children.[56] Development of significant pulmonary disease later in life is then the result of loss of immune defense and growth of the fungus. More recent animal studies suggest that *P. jirovecii* can be transmitted by the airborne route and that individuals could go through cycles of transient colonization of one strain followed by loss of that strain and acquisition of a new strain. Genotyping studies support the concept that transmission from person-to-person does occur and that an individual can harbor multiple strains of *P. jirovecii* over time. Disease development may therefore not be the result of latency and reactivation but rather acquisition and transient colonization of a strain at the time of immune compromise.[57,58]

Clinical Presentation

In socioeconomically challenged countries, *P. jirovecii* disease can manifest itself in undernourished, debilitated children in the form of interstitial plasma cell pneumonia, which can progress to respiratory distress and cyanosis. In immunocompromised patients presenting symptoms are fever, shortness of breath, and a nonproductive cough. Tachypnea and hypoxia may be seen. Chest films may reveal diffuse, bilateral infiltrates and ground glass opacifications. The presentation of *Pneumocystis jirovecii* pneumonia (PjP) is variable and can differ among patient groups (AIDS vs lung allograft patients). In HIV patients who received HAART, immune reconstitution inflammatory syndrome can occur as a result of improved $CD4^+$ counts resulting in the need to treat with antiinflammatory agents rather than anti-*P. jirovecii* drugs.

Pathogenesis

Development of PjP involves multiple factors. A discussion of these is beyond the scope of this review. Attachment of *P. jirovecii* to host lung epithelial cells is critical and results in an inflammatory response, which can limit progression of disease. Impaired cell immunity (especially loss of $CD4^+$ cells) can alter the inflammatory response and allow the organism to grow and fill alveoli.

Laboratory Diagnosis

In vitro cultivation is not an option; thus laboratories must rely on less direct methods for detection. Before molecular methods for diagnosis, methods used in the clinical laboratory have included stains, such as toluidine O, methenamine silver, Wright-Giemsa, and calcofluor white. Specimens include BAL fluids, sputa, and tissue. These stains are not particularly sensitive with the exception of perhaps calcofluor white. Direct fluorescent antibody stains are commercially available and can improve sensitivity over standard stains. However, the ability to distinguish organisms from debris and other nonorganism material requires an experienced eye. Of the many direct fluorescent antibody (DFA)/indirect fluorescent antibody assays used in the clinical microbiology laboratory, the *P. jirovecii* DFA is, in this author's opinion, the most difficult to interpret.

Molecular methods for detection of *P. jirovecii* in patients with respiratory disease have progressed over the past 20 years, essentially advancing in step with improvements to molecular technology (**Table 1**). Several specimen types have been investigated. As with many respiratory pathogens, the best specimen is the one directly associated with the organism, that is, tissue. Fortunately, BALs and induced sputa have proved to be excellent specimens for detection of *P. jirovecii* by molecular methods. Oral rinses (50 mL of saline agitated inside the mouth for 10–30 seconds) have also been studied and found to be useful for diagnosing PjP; however adjustment of cut-off values compared to other specimens may be necessary to improve specificity.[59–61]

Several issues with molecular tests are predicated on the observation that patients exposed or colonized with *P. jirovecii* may not manifest symptoms and that the assays must be able to detect levels of organism lower than current diagnostic methods. Inherent in the latter criterion is the problem of comparing a molecular-based assay with a "gold standard" diagnostic method when the gold standard is, by its design, inferior. These "gold standard" criteria may include one or more indications of disease

Table 1
Example PCR assays for *Pneumocystis jirovecii* pneumonia and their performance characteristics

PCR Assay	Sample Type	Target	Internal Control (Y/N/What)	Reported Sensitivity	Reported Specificity	"Gold Standard" for Positive	Reference
Conventional PCR	BAL	mt LSU	N	91%	88%	None	69
Conventional PCR	Induced sputum	ITS2	N	88.2%	81.2%	Clinical, radiographic, therapeutic response	63
Nested PCR	Lung biopsy and BAL	mt LSU	N	100 (AIDS patients)	100 (AIDS patients)	Clinical, radiographic, therapeutic response, lactate dehydrogenase	70
Touch-down nested PCR	BAL	DHPS	N	94%	81%	Clinical, radiographic, microscopic	71
Touch-down real-time PCR	Induced sputum, BAL	MSG	Y (tet^R gene)	100%	67%[a]	Immunofluorescence or standard stain	61
Touch-down real-time PCR	BAL	MSG	Y (human beta-globulin gene)	100% (C$_t$ <28 cycles)	98.1%	Immunofluorescence	72
Real-time PCR	Induced sputum, BAL	MSG	Y (tet^R gene)	95%	64%	Immunofluorescence or standard stain	61
Real-time PCR	Induced sputum	ITS2	N	82.4% (positive = 1500 copies/ml	98.6%	Clinical, radiographic, therapeutic response	63
Real-time PCR	BAL	DHPS	Unclear	94%	96%	Clinical, radiographic, microscopic	71
Real-time PCR	BAL	cdc2	N	100%	96.9%	Calcofluor white stain	73
Real-time PCR	Induced sputum, BAL	mt LSU	Y	100% (cut-off ≥120 trophic form equivalents/ml)	96.9%	Immunofluorescence and Giemsa stain	62

Abbreviations: BAL, bronchoalveolar lavage; Cdc2, cell division cycle 2 gene; DHPS, dihydropteroate synthase gene; ITS2, internal transcribed sequence 2; MSG, multicopy major surface glycoprotein gene; mt LSU, mitochondrial large subunit.
[a] Specimens were biased toward higher false positivity, thus increasing the chance for poor specificity.

such as radiographic appearance, response to therapy, and symptoms plus underlying diagnosis. A more definitive gold standard is to use microscopic detection of organisms in specimens, but this lends itself toward a poor specificity bias.

Quantitative real-time PCR (qrt-PCR) has been exploited to address the problem of distinguishing colonization from infection.[61–63] To create a calibration curve, investigators have used trophic forms from human BAL specimens and cloned plasmids containing target sequence. In none of the cited studies was an effort made to determine limits of detection and quantification for a given specimen type. The qrt-PCR studies demonstrated that there is no absolute cut-off that distinguishes infection from noninfection, that is, achieving 100% specificity without sacrificing sensitivity. For this reason, quantitative assays appear to best used as an adjunct diagnostic test weighed with the totality of clinical evidence supporting the diagnosis when low-levels of organism are detected. As with all DNA target PCR assays, these tests do not distinguish live from dead organisms, and therefore may not provide useful information for guiding therapeutic success.

PCR or Antigen Tests

Similar to studies with *Aspergillus* spp. and galactomannan, interest exists in whether an antigen test, namely detection of β-D-1,3-glucan, could be used to indicate PjP.[64–68] β-D-1,3-glucan is a polysaccharide found in the cell walls of many fungi. As such, detection of it in serum or plasma in the absence of other signs or symptoms of PjP suggests only that a fungal cause may be involved. Desmet and colleagues[64] studied 2 patient populations that are susceptible to PjP: HIV patients and hematologic malignancy patients. Diagnosis of PjP was confirmed by PCR (real-time PCR using mitochondrial rRNA as the target). Using a higher β-D-1,3-glucan cut-off for positivity than recommended by the manufacturer (100 vs 80 pg/mL), the sensitivity and specificity of the assay was 100% and 96.4%, respectively. These results suggest that β-D-1,3-glucan detection is a useful adjunct test for diagnosis of PjP in both patient populations. The study was, however, retrospective. Whether antigen testing is equivalent to PCR testing for diagnosis of suspected PjP prospectively is not clear.

Treatment

Several effective agents to treat *Pneumocystis* infection are available. These include trimethoprim-sulfamethoxazole, clindamycin and primaquine in combination, atovaquone, and pentamidine. The presence of β-D-1,3-glucan suggests the echinocandins may also be effective, but mixed results have been seen.

SUMMARY

Laboratory diagnosis of fungal respiratory infections is challenging not only because the etiologic agents can take days to weeks to grow in culture but also because many, although not all, of the agents causing disease in immunocompromised patients are common environmental contaminants and some may transiently reside in the upper airway and in the oral cavity. Molecular methods certainly can overcome the problem of poor turnaround time but may not correspondingly eliminate the problem of equivocation of clinical significance. Quantitative molecular assays (such as those afforded by real-time PCR) have the potential to help with this issue as has been demonstrated with some of the assays developed for aspergillosis and pneumocystosis. Molecular assays are therefore a potential additional and sensitive weapon that can be added to the diagnostic arsenal used by physicians to determine whether a fungus is definitively, probably, or possibly causing infection in a patient.

REFERENCES

1. Limper AH. The changing spectrum of fungal infections in pulmonary and critical care practice: clinical approach to diagnosis. Proc Am Thorac Soc 2010; 7(3):163–8.
2. De Pauw B, Walsh TJ, Donnelly JP, et al. Revised definitions of invasive fungal disease from the European Organization for Research and Treatment of Cancer/Invasive Fungal Infections Cooperative Group and the National Institute of Allergy and Infectious Diseases Mycoses Study Group (EORTC/MSG) Consensus Group. Clin Infect Dis 2008;46(12):1813–21.
3. Ghannoum MA, Jurevic RJ, Mukherjee PK, et al. Characterization of the oral fungal microbiome (mycobiome) in healthy individuals. PLoS Pathog 2010; 6(1):e1000713.
4. Dannaoui E, Schwarz P, Slany M, et al. Molecular detection and identification of zygomycetes species from paraffin-embedded tissues in a murine model of disseminated zygomycosis: a collaborative European Society of Clinical Microbiology and Infectious Diseases (ESCMID) Fungal Infection Study Group (EFISG) evaluation. J Clin Microbiol 2010;48(6):2043–6.
5. Hammond SP, Bialek R, Milner DA, et al. Molecular methods to improve diagnosis and identification of mucormycosis. J Clin Microbiol 2011;49(6):2151–3.
6. Hata DJ, Buckwalter SP, Pritt BS, et al. Real-time PCR method for detection of zygomycetes. J Clin Microbiol 2008;46(7):2353–8.
7. Kobayashi M, Togitani K, Machida H, et al. Molecular polymerase chain reaction diagnosis of pulmonary mucormycosis caused by *Cunninghamella bertholletiae*. Respirology 2004;9(3):397–401.
8. Babady NE, Buckwalter SP, Hall L, et al. Detection of *Blastomyces dermatitidis* and *Histoplasma capsulatum* from culture isolates and clinical specimens by use of Real-Time PCR. J Clin Microbiol 2011;49(9):3204–8.
9. Binnicker MJ, Buckwalter SP, Eisberner JJ, et al. Detection of *Coccidioides* species in clinical specimens by Real-Time PCR. J Clin Microbiol 2007;45(1):173–8.
10. Buitrago MJ, Merino P, Puente S, et al. Utility of real-time PCR for the detection of *Paracoccidioides brasiliensis* DNA in the diagnosis of imported paracoccidioidomycosis. Med Mycol 2009;47(8):879–82.
11. Harun A, Blyth CC, Gilgado F, et al. Development and validation of a multiplex PCR for detection of *Scedosporium* spp. in respiratory tract specimens from patients with cystic fibrosis. J Clin Microbiol 2011;49(4):1508–12.
12. Muñoz C, Gómez BL, Tobón A, et al. Validation and clinical application of a molecular method for identification of *Histoplasma capsulatum* in human specimens in Colombia, South America. Clin Vaccine Immunol 2010;17(1):62–7.
13. Sampaio ID, Freire AK, Ogusko MM, et al. Selection and optimization of PCR-based methods for the detection of *Histoplasma capsulatum* var. *capsulatum*. Rev Iberoam Micol 2012;29(1):34–9.
14. Schabereiter-Gurtner C, Selitsch B, Rotter ML, et al. Development of novel real-time PCR assays for detection and differentiation of eleven medically important *Aspergillus* and *Candida* species in clinical specimens. J Clin Microbiol 2007; 45(3):906–14.
15. Vucicevic D, Blair JE, Binnicker MJ, et al. The utility of *Coccidioides* polymerase chain reaction testing in the clinical setting. Mycopathologia 2010;170(5): 345–51.
16. Barton RC. Laboratory diagnosis of invasive aspergillosis: from diagnosis to prediction of outcome. Scientifica (Cairo) 2013;2013:29.

17. Hsu JL, Ruoss SJ, Bower ND, et al. Diagnosing invasive fungal disease in critically ill patients. Crit Rev Microbiol 2011;37(4):277–312.
18. Kourkoumpetis TK, Fuchs BB, Coleman JJ, et al. Polymerase chain reaction-based assays for the diagnosis of invasive fungal infections. Clin Infect Dis 2012;54(9):1322–31.
19. Ostrosky-Zeichner L. Invasive mycoses: diagnostic challenges. Am J Med 2012;125(Suppl 1):S14–24.
20. Putignani L, D'Arezzo S, Paglia MG, et al. DNA-based detection of human pathogenic fungi: dermatophytes, opportunists, and causative agents of deep mycoses. In: Gherbawy Y, Voigt K, editors. Molecular identification of fungi. Berlin: Springer-Verlag; 2010. p. 357–415.
21. Tuon FF. A systematic literature review on the diagnosis of invasive aspergillosis using polymerase chain reaction (PCR) from bronchoalveolar lavage clinical samples. Rev Iberoam Micol 2007;24(2):89–94.
22. de Aguirre L, Hurst SF, Choi JS, et al. Rapid differentiation of *Aspergillus* species from other medically important opportunistic molds and yeasts by PCR-enzyme immunoassay. J Clin Microbiol 2004;42(8):3495–504.
23. Faber J, Moritz N, Henninger N, et al. Rapid detection of common pathogenic *Aspergillus* species by a novel real-time PCR approach. Mycoses 2009;52(3): 228–33.
24. Halliday C, Wu QX, James G, et al. Development of a nested qualitative real-time PCR assay to detect *Aspergillus* species DNA in clinical specimens. J Clin Microbiol 2005;43(10):5366–8.
25. Hansen D, Healy M, Reece K, et al. Repetitive-sequence-based PCR using the DiversiLab system for identification of *Aspergillus* species. J Clin Microbiol 2008;46(5):1835–9.
26. Healy M, Reece K, Walton D, et al. Identification to the species level and differentiation between strains of *Aspergillus* clinical isolates by automated repetitive-sequence-based PCR. J Clin Microbiol 2004;42(9):4016–24.
27. Henry T, Iwen PC, Hinrichs SH. Identification of *Aspergillus* species using internal transcribed spacer regions 1 and 2. J Clin Microbiol 2000;38(4):1510–5.
28. Kami M, Fukui T, Ogawa S, et al. Use of real-time PCR on blood samples for diagnosis of invasive aspergillosis. Clin Infect Dis 2001;33(9):1504–12.
29. Loeffler J, Hebart H, Brauchle U, et al. Comparison between plasma and whole blood specimens for detection of *Aspergillus* DNA by PCR. J Clin Microbiol 2000;38(10):3830–3.
30. Makimura K, Murayama SY, Yamaguchi H. Specific detection of *Aspergillus* and *Penicillium* species from respiratory specimens by polymerase chain reaction (PCR). Jpn J Med Sci Biol 1994;47:141–56.
31. Mancini N, Clerici D, Diotti R, et al. Molecular diagnosis of sepsis in neutropenic patients with haematological malignancies. J Med Microbiol 2008;57(Pt 5):601–4.
32. Pham AS, Tarrand JJ, May GS, et al. Diagnosis of invasive mold infection by real-time quantitative PCR. Am J Clin Pathol 2003;119(1):38–44.
33. Sanguinetti M, Posteraro B, Pagano L, et al. Comparison of real-time PCR, conventional PCR, and galactomannan antigen detection by enzyme-linked immunosorbent assay using bronchoalveolar lavage fluid samples from hematology patients for diagnosis of invasive pulmonary aspergillosis. J Clin Microbiol 2003;41(8):3922–5.
34. Zhao J, Kong F, Li R, et al. Identification of and related species by nested PCR targeting ribosomal DNA internal transcribed spacer regions. J Clin Microbiol 2001;39(6):2261–6.

35. Bretagne S, Costa J, Marmorat-Khuong A, et al. Detection of *Aspergillus* species DNA in bronchoalveolar lavage samples by competitive PCR. J Clin Microbiol 1995;33(5):1164–8.
36. Costa C, Costa JM, Desterke C, et al. Real-time PCR coupled with automated DNA extraction and detection of galactomannan antigen in serum by enzyme-linked immunosorbent assay for diagnosis of invasive aspergillosis. J Clin Microbiol 2002;40(6):2224–7.
37. Costa C, Vidaud D, Olivi M, et al. Development of two real-time quantitative Taq-Man PCR assays to detect circulating *Aspergillus fumigatus* DNA in serum. J Microbiol Methods 2001;44(3):263–9.
38. Rickerts V, Just-Nubling G, Konrad F, et al. Diagnosis of invasive aspergillosis and mucormycosis in immunocompromised patients by seminested PCR assay of tissue samples. Eur J Clin Microbiol Infect Dis 2006;25(1):8–13.
39. Spiess B, Seifarth W, Hummel M, et al. DNA microarray-based detection and identification of fungal pathogens in clinical samples from neutropenic patients. J Clin Microbiol 2007;45(11):3743–53.
40. Duval SM, Donnelly JP, Barnes R, et al. PCR-based methods with aspergillosis as a model. J Invasive Fungal Infect 2008;2(2):46–51.
41. White PL, Bretagne S, Klingspor L, et al. *Aspergillus* PCR: one step closer to standardization. J Clin Microbiol 2010;48(4):1231–40.
42. White PL, Mengoli C, Bretagne S, et al. Evaluation of *Aspergillus* PCR protocols for testing serum specimens. J Clin Microbiol 2011;49(11):3842–8.
43. White PL, Perry MD, Loeffler J, et al. Critical stages of extracting DNA from *Aspergillus fumigatus* in whole-blood specimens. J Clin Microbiol 2010; 48(10):3753–5.
44. Lyon GM, Abdul-Ali D, Loeffler J, et al. Development and evaluation of a calibrator material for nucleic acid-based assays for diagnosing aspergillosis. J Clin Microbiol 2013;51(7):2403–5.
45. White PL, Barton R, Guiver M, et al. A consensus on fungal polymerase chain reaction diagnosis?: a United Kingdom-Ireland evaluation of polymerase chain reaction methods for detection of systemic fungal infections. J Mol Diagn 2006;8(3):376–84.
46. Springer J, Morton CO, Perry M, et al. Multicenter comparison of serum and whole-blood specimens for detection of *Aspergillus* DNA in high-risk hematological patients. J Clin Microbiol 2013;51(5):1445–50.
47. Cahill BC, Hibbs JR, Savik K, et al. *Aspergillus* airway colonization and invasive disease after lung transplantation. Chest 1997;112(5):1160–4.
48. Mengoli C, Cruciani M, Barnes RA, et al. Use of PCR for diagnosis of invasive aspergillosis: systematic review and meta-analysis. Lancet Infect Dis 2009; 9(2):89–96.
49. Lopes da Silva R, Ribeiro P, Abreu N, et al. Early diagnosis of invasive aspergillosis in neutropenic patients. comparison between serum galacto-mannan and polymerase chain reaction. Clin Med Insights Oncol 2010;4: 81–8.
50. Luong ML, Clancy CJ, Vadnerkar A, et al. Comparison of an *Aspergillus* real-time polymerase chain reaction assay with galactomannan testing of bronchoalvelolar lavage fluid for the diagnosis of invasive pulmonary aspergillosis in lung transplant recipients. Clin infect Dis 2011;52(10):1218–26.
51. Suzuki M, Fukazawa Y. Immunochemical characterization of *Candida albicans* cell wall antigens: specific determinant of *Candida albicans* serotype A mannan. Microbiol Immunol 1982;26(5):387–402.

52. Suzuki S. Immunochemical study on mannans of genus *Candida*. I. Structural investigation of antigenic factors 1,4,5,6,8,9,11,13,13b and 34. Curr Top Med Mycol 1997;8:57–70.

53. Avni T, Levy I, Sprecher H, et al. Diagnostic accuracy of PCR alone compared to galactomannan in bronchoalveolar lavage fluid for diagnosis of invasive pulmonary aspergillosis: a systematic review. J Clin Microbiol 2012;50(11): 3652–8.

54. Chagas C. Nova tripanozomiase humana: Estudos sobre a morfologia e o ciclo evolutivo do *Schizotrypanum cruzi* n. gen., n. sp., ajente etiologico de nova entidade mobido do homen. Memórias do Instituto Oswaldo Cruz 1909;1(2): 159–218.

55. Hibbett DS, Binder M, Bischoff JF, et al. A higher-level phylogenetic classification of the Fungi. Mycol Res 2007;111(Pt 5):509–47.

56. Larsen HH, von Linstow ML, Lundgren B, et al. Primary pneumocystis infection in infants hospitalized with acute respiratory tract infection. Emerg Infect Dis 2007;13(1):66–72.

57. Keely SP, Baughman RP, Smulian AG, et al. Source of *Pneumocystis carinii* in recurrent episodes of pneumonia in AIDS patients. AIDS 1996;10(8):881–8.

58. Huang L, Beard CB, Creasman J, et al. Sulfa or sulfone prophylaxis and geographic region predict mutations in the *Pneumocystis carinii* dihydropteroate synthase gene. J Infect Dis 2000;182(4):1192–8.

59. Fischer S, Gill VJ, Kovacs J, et al. The use of oral washes to diagnose *Pneumocystis carinii* pneumonia: a blinded prospective study using a polymerase chain reaction-based detection system. J Infect Dis 2001;184(11):1485–8.

60. Larsen HH, Huang L, Kovacs JA, et al. A prospective, blinded study of quantitative touch-down polymerase chain reaction using oral-wash samples for diagnosis of *Pneumocystis* pneumonia in HIV-infected patients. J Infect Dis 2004; 189(9):1679–83.

61. Larsen HH, Masur H, Kovacs JA, et al. Development and evaluation of a quantitative, touch-down, real-time PCR assay for diagnosing *Pneumocystis carinii* pneumonia. J Clin Microbiol 2002;40(2):490–4.

62. Alanio A, Desoubeaux G, Sarfati C, et al. Real-time PCR assay-based strategy for differentiation between active *Pneumocystis jirovecii* pneumonia and colonization in immunocompromised patients. Clin Microbiol Infect 2011;17(10):1531–7.

63. Fujisawa T, Suda T, Matsuda H, et al. Real-time PCR is more specific than conventional PCR for induced sputum diagnosis of *Pneumocystis* pneumonia in immunocompromised patients without HIV infection. Respirology 2009;14(2): 203–9.

64. Desmet S, Van Wijngaerden E, Maertens J, et al. Serum (1-3)-β-d-glucan as a tool for diagnosis of *Pneumocystis jirovecii* pneumonia in patients with Human Immunodeficiency Virus infection or hematological malignancy. J Clin Microbiol 2009;47(12):3871–4.

65. Sax PE, Komarow L, Finkelman MA, et al. Blood (1->3)-beta-D-glucan as a diagnostic test for HIV-related *Pneumocystis jirovecii* pneumonia. Clin Infect Dis 2011;53(2):197–202.

66. Kawagishi N, Miyagi S, Satoh K, et al. Usefulness of beta-D glucan in diagnosing *Pneumocystis carinii* pneumonia and monitoring its treatment in a living-donor liver-transplant recipient. J Hepatobiliary Pancreat Surg 2007; 14(3):308–11.

67. Tasaka S, Hasegawa N, Kobayashi S, et al. Serum indicators for the diagnosis of pneumocystis pneumonia. Chest 2007;131(4):1173–80.

68. Watanabe T, Yasuoka A, Tanuma J, et al. Serum (1–>3) beta-D-glucan as a noninvasive adjunct marker for the diagnosis of *Pneumocystis* pneumonia in patients with AIDS. Clin Infect Dis 2009;49(7):1128–31.

69. Wakefield AE, Pixley FJ, Banerji S, et al. Detection of *Pneumocystis carinii* with DNA amplification. Lancet 1990;336(8713):451–3.

70. Weig M, Brown AJ. Genomics and the development of new diagnostics and anti-Candida drugs. Trends Microbiol 2007;15(7):310.

71. Alvarez-Martinez MJ, Miro JM, Valls ME, et al. Sensitivity and specificity of nested and real-time PCR for the detection of *Pneumocystis jiroveci* in clinical specimens. Diagn Microbiol Infect Dis 2006;56(2):153–60.

72. Fillaux J, Malvy S, Alvarez M, et al. Accuracy of a routine real-time PCR assay for the diagnosis of *Pneumocystis jirovecii* pneumonia. J Microbiol Methods 2008; 75(2):258–61.

73. Arcenas RC, Uhl JR, Buckwalter SP, et al. A real-time polymerase chain reaction assay for detection of *Pneumocystis* from bronchoalveolar lavage fluid. Diagn Microbiol Infect Dis 2006;54(3):169–75.

Rapid Diagnosis of Influenza: State of the Art

David R. Peaper, MD, PhD[a,b], Marie L. Landry, MD[a,c],*

KEYWORDS

- Influenza • Rapid diagnosis • Antigen • Direct immunofluorescence assays
- Polymerase chain reaction • Nucleic acid amplification tests • Respiratory virus

KEY POINTS

- Rapid influenza antigen tests have lower sensitivity compared to other methods, but newer assays control for some of the factors that may contribute to poor performance.
- Nucleic acid amplified tests are now available that allow for the identification of infection with influenza and other respiratory viruses with high sensitivity in as little 1 hour.
- The best way to clinically implement these assays remains unclear, and many different factors must be considered when choosing an optimal testing algorithm including: patient population tested, required turn-around-time, and testing-driven clinical interventions.
- To help guide both laboratory and provider decision making, studies are urgently needed to determine the clinical utility, impact on outcomes, and cost-effectiveness of rapid antigen and nucleic acid amplification tests for influenza and other respiratory viruses in different patient groups and clinical settings.

INFLUENZA VIRUSES

Influenza viruses are members of the family Orthomyxoviridae. Based on antigenic differences in the matrix (M) protein and the nucleoprotein (NP), influenza viruses are separated into 3 genera: Influenzavirus A, Influenzavirus B, and Influenzavirus C. Because influenza type C causes only mild illness, it is not further considered in this review. Influenza A is further classified into subtypes based on surface proteins hemagglutinin (HA) and neuraminidase (NA). Sixteen HA and 9 NA subtypes are now recognized. Strains have been identified within subtypes, and lineages or clades within strains. Aquatic birds are considered the reservoir of influenza A in nature.[1]

The authors have no conflicts of interest.

[a] Department of Laboratory Medicine, Yale University School of Medicine, 333 Cedar Street, New Haven, CT, USA; [b] Section of Pathology and Laboratory Medicine, VA Connecticut Healthcare System, 950 Campbell Avenue, West Haven, CT 06516, USA; [c] Department of Internal Medicine, Yale University School of Medicine, 333 Cedar Street, New Haven, CT, USA
* Corresponding author. Yale University School of Medicine, PO Box 208035, 333 Cedar Street, New Haven, CT 06520-8035.
E-mail address: marie.landry@yale.edu

Clin Lab Med 34 (2014) 365–385
http://dx.doi.org/10.1016/j.cll.2014.02.009   labmed.theclinics.com
0272-2712/14/$ – see front matter © 2014 Elsevier Inc. All rights reserved.

Influenza A and B genomes have 8 RNA segments encoding structural and nonstructural proteins. When 2 viruses infect the same cell, genetic reassortment can occur with generation of new strains or subtypes. Such reassortment between human and avian virus strains gave rise to the influenza A pandemics of 1957 (H2N2), 1968 (H3N2), and, to some degree, 2009 (H1N1). Swine can be infected with both human and avian viruses, and thus serve as a mixing vessel facilitating emergence of new subtypes that may or may not readily transmit. Some highly pathogenic avian viruses (H5N1 and H7N9) have been transmitted directly from birds to humans, resulting in high mortality but, fortunately to date, low transmissibility.[2] In addition, mutations occur during routine replication that can lead to antigenic change in both influenza types A and B.

The unique ability of influenza viruses to change their genetic and antigenic makeup leads to annual epidemics of illness, hospitalizations, and excess mortality, as well as the continual threat of a new pandemic, with potentially higher morbidity and mortality. For diagnostic laboratories, the challenge is providing assays that detect all circulating strains from year to year. Although tests typically target conserved M or NP genes or proteins, test performance should be validated annually, especially when new viruses emerge.

Pathogenesis

Influenza is transmitted primarily by droplets spread by sneezing and coughing but also by contact with infected surfaces and via small-particle aerosols. After entering the respiratory tract, influenza virions attach via HA envelope proteins to sialic acid receptors on ciliated columnar epithelial cells. After cleavage of the HA by cellular proteases, the virus is endocytosed and replication ensues. An essential step in viral release and infectivity is removal of sialic acid residues from the envelopes of new virions by viral neuraminidase. After an incubation of 1 to 4 days, virus shedding and symptoms appear. Viral shedding lasts for 5 to 10 days, but begins to decrease within 3 to 5 days after symptom onset.[3]

Clinical Presentation

Uncomplicated influenza is characterized by the abrupt onset of malaise, headache, myalgia, and fever, followed by sore throat and nonproductive cough. Children may also develop otitis media, nausea, and vomiting. Influenza typically causes a tracheobronchitis that resolves within a week, but cough and malaise can persist for weeks longer. Complications include febrile seizures in young children, sinusitis, viral pneumonia, secondary bacterial pneumonia, myocarditis, pericarditis, and encephalopathy. Older adults may not present with fever, but rather with decompensation of underlying cardiac or pulmonary conditions. The main focus of influenza management is prevention through vaccination, and annual vaccination is now recommended for all persons older than 6 months.[4]

Treatment

When indicated, treatment should be begun as soon as possible, ideally within 48 hours of onset of symptoms. Thus when suspicion is high, antiviral therapy should be administered without waiting for laboratory confirmation.[5] For severe disease, treatment may still be useful when initiated after 48 hours, and should not be withheld. The adamantanes, amantadine and rimantidine, block the influenza A M2 protein ion channel and thus prevent viral uncoating. However, because of widespread resistance, the adamantanes are no longer recommended for routine use. The neuraminidase inhibitors, oseltamivir and zanamivir, are active against both influenza A and

B. Although resistance has been reported with oseltamivir, most viruses are susceptible at present. Zanamivir is administered via inhalation and, owing to the risk of bronchospasm, is contraindicated in persons with underlying pulmonary disease. For the latest information on treatment of circulating strains, the reader is referred to the Centers for Disease Control and Prevention (CDC) Web site at http://www.cdc.gov/flu/professionals/antivirals/.

GENERAL PRINCIPLES OF LABORATORY DIAGNOSIS OF INFLUENZA INFECTION

For patients with influenza-like illness (ILI), clinical diagnostic efforts should be focused on detection of the virus rather than on antibody response. Samples should be collected ideally within 12 to 36 hours after onset of illness, to initiate antiviral therapy within the recommended 48-hour time frame, and within 72 hours for maximum detection. Factors affecting the performance of influenza diagnostic assays are briefly discussed in **Box 1**.

Viral diagnostic methods have evolved dramatically in the past 20 years, as summarized in **Table 1**. The traditional gold standard of viral diagnostics, conventional cell culture, can require up to 10-14 days to generate final results. Thus the introduction of rapid centrifugation culture, with results in 1 to 2 days, was a great advance. Viral antigen assays such as immunochromatography (IC) or direct immunofluorescence assays (DFA) are capable of yielding results in 10 minutes to 2 hours and are widely

---

Box 1
Factors affecting detection of influenza viruses

Viral Factors

- Genetic variation: primer/probe mismatches; variations in antigens detected by rapid influenza diagnostic tests (RIDTs)

- Site of infection: lower respiratory tract specimens may be optimal for emerging viral strains

Sample Collection Factors

- Inadequate specimen: correct site, but few respiratory cells collected

- Improper specimen: nasopharyngeal swabs are recommended/approved, and other specimens may be suboptimal or nonvalidated

- Improper time of collection: collecting too early (<12 hours) or too late (>72 hours) after symptom onset

Storage and Transport Factors

- Incorrect transport medium: formulations vary, laboratory may have to reject if incorrect

- Improper transport or storage: freezing or prolonged storage reduces viral titers and can promote nucleic acid degradation

- Dilution: samples for RIDT should be minimally diluted in transport media

Testing Factors

- Test choice: different sensitivity of assay classes and assays within class

- Workflow: Storage of specimens before batch testing

- Workload: Suboptimal performance during periods of high testing intensity

- Interpretation: RIDT must be read at specific time for valid results; direct fluorescence assay requires subjective assessment

Table 1
Summary of methods for influenza diagnosis with advantages and limitations

Technique		Assay Time	Advantages	Limitations
Viral isolation	Conventional culture	1–14 d	Allows isolation of many viruses; can detect unexpected or novel viruses; more sensitive than antigen detection	Requires expertise to interpret CPE and maintain cell cultures; some viruses do not grow in routine cultures; biosafety concerns for zoonotic and emerging viruses
	Rapid culture	1–5 d	Most results in 1–2 d; requires less training to interpret IF staining than CPE; use of mixed-cell cultures allows detection of multiple viruses in a single vial	Requires cell culture and IF expertise; detects only targeted viruses; less sensitive than conventional culture; biosafety concerns
Antigen detection	DFA	1–2 h	Can be done on demand as samples arrive in the laboratory; reagents available for 8 respiratory and 4 herpes viruses; can assess sample quality	Requires substantial expertise for accurate results; manual and labor-intensive; requires an adequate number of target cells for valid results
	IC	<30 min	Requires no equipment and little expertise; simply add sample and set timer; approved for use at point of care	Less sensitive than other methods; limited test menu
NAAT	General comments		Most sensitive method; detects viruses that do not grow in culture; more rapid than culture; safer than culture because pathogens are inactivated and disrupted before testing; potential for automation and quantification	Requires specialized equipment and expertise; results variable across laboratories; inhibitors can prevent amplification; cross-contamination leads to false positives; can detect clinically irrelevant viruses; genetic variability can lead to false negative results; few FDA-approved assays
	End-point PCR	5–9 h	Uses inexpensive conventional thermocyclers; less affected by genome variability; highly multiplexed respiratory pathogen assays commercially available	Prone to carryover contamination from amplified products because tube is opened after amplification; slower than real-time methods; expensive and complex detection methods for multiplexed assays
	Real-time PCR	0.5–5 h	Faster, less prone to cross-contamination, readily quantified; laboratory-developed assays can be readily updated; more commercial kits becoming available, including walk-away tests	More prone to falsely negative or low values owing to genetic variations in viral strains; lack of standardization; limited capacity to multiplex

Abbreviations: CPE, cytopathic effect; DFA, direct immunofluorescence assay; FDA, Food and Drug Administration; IC, immunochromatography; IF, immunofluorescence; NAAT, nucleic acid amplification technique; PCR, polymerase chain reaction.

used. Molecular tests are now available that provide high sensitivity with a turnaround time (TAT) of approximately 1 hour. Thus, advancing technology has allowed clinicians to redefine what is considered as rapid testing. Although IC assays are most frequently referred to as rapid flu tests, in this article rapid testing is defined as those assays capable of providing a result in less than 3 hours. This time frame was selected based on recently released nucleic acid amplified tests (NAATs) that can, theoretically, be performed round the clock by core laboratory staff. In considering such assays it will be important to establish their performance characteristics in reference to the gold-standard methods of conventional culture and conventional reverse transcriptase–polymerase chain reaction (RT-PCR) assays.

SAMPLE COLLECTION AND TRANSPORT

Laboratories should provide collection guidelines appropriate to the tests that they offer, including sample type and volume, proper container, transport media or stabilizers if needed, transport temperature, and other special instructions, especially for commercial kits. For optimal results, sample-collection instructions should be strictly followed.

A variety of sample types have been studied for influenza testing (**Box 2**), but nasopharyngeal (NP) swabs were recommended by a recent consensus conference on respiratory virus testing.[6] Increased sensitivity may be seen with NP aspirates and

---

Box 2
Types of specimens for influenza testing

Laboratories validate assays for specific specimen types. Deviation from recommended specimens may lead to test cancellation.

Nasopharyngeal (NP) Swabs

- Insert swab deep into nasopharynx past the point of resistance to collect ciliated respiratory epithelial cells

- Most widely accepted specimen; approved for all assays cleared by Food and Drug Administration (FDA)

- Less expertise to collect, but inadequate specimens not uncommon

- Swab type (flocked or unflocked) and transport media vary by institution

Nasal Washes/Aspirates

- Requires equipment and expertise to collect; more uncomfortable for patient

- Approved for use with some FDA-cleared assays

- Increased sensitivity compared with NP swabs

- May be required for young children

Lower Respiratory Specimens (Bronchoalveolar Lavage, Bronchial Brushing, Induced Sputum)

- Invasive techniques requiring specialized expertise and equipment

- Can help establish cause of pneumonia

- No commercially available FDA-approved tests; requires local validation

Others (Sputum, Throat Swab, Nares Swab)

- Much less well studied

- Variable sensitivity compared with NP swabs/washes/aspirates

NP washes, but these are relatively more invasive and require more expertise to collect.[7] Other specimen types are less widely used.

Once collected, swabs and tissues are usually placed into transport media that may vary with the test method or kit used. Factors associated with specimen transport and storage are summarized in **Box 1**. For laboratories performing tests that have undergone regulatory approval, manufacturers' guidelines for sample type, collection device, and transport should be followed.

DIAGNOSTIC METHODS
Viral Culture

Conventional viral culture has been the traditional gold standard for influenza diagnosis, and remains the comparator method for many commercial assays. Rapid culture techniques have been widely applied for respiratory viruses.[8–10] Culture techniques are discussed in **Box 3**, and have been recently reviewed.[11]

Viral Antigen Detection

Antigen-detection methods do not amplify the virus and are thus less sensitive than culture or NAAT. In addition, assay performance for influenza viruses can vary from year to year because of antigenic variation in circulating strains.[12–14]

Immunofluorescence
For DFA, cells are affixed to glass slides, stained with antibodies coupled to fluorophores, and examined under a fluorescence microscope to visualize viral proteins in infected cells. Cytospin preparation of slides improves results.[15] For respiratory

---

Box 3
Viral culture methods

Conventional Culture

- Multiple cell lines inoculated to increase number of viruses detected
- Examined for 10 to 14 days for the presence of viral cytopathic effect (CPE)
- Time to CPE, CPE morphology, cell line(s) infected suggest potential virus
- Viral identification, usually by immunofluorescence (IF)
- Advantages: Traditional gold standard, sensitive for cultivatable viruses, comprehensive, can detect unexpected or unknown viruses, isolate obtained for further testing (eg, subtype or strain identification, antiviral susceptibility)
- Disadvantages: Requires expertise, potentially long turnaround time, some viruses are noncultivable in common cell cultures, some BSL-3 or BSL-4 pathogens may be inadvertently grown in culture

Rapid Culture

- Mixture of cell lines in a shell vial to increase viruses detected
- IF staining at 24 to 48 hours to assess for cells infected by virus present in specimen
- Pool of IF reagents → up to 8 respiratory pathogens
- Advantages: Detect viruses before CPE is apparent, less expertise than conventional culture
- Disadvantages: Limited number of viruses, requires some expertise, requires cell culture facility and IF microscope, some BSL-3 or BSL-4 pathogens may be inadvertently grown in culture

viruses, a pool of antibodies to several different pathogens can be used to screen a single cell spot for multiple viruses including 7 or 8 respiratory viruses (respiratory syncytial virus [RSV], influenza A and B, parainfluenza types 1, 2, 3, adenovirus, and human metapneumovirus).[16] For samples that screen positive, additional testing is required to identify infecting viruses.

Compared with lateral flow IC (see later discussion), DFA is more sensitive, allows for an assessment of sample adequacy (ie, sufficient numbers of target cells), and can detect multiple viruses in a single test.[17] However, application of DFA is limited by technical requirements (eg, a fluorescence microscope, dark room, and technical expertise),[14] and assay time is one to two hours, which is longer than simpler rapid tests.[18]

Lateral flow IC

IC assays are widely used for the detection of influenza A and B, and separate assays are available for RSV. When used for influenza, these are referred to as rapid influenza diagnostic tests (RIDT), some of which are approved as point-of-care tests. These assays are simple to perform and amenable to round-the-clock testing by laboratory generalists. Samples are minimally manipulated, added to the test kit, and read at 10 to 20 minutes (**Fig. 1**). RIDTs have reduced sensitivity in comparison with other techniques. Factors contributing to reduced test performance are outlined in **Box 1**.

Performance of RIDTs

In a seminal article from the onset of the 2009 H1N1 influenza A pandemic, Ginocchio and colleagues[12] reported the real-world performance of 2 RIDTs compared with DFA, rapid culture, and xTag RVP. The sensitivity of the RIDTs for influenza A was 18%, DFA

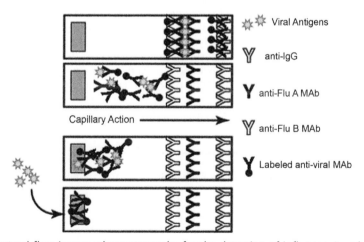

Fig. 1. Lateral flow immunochromatography for the detection of influenza A and B. (*Bottom left*) The patient specimen is applied to a defined area that contains antiviral antibodies labeled with a detection molecule. Next, labeled antibodies with or without bound antigen are drawn along the test strip through capillary action. Antiviral monoclonal antibody and anti–immunoglobulin G (IgG) are immobilized at the distal end of the test strip in well-demarcated areas corresponding to influenza A or influenza B. Viral antigens mediate the retention of labeled antiviral antibodies at the test strip, and anti-IgG binds residual labeled antibodies present. (*Top right*) Visible or fluorescent lines appear at both the test and control locations when viral antigens are present (positive test), or the control location only when antigens are absent (negative test).

was 47% sensitive, and R-mix (Diagnostic Hybrids/Quidel Corp) rapid culture was 89% sensitive compared with RVP. Several factors could have contributed to the reduced sensitivity of RIDT and DFA in this study, including: (1) antigenic variation in viruses; (2) high workload leading to suboptimal performance and interpretation; (3) poor sample quality owing to collection by inexperienced staff; and (4) inherent insensitivity of the assays.

To address the contribution of antigenic variation to analytical sensitivity of RIDTs, the CDC coordinated a study of 11 different RIDTs available in the United States.[19] The CDC prepared stocks of influenza A and B strains recently circulated in the United States. At high concentrations (a 1:10 dilution of stock), all viruses were detected by most of the RIDTs tested, but on further dilution performance quickly fell off such that less than half of the RIDTs were positive for 6 of 23 viruses tested at approximately a 1:30 dilution. At 1:100, some viruses were not detected by any of the 11 RIDTs. This study revealed the marked variability in RIDT detection of different influenza subtypes and strains, and confirmed the need for annual assessment of RIDT performance against circulating viruses.

These differences were further emphasized when the CDC examined the performance of RIDT for the influenza A H3N2v that emerged in the summer of 2012.[20] Several of the assays were able to detect all of the strains tested, but RIDT performance was highly variable.

Three meta-analyses of RIDTs have recently been published (**Table 2**).[21–23] Among these, Chartrand and colleagues[23] looked at 159 studies comparing the performance of 26 different RIDTs with either RT-PCR or culture as the gold standard, and specifically pulled out several different factors from the included studies to perform a comprehensive analysis of RIDT sensitivity and specificity.

Higher sensitivity was seen in studies of children (66.6%) in comparison with adults (53.9%, $P<.001$). Sensitivity was lower for studies using RT-PCR as the gold standard (53.9%) than those using culture (72.3%, $P<.001$). Factors that did not significantly affect RIDT sensitivity were specimen type or testing at the point of care. In reviewing studies in which the duration of patient symptoms were tracked, the highest sensitivity was seen for patients tested between 1 and 3 days from the time of symptom onset.

Two studies performed during the 2009 pandemic found substantially lower specificities than expected.[24,25] However, specificity increased during the course of the flu season, as the nonlaboratory staff performing and interpreting the tests gained expertise.

Table 2
Summary of recent meta-analyses of rapid influenza diagnostic test (RIDT) performance

Authors,[Ref.] Year	Time Period (% Studies)	No. of Studies	No. of RIDTs Studied	Pooled Sensitivity (95% CI) (%)	Pooled Specificity (95% CI) (%)	Reference Method(s)
Babin et al,[21] 2011	2009[a] (100)	14	7	67.5 (66.2–68.9)	80.7 (80.0–81.4)	RT-PCR[b]
Chu et al,[22] 2012	2009[a] (100)	17	7	51 (41–60)	98 (94–99)	RT-PCR[b]
Chartrand et al,[23] 2012	2009[a,c] (35) Non-2009[c] (65)	159	26	62.3 (57.9–66.6)	98.2 (97.5–98.7)	RT-PCR or Culture

Abbreviations: CI, confidence interval; RT-PCR, reverse transcriptase–polymerase chain reaction.
[a] Predominantly pandemic H1N1 influenza A.
[b] RT-PCR was the predominant method.
[c] Study period not specified in 44 studies.

Several manufacturers have developed systems that automate the reading of RIDTs (**Table 3**). Both the Sofia Influenza A + B fluorescent immunoassay (FIA) (Quidel) and the 3M Rapid Detection Flu A + B test use antibodies coupled to fluorescent compounds, whereas the BD Veritor System uses a proprietary enhanced colloidal-gold particle for detection. All 3 devices standardize interpretation among personnel, but the BD Veritor does not have a walk-away function, such that reading time could still vary. Several independent studies of the Sofia,[26–29] Veritor,[30] and 3M Rapid Detection system[12,31,32] have been published.

Taken together, these studies confirm, to a high degree of certainty, what had previously been reported, namely that both the clinical and analytical sensitivities of RIDTs are less than those of other methods including DFA, culture, and RT-PCR. These studies did not address the clinical utility or cost-effectiveness of RIDTs. Because of the low sensitivity of RIDTs, there has been an impetus to develop molecular assays that can provide both high sensitivity and a relatively rapid TAT.

Nucleic Acid Detection

Molecular methods for virus detection have gained favor because (1) their sensitivity is equal to or exceeds that of culture, (2) they can be quantitative, (3) they can detect viruses that are otherwise unculturable, (4) their TAT is a day or less, (5) multiplexed methods allow for the detection of multiple analytes in a single test, and (6) extraction renders the virus noninfectious. NAATs have been historically restricted to larger academic centers and reference laboratories, but the recent development of kits approved by the Food and Drug Administration (FDA) and less complex assays has allowed for these highly sensitive methods to become more widely used.

Conventional PCR

Conventional PCR consists of 3 steps: extraction and purification of nucleic acid, amplification of target sequences using specific primers and DNA polymerase, and detection of amplified fragments (**Box 4**, **Fig. 2**). The 3 steps must be performed in separate spaces with unidirectional workflow so as to limit cross-contamination and false-positive results. For RNA viruses such as influenza viruses, viral RNA must first be reverse transcribed to cDNA before PCR amplification (ie, RT-PCR). Assays in which amplified products are analyzed independently of the amplification step are

		Flu A Sensitivity[b] (95% CI) (%)	Flu A Specificity[b] (95% CI) (%)	Flu B Sensitivity[b] (95% CI) (%)	Flu B Specificity[b] (95% CI) (%)	Walk-Away
Assay	Comparator					
Quidel Sofia Influenza A + B	Culture	97 (91–99)	95 (93–96)	90 (83–95)	97 (95–98)	Yes
BD Veritor	RT-PCR	81.3[c] (70.0–88.9)	97.4[c] (94.4–98.8)	85.6[c] (76.8–91.4)	99.0[c] (96.5–99.7)	No
3M Direct Detection Flu A+ B	Culture	80.3 (68.7–89.1)	96.6 (94.8–97.9)	58.3 (27.7–84.8)	98.0 (96.6–99.0)	Yes

Table 3
Performance of RIDTs with automated readers[a]

[a] Data derived from product inserts accessed from company Web sites, October 2013.
[b] Sensitivity and specificity shown for nasopharyngeal swabs.
[c] Positive percent agreement and negative percent agreement shown on product insert.

Box 4
Conventional nucleic acid amplification steps

Extraction: Isolate nucleic acids and remove inhibitors

- Automated extractors commonly used for high-volume testing
- Multiple parameters vary: extracted volume, washing, elution volume, DNA, RNA, or total nucleic acid recovery
- Extraction protocols may vary among laboratories using same assay, thus must interpret literature carefully

Amplification: Increase amount of target nucleic acids to facilitate detection

- Polymerase chain reaction is the most common technique
- Sensitivity and specificity are strongly affected by primers used
- Targeted genes can be specific for subtypes (eg, influenza A hemagglutinin) or broadly reactive (eg, influenza A matrix)
- Primer mismatches and falsely negative results may occur in evolving/mutating viruses

Detection: Detect amplified nucleic acids

- Agarose gel electrophoresis with ethidium staining or dot-blot hybridization
- New highly multiplexed conventional methods use novel detection methods

---

end-point PCR assays, whereas those whereby amplification and detection occur simultaneously are said to be real-time PCR assays. The advantages and disadvantages of these assay formats are listed in **Table 1**. Laboratories have generally moved from end-point to real-time PCR assays, but several highly multiplexed commercial kits for the detection of respiratory viruses use end-point methods.

Real-time PCR
Real-time PCR methods have had a major impact on diagnostic testing by combining amplification and detection into one step (see **Fig. 2**). This combination shortens assay

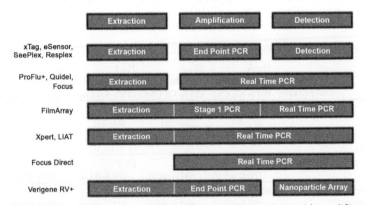

Fig. 2. Workflow of commercially available influenza virus nucleic acid amplification test. Proprietary detection methods are used by xTag, eSensor, SeePlex, and Resplex assays. Black boxes indicate steps performed on a single instrument, white spaces indicate requirement to move samples to new instrument, and white lines indicate discrete processes occurring on a single instrument. Processes are not drawn to scale. PCR, polymerase chain reaction.

time, reduces amplicon cross-contamination because the reaction tube is not opened, and allows visualization of amplification results as they are unfolding in real time. All steps can be performed in one room. Real-time PCR methods use nonsequence specific fluorescent DNA binding dyes such as SYBR Green or sequence-specific fluorescent DNA probes. Thus, real-time assays require the use of thermocyclers with built-in light sources, filters, and detectors.

Assays using SYBR dyes gain their specificity through a melt-curve analysis wherein fluorescence is monitored with increasing temperature after completion of a certain number of cycles. The melting of double-stranded DNA occurs in a sequence-specific manner, and this is associated with a change in detectable fluorescence. One of the most common real-time PCR assays uses hydrolysis probes (eg, TaqMan probes) that contain a reporter fluorophore and quencher in close proximity. When the probe is intact, fluorescence from the reporter is quenched, but when the probe binds to a DNA segment undergoing amplification, the 5'-3' nuclease activity of Taq polymerase degrades the probe, releasing the reporter from the quencher and leading to detectable fluorescence. For assays using this design, specificity is determined by both primer and probe sequences, and although a product may be amplified, mismatches in the probe might lead to failed hydrolysis and no detectable fluorescence. Other real-time assay designs circumvent this problem by incorporating the fluorescent reporter and quencher into the primer itself.

Several different thermocyclers are commercially available. These devices differ in the mechanism by which temperature cycling occurs (eg, metal blocks, heated air), reaction vessels (eg, 96-well plates, capillary tubes, proprietary cartridges), and fluorescent channels available, among other parameters. These factors determine how quickly reactions can take place, the number of analytes that may be detected, and compatibility with commercial assays.

Multiplex methods

Multiplexing refers to the detection of more than 1 analyte in a sample in a single test reaction. Real-time PCR instruments contain several different filters and/or light sources that allow for the detection of up to 6 different fluorophores, but given the need for internal controls and a reference dye, these instruments are limited to only 3- or 4-plexing. There are several different assays commercially available capable of detecting influenza A, influenza B, and RSV, as well as an internal control.[13,14]

Several manufacturers have developed novel methods to multiplex up to 20 different targets. For respiratory pathogens, BioFire, Luminex, and GenMark have FDA-cleared highly multiplexed assays. Other companies including Seegene, Qiagen, and Nanosphere have highly multiplexed respiratory pathogen panels that may be available for in vitro diagnostics (IVD) or as research-use only (RUO) tests depending on laboratory location. The BioFire FilmArray and Nanosphere Verigene are discussed herein, and recent reviews in *Clinics in Laboratory Medicine* discussed the Luminex and Genmark systems.[33]

RAPID NAAT FOR THE DETECTION OF INFLUENZA VIRUSES

TAT for current molecular assays can vary from 30 minutes to 9 hours from start to finish, and many real-time PCR assays can go from sample to result in approximately 5 hours. However, this does not likely reflect true clinical TAT because the assay workflow is not compatible with random access/on-demand processing and testing. Extraction and amplification/detection instruments are often not designed to be used for a single specimen, and laboratory protocols often require several controls for each assay run, leading to rapidly escalating reagent costs for each single sample run. Because of this, most laboratories perform NAAT for influenza viruses in batches with the frequency of runs determined by staffing, workload, and clinical need. This strategy delays clinical TAT beyond the actual time required to perform the assays.

Description of the Systems

In the past 3 years, 5 NAATs designed to be random-access and capable of giving results in less than 3 hours have been cleared by the FDA for the detection of influenza A and B (**Table 4**). These assays use several unique modifications to the traditional extraction/amplification/detection workflow required for conventional NAATs (see **Fig. 2**). Most test systems are not amenable to the implementation of laboratory-developed tests (LDTs) because of their proprietary disposables. However, all are classified as moderately complex, allowing for performance by a much broader spectrum of laboratory personnel, and hands-on requirements are minimal regarding both time and manipulation.

Focus Diagnostics released an FDA-cleared highly complex multiplexed real-time RT-PCR assay for the detection of influenza A, influenza B, and RSV in 2011 that required a separate extraction step, but Focus has subsequently received FDA clearance for a Flu A/B & RSV Direct (no extraction) assay that uses a larger sample input volume than is possible on its previous assay. Focus has several other FDA-cleared assays available for this platform, and several analyte-specific reagent assays are available for bacterial and viral targets. The platform is amenable to implementation of LDTs including fully home-brew assays, but adapting existing assays to new platforms may not be straightforward.

The GeneXpert Flu assay components are found in a self-contained cartridge in which a series of chambers house appropriate reagents and are used for different assay functions. There are several other assays available for use on the GeneXpert system, including viral, bacterial, and other tests.

The FilmArray uses a series of different chambers in a mylar pouch to separate extraction, first-stage amplification, and second-stage amplification/real-time detection of respiratory pathogens. It uses a nested PCR approach whereby products from a first-stage PCR reaction that amplifies targets from several pathogens are diluted into a pathogen-specific second-stage PCR array. During second-stage PCR, amplification is detected in real time through a target-independent DNA-binding dye, and amplification specificity is confirmed by melt-curve analysis. Throughput is limited to 1 specimen per instrument. A highly multiplexed assay for the detection of bacterial and fungal pathogens from blood cultures was recently FDA-cleared on the BioFire instrument.

The Verigene system uses gold nanoparticles as a novel means to detect amplified nucleic acids. Samples undergo extraction, RT-PCR, and incubation with slide-immobilized gold nanoparticles in a single-use cartridge in the Verigene processor. Slides are then removed from the processor, and the presence of analytes is detected by the reader. A processor is occupied continuously by a specimen, potentially limiting throughput. A highly multiplexed respiratory virus assay with an additional 9 respiratory pathogens is currently an RUO test. Verigene has other clinical diagnostics assays, for both microbiology and human genetics/pharmacogenetics applications, all FDA-cleared on this platform.

Like the GeneXpert, the iQuum LIAT influenza A/B assay is performed in a self-contained test cartridge, and the influenza A/B assay is the only test currently available on this platform. Like the FilmArray and Verigene, each LIAT analyzer can handle only 1 test at a time, potentially limiting throughput.

Table 4
Rapid nucleic acid amplification test for influenza (TAT <3 hours)

Assay	Manufacturer	Pathogens Detected	Unique Instrumentation (Other Assays)	TAT (h)	Throughput	Refs.
Flu A/B/RSV Direct	Focus	Influenza A, influenza B, RSV	3M Integrated Cycler (Yes)	1.25	Up to 8 samples/instrument/run	34
Xpert Flu	Cepheid	Influenza A, influenza A 2009 H1, influenza B	Gene Xpert (Yes)	1.25	Variable[a]	35–39
FilmArray	BioFire	Influenza A (H1, H3, 2009 H1), influenza B, adenovirus, parainfluenza 1, 2, 3, 4, RSV, hMPV, rhinovirus/enterovirus, coronaviruses HKU1, NL63, 229E, OC43, Bordetella pertussis, Chlamydophila pneumoniae, Mycoplasma pneumoniae	FilmArray (Yes)	1.25	1 sample/instrument/run[b]	31–33,40–46
Respiratory Virus Plus	Nanosphere	Influenza A (H1, H3, 2009 H1), influenza B, RSV (A & B)[c]	Verigene Processor & Reader (Yes)	2.5	1 sample/processor/run[b]	46–48
LIAT	IQuum	Influenza A, influenza B	LIAT Analyzer (No)	0.5	1 sample/instrument/run[b]	None

Abbreviations: hMPV, human metapneumovirus; RSV, respiratory syncytial virus; TAT, turnaround time.
[a] Modular instrumentation with 1, 4, 16, or 80 possible positions.
[b] Instruments with small footprints to facilitate placement of multiple instruments to increase throughput.
[c] Oseltamivir call-out is available outside the United States.

Assay Performance

These newly developed assays have been available for only a short time, and comparison studies are limited. All have been subjected to FDA review, and the publicly available results from their FDA-clearance documents and product inserts suggest sensitivity and specificity consistent with many NAATs. However, for regulatory approval only the GeneXpert Flu was compared with a NAAT, and all others were compared with culture. NAATs are generally more sensitive than culture, thus this would lead to an overestimation of the sensitivity of these assays. Finally, all data from FDA trials are likely obtained under ideal circumstances and may not represent real-world performance. Thus, the sensitivities and specificities determined during FDA trials may not be borne out by subsequent postmarketing studies using NAAT as the gold standard (see later discussion).

The performance of the FilmArray has been the most thoroughly assessed, with at least 10 different comparison studies published.[35–39,42–46] Among these, only Van Wesenbeeck and colleagues[39] compared 2 assays with a TAT of less than 3 hours, the FilmArray and Verigene RV+. Five of the studies compared the FilmArray with other highly multiplexed assays including the Luminex RVP and RVP Fast, Qiagen ResPlex II, and GenMark eSensor. Others used LDTs or the Prodesse ProFlu+ as their comparator method. Not all studies differentiated among influenza A subtypes. The sensitivity of the influenza A assay ranged from 90.2% to 100%, and specificity was 100% in all studies. Detection of influenza B was between 77.3% and 100% sensitive, with 100% specificity across all studies. Performance of the FilmArray for influenza A subtypes was variable. Nearly all of these reports also compared the performance of the other analytes contained in the FilmArray panel either through comparison with other highly multiplexed tests, other commercial assays, or LDTs.

The Xpert Flu assay has been examined in several studies in comparison with the xTag RVP, several different LDTs, the ProFlu+, and/or culture.[34,47–50] These studies found sensitivity between 78.8% and 100% with 99.4% to 100% specificity for influenza A, and sensitivity between 76.5% and 100% and specificity of 100% for influenza B. However, the original Xpert Flu assay was released in 2011, and a reformulated version of the assay with an additional primer pair for influenza A was released in late 2012/early 2013; the published studies do not specify which version of the assay was used.

Three studies have examined the performance of the Verigene RV+ in comparison with other NAATs including the extracted Focus Flu A/B & RSV and ProFlu+, among others.[39,51,52] Sensitivity in 2 studies exceeded 96.6% with 100% specificity for influenza A, but a third study found sensitivity of only 84.7% with a high invalid rate.[39] Performance of the RV+ for influenza B was only assessed in one study, and was 100% sensitive and 99.4% specific.[52]

No studies examining the performance of the iQuum LIAT have been published, and only one study of the Focus Flu A/B & RSV Direct kit has been published. Woodberry and colleagues[53] found only an 86.4% positive agreement for influenza A and 36.8% for influenza B, but the investigators suspected a thermocycler malfunction could have negatively affected assay performance, especially that of influenza B. Two studies compared the performance of the 96-well Focus Flu A/B & RSV kit without extraction, and found much higher sensitivities and specificities for both influenza A and B.[54,55] However, Alby and colleagues[51] used the FDA-cleared extracted protocol and assay, and found sensitivities of 82.8% and 76.2% for influenza A and B, respectively.

These studies are of varying quality and sample size, mixture of prospective and retrospective designs, and performance during years with limited circulating strains.

Nonetheless, they demonstrate the potential real-world performance of assays. With only a few exceptions, these studies fail to address an important question: how does the performance compare among influenza NAAT with rapid TAT? Few head-to-head comparisons of rapid NAATs have been performed, and these studies are needed to help laboratories make informed decisions about assay selection.

Limitations and Future Developments

There are no currently available NAATs capable of delivering high-order multiplexing, TAT of less than 3 hours, and high throughput. Reagent and instrumentation costs are also substantial for many of these assays. Furthermore, influenza test volumes are fairly seasonal, and instrumentation dedicated to only influenza testing will likely sit idle for many months of the year. Most of the testing platforms discussed here have limited test menus that may not have assays with sufficient volumes to be performed year-round. Conversely, instruments with appropriate demand throughout the year may be unable to handle the increased volume associated with influenza season.

The GeneXpert, Focus Diagnostics, and LIAT assays all rely on real-time PCR, and the degree of multiplexing available on these platforms is intrinsically limited to the ability of their instruments to detect multiple fluorophores. Changing the viruses detected is possible (eg, RSV instead of 2009 H1 influenza A), but this would require new regulatory approval. By contrast, the Verigene and FilmArray systems are capable of high-order multiplexing for the simultaneous detection of 15 to 20 respiratory pathogens and/or pathogen subtypes, but throughput can be limiting on these instruments.

FACTORS TO CONSIDER

In selecting an assay, it is essential to identify why testing will be performed and whether multiplexed testing may be appropriate (**Table 5**). Several studies have been performed to assess the clinical impact of rapid influenza testing, and these

Table 5 Considerations for adoption of rapid respiratory virus testing		
Testing Rationale	**Focused Influenza Testing**	**Multiplexed Testing**
Limit unnecessary testing	Known pathogen capable of causing severe disease Evidence to support	Theoretically better to detect more pathogens Unclear significance of coronaviruses, rhinoviruses No data to support
Patient cohorting	Need sensitive test May miss other pathogens requiring precautions	More pathogens detected limiting nosocomial spread Detection of coinfections Unclear how to respond to coronaviruses, rhinoviruses
Limit antibiotics	Known pathogen capable of causing severe disease Evidence to support	Theoretically better to detect more pathogens Unclear how to respond to coronaviruses, rhinoviruses No data to support
Targeted anti-influenza therapy	Theoretical benefit Empiric/clinician-guided therapy may be more cost-effective	No benefit

are split between asking 2 related, but different questions: (1) does the immediate availability of a rapid influenza test affect care, or (2) does a positive rapid influenza test affect care?

Several randomized studies compared triage-based protocol testing (ie, test results were available before the patient was seen) with standard care, and, although the results of these trials were mixed, they suggest that the availability of a rapid influenza test can decrease diagnostic evaluation, antibiotic utilization, and both the length and cost of visit in the emergency room.[56–61] Results were most pronounced for individuals testing positive for influenza, but not all studies performed this analysis, and trials were not necessarily powered to make these comparisons. All of these studies looked at only pediatric patients in an emergency room/urgent care setting. A recent meta-analysis of 5 studies recently concluded that RIDT use can reduce some diagnostic testing, but larger adequately powered studies are needed to fully address this issue.[62]

Several nonrandomized studies included adults and inpatients and used chart review to compare individuals testing positive for influenza with those testing negative.[63–67] These studies found decreased antibiotic usage and reduced length of visit/length of stay among individuals testing influenza positive. In one study among hospitalized adults with cardiopulmonary disease, a positive RIDT led to reduced antibiotic use and increased antiviral therapy. However, several influenza-positive adults continued to receive antibiotics, leading the investigators to conclude that better tools are needed to exclude bacterial infections and further reduce antibiotic utilization.[64]

Very few studies assessed whether rapid influenza testing availability or result affected the prescription of antivirals, which is likely due to the number of studies that examined only children. Two studies showed that antiviral prescriptions were appropriately increased among patients testing positive for influenza.[59,64] No studies examined the impact of rapid influenza testing on bed-management decisions beyond admission to hospital or discharge from the emergency department in a systematic manner.

All of the previously cited studies used either an RIDT or a 7-virus DFA for rapid testing, and studies of molecular tests are limited. Oosterheert and colleagues[68] examined the contribution of a PCR panel for viral and atypical bacterial pathogens on hospitalized adults, and although PCR increased the diagnostic yield and cost of care, there was no difference in antibiotic utilization for patients with available PCR results. The clinical impact of the BioFire FilmArray has been reported in one study that found decreased TAT compared with previous years, and timely prescription of oseltamivir.[69]

Many of the arguments put forth to rationalize rapid influenza testing also hold true for highly multiplexed assays, but this has not been studied in depth. Testing specifically for adenovirus by DFA affected the differential diagnosis, diagnostic evaluation, and management of hospitalized children.[70] Byington and colleagues[65] found that results of RSV testing in a 7-virus DFA also affect patient care. For well-characterized respiratory pathogens, identification of a potentially causative agent could be beneficial, but sensitive multiplex assays lead to higher rates of identification of coinfection and infection with agents associated with the common cold such as rhinovirus or human coronaviruses. In the former cases, it can be difficult to determine the virus responsible for the patient's current presentation. Rhinoviruses and coronaviruses can cause more severe disease, especially in immunocompromised hosts, yet may be disregarded as normal flora by some providers. Alternatively, symptoms may be ascribed to these viruses when other processes may be contributing to disease.

SUMMARY

It is now possible to identify infection with influenza and other respiratory viruses with high sensitivity in as little 1 hour. Manufacturers are also developing more advanced point-of-care IC assays that seek to minimize the known limitations of many RIDTs. Thus, laboratories and institutions have a wide variety of assays and platforms from which to choose when implementing rapid influenza testing.

The best way to clinically implement these assays remains unclear, and many different factors must be considered when choosing an optimal testing algorithm. The use, interpretation, and impact of rapid respiratory virus assays vary among children, adults, outpatients, inpatients, the immunosuppressed, and so forth. The patient population served is among the most important considerations when deciding whether to test, and clinician guidance and education are needed if optimal interventions are to occur. To help guide both laboratory and provider decision making, studies are urgently needed to determine the clinical utility, impact on outcomes, and cost-effectiveness of rapid antigen and NAATs for influenza and other respiratory viruses in different patient groups and clinical settings.

REFERENCES

1. Altmar RL, Lindstrom SE. Influenza viruses. In: Versalovic J, Carroll KC, Funke G, et al, editors. Manual of clinical microbiology. 10th edition. Washington, DC: ASM Press; 2011. p. 1333–46.
2. Yu H, Cowling BJ, Feng L, et al. Human infection with avian influenza A H7N9 virus: an assessment of clinical severity. Lancet 2013;382(9887): 138–45.
3. Hayden FG, Palese P. Influenza virus. In: Richman DD, Whitley RJ, Hayden FG, editors. Clinical virology. Washington, DC: ASM Press; 2009. p. 943–76.
4. Centers for Disease Control and Prevention (CDC). Prevention and control of seasonal influenza with vaccines. Recommendations of the Advisory Committee on Immunization Practices—United States, 2013-2014. MMWR Recomm Rep 2013;62(RR-07):1–43.
5. Harper SA, Bradley JS, Englund JA, et al. Seasonal influenza in adults and children—diagnosis, treatment, chemoprophylaxis, and institutional outbreak management: clinical practice guidelines of the Infectious Diseases Society of America. Clin Infect Dis 2009;48(8):1003–32.
6. Ginocchio CC, McAdam AJ. Current best practices for respiratory virus testing. J Clin Microbiol 2011;49(Suppl 9):S44–8.
7. Debyle C, Bulkow L, Miernyk K, et al. Comparison of nasopharyngeal flocked swabs and nasopharyngeal wash collection methods for respiratory virus detection in hospitalized children using real-time polymerase chain reaction. J Virol Methods 2012;185(1):89–93.
8. Fong CK, Lee MK, Griffith BP. Evaluation of R-Mix FreshCells in shell vials for detection of respiratory viruses. J Clin Microbiol 2000;38(12):4660–2.
9. Huang YT, Turchek BM. Mink lung cells and mixed mink lung and A549 cells for rapid detection of influenza virus and other respiratory viruses. J Clin Microbiol 2000;38(1):422–3.
10. Weinberg A, Brewster L, Clark J, et al. Evaluation of R-Mix shell vials for the diagnosis of viral respiratory tract infections. J Clin Virol 2004;30(1): 100–5.
11. Leland DS, Ginocchio CC. Role of cell culture for virus detection in the age of technology. Clin Microbiol Rev 2007;20(1):49–78.

12. Ginocchio CC, Zhang F, Manji R, et al. Evaluation of multiple test methods for the detection of the novel 2009 influenza A (H1N1) during the New York City outbreak. J Clin Virol 2009;45(3):191–5.

13. Centers for Disease Control and Prevention. Performance of rapid influenza diagnostic tests during two school outbreaks of 2009 pandemic influenza A (H1N1) virus infection—Connecticut, 2009. MMWR Morb Mortal Wkly Rep 2009;58(37):1029–32.

14. Landry ML, Ferguson D. Cytospin-enhanced immunofluorescence and impact of sample quality on detection of novel swine origin (H1N1) influenza virus. J Clin Microbiol 2010;48(3):957–9.

15. Doing KM, Jerkofsky MA, Dow EG, et al. Use of fluorescent-antibody staining of cytocentrifuge-prepared smears in combination with cell culture for direct detection of respiratory viruses. J Clin Microbiol 1998;36(7):2112–4.

16. Landry ML, Ferguson D. SimulFluor respiratory screen for rapid detection of multiple respiratory viruses in clinical specimens by immunofluorescence staining. J Clin Microbiol 2000;38(2):708–11.

17. Chan EL, Brandt K, Horsman GB. Comparison of Chemicon SimulFluor direct fluorescent antibody staining with cell culture and shell vial direct immunoperoxidase staining for detection of herpes simplex virus and with cytospin direct immunofluorescence staining for detection of varicella-zoster virus. Clin Diagn Lab Immunol 2001;8(5):909–12.

18. Landry ML. Developments in immunologic assays for respiratory viruses. Clin Lab Med 2009;29(4):635–47.

19. Centers for Disease Control and Prevention. Evaluation of 11 commercially available rapid influenza diagnostic tests—United States, 2011-2012. MMWR Morb Mortal Wkly Rep 2012;61(43):873–6.

20. Balish A, Garten R, Klimov A, et al. Analytical detection of influenza A(H3N2)v and other A variant viruses from the USA by rapid influenza diagnostic tests. Influenza Other Respir Viruses 2013;7(4):491–6.

21. Babin SM, Hsieh YH, Rothman RE, et al. A meta-analysis of point-of-care laboratory tests in the diagnosis of novel 2009 swine-lineage pandemic influenza A (H1N1). Diagn Microbiol Infect Dis 2011;69(4):410–8.

22. Chu H, Lofgren ET, Halloran ME, et al. Performance of rapid influenza H1N1 diagnostic tests: a meta-analysis. Influenza Other Respir Viruses 2012;6(2):80–6.

23. Chartrand C, Leeflang MM, Minion J, et al. Accuracy of rapid influenza diagnostic tests: a meta-analysis. Ann Intern Med 2012;156(7):500–11.

24. Likitnukul S, Boonsiri K, Tangsuksant Y. Evaluation of sensitivity and specificity of rapid influenza diagnostic tests for novel swine-origin influenza A (H1N1) virus. Pediatr Infect Dis J 2009;28(11):1038–9.

25. Sambol AR, Abdalhamid B, Lyden ER, et al. Use of rapid influenza diagnostic tests under field conditions as a screening tool during an outbreak of the 2009 novel influenza virus: practical considerations. J Clin Virol 2010;47(3):229–33.

26. Lee CK, Cho CH, Woo MK, et al. Evaluation of Sofia fluorescent immunoassay analyzer for influenza A/B virus. J Clin Virol 2012;55(3):239–43.

27. Lewandrowski K, Tamerius J, Menegus M, et al. Detection of influenza A and B viruses with the Sofia analyzer: a novel, rapid immunofluorescence-based in vitro diagnostic device. Am J Clin Pathol 2013;139(5):684–9.

28. Rath B, Tief F, Obermeier P, et al. Early detection of influenza A and B infection in infants and children using conventional and fluorescence-based rapid testing. J Clin Virol 2012;55(4):329–33.

29. Leonardi GP, Wilson AM, Zuretti AR. Comparison of conventional lateral-flow assays and a new fluorescent immunoassay to detect influenza viruses. J Virol Methods 2013;189(2):379–82.

30. Peters TR, Blakeney E, Vannoy L, et al. Evaluation of the limit of detection of the BD Veritor™ system flu A+B test and two rapid influenza detection tests for influenza virus. Diagn Microbiol Infect Dis 2013;75(2):200–2.

31. Ginocchio CC, Lotlikar M, Falk L, et al. Clinical performance of the 3M Rapid Detection Flu A+B Test compared to R-Mix culture, DFA and BinaxNOW Influenza A&B test. J Clin Virol 2009;45(2):146–9.

32. Dale SE, Mayer C, Mayer MC, et al. Analytical and clinical sensitivity of the 3M rapid detection influenza A+B assay. J Clin Microbiol 2008;46(11):3804–7.

33. Buller RS. Molecular detection of respiratory viruses. Clin Lab Med 2013;33(3): 439–60.

34. Salez N, Ninove L, Thirion L, et al. Evaluation of the Xpert Flu test and comparison with in-house real-time RT-PCR assays for detection of influenza virus from 2008 to 2011 in Marseille, France. Clin Microbiol Infect 2012;18(4):E81–3.

35. Hammond SP, Gagne LS, Stock SR, et al. Respiratory virus detection in immunocompromised patients with FilmArray respiratory panel compared to conventional methods. J Clin Microbiol 2012;50(10):3216–21.

36. Renaud C, Crowley J, Jerome KR, et al. Comparison of FilmArray Respiratory Panel and laboratory-developed real-time reverse transcription-polymerase chain reaction assays for respiratory virus detection. Diagn Microbiol Infect Dis 2012;74(4):379–83.

37. Couturier MR, Barney T, Alger G, et al. Evaluation of the FilmArray® Respiratory Panel for clinical use in a large children's hospital. J Clin Lab Anal 2013;27(2): 148–54.

38. Popowitch EB, O'Neill SS, Miller MB. Comparison of the Biofire FilmArray RP, Genmark eSensor RVP, Luminex xTAG RVPv1, and Luminex xTAG RVP fast multiplex assays for detection of respiratory viruses. J Clin Microbiol 2013; 51(5):1528–33.

39. Van Wesenbeeck L, Meeuws H, Van Immerseel A, et al. Comparison of the FilmArray RP, Verigene RV+, and Prodesse ProFLU+/FAST+ multiplex platforms for detection of influenza viruses in clinical samples from the 2011-2012 influenza season in Belgium. J Clin Microbiol 2013;51(9):2977–85.

40. Legoff J, Kara R, Moulin F, et al. Evaluation of the one-step multiplex real-time reverse transcription-PCR ProFlu-1 assay for detection of influenza A and influenza B viruses and respiratory syncytial viruses in children. J Clin Microbiol 2008;46(2):789–91.

41. Liao RS, Tomalty LL, Majury A, et al. Comparison of viral isolation and multiplex real-time reverse transcription-PCR for confirmation of respiratory syncytial virus and influenza virus detection by antigen immunoassays. J Clin Microbiol 2009; 47(3):527–32.

42. Rand KH, Rampersaud H, Houck HJ. Comparison of two multiplex methods for detection of respiratory viruses: FilmArray RP and xTAG RVP. J Clin Microbiol 2011;49(7):2449–53.

43. Loeffelholz MJ, Pong DL, Pyles RB, et al. Comparison of the FilmArray Respiratory Panel and Prodesse real-time PCR assays for detection of respiratory pathogens. J Clin Microbiol 2011;49(12):4083–8.

44. Pierce VM, Elkan M, Leet M, et al. Comparison of the Idaho Technology FilmArray system to real-time PCR for detection of respiratory pathogens in children. J Clin Microbiol 2012;50(2):364–71.

45. Hayden RT, Gu Z, Rodriguez A, et al. Comparison of two broadly multiplexed PCR systems for viral detection in clinical respiratory tract specimens from immunocompromised children. J Clin Virol 2012;53(4):308–13.

46. Babady NE, Mead P, Stiles J, et al. Comparison of the Luminex xTAG RVP Fast assay and the Idaho Technology FilmArray RP assay for detection of respiratory viruses in pediatric patients at a cancer hospital. J Clin Microbiol 2012;50(7): 2282–8.

47. Sambol AR, Iwen PC, Pieretti M, et al. Validation of the Cepheid Xpert Flu A real time RT-PCR detection panel for emergency use authorization. J Clin Virol 2010; 48(4):234–8.

48. Popowitch EB, Rogers E, Miller MB. Retrospective and prospective verification of the Cepheid Xpert influenza virus assay. J Clin Microbiol 2011;49(9):3368–9.

49. Novak-Weekley SM, Marlowe EM, Poulter M, et al. Evaluation of the Cepheid Xpert Flu Assay for rapid identification and differentiation of influenza A, influenza A 2009 H1N1, and influenza B viruses. J Clin Microbiol 2012;50(5): 1704–10.

50. Li M, Brenwald N, Bonigal S, et al. Rapid diagnosis of influenza: an evaluation of two commercially available RT-PCR assays. J Infect 2012;65(1):60–3.

51. Alby K, Popowitch EB, Miller MB. Comparative evaluation of the Nanosphere Verigene RV+ assay and the Simplexa Flu A/B & RSV Kit for detection of influenza and respiratory syncytial viruses. J Clin Microbiol 2013;51(1):352–3.

52. Boku S, Naito T, Murai K, et al. Near point-of-care administration by the attending physician of the rapid influenza antigen detection immunochromatography test and the fully automated respiratory virus nucleic acid test: contribution to patient management. Diagn Microbiol Infect Dis 2013;76(4):445–9.

53. Woodberry MW, Shankar R, Cent A, et al. Comparison of the Simplexa FluA/B & RSV direct assay and laboratory-developed real-time PCR assays for detection of respiratory virus. J Clin Microbiol 2013;51(11):3883–5.

54. Ko SY, Jang JW, Song DJ, et al. Evaluation of the Simplexa Flu A/B and RSV test for the rapid detection of influenza viruses. J Med Virol 2013;85(12): 2160–4.

55. Hindiyeh M, Kolet L, Meningher T, et al. Evaluation of Simplexa™ Flu A/B & RSV for the direct detection of influenza viruses (A, B) and respiratory syncytial virus in patient clinical samples. J Clin Microbiol 2013;51(7):2421–4.

56. Poehling KA, Zhu Y, Tang YW, et al. Accuracy and impact of a point-of-care rapid influenza test in young children with respiratory illnesses. Arch Pediatr Adolesc Med 2006;160(7):713–8.

57. Abanses JC, Dowd MD, Simon SD, et al. Impact of rapid influenza testing at triage on management of febrile infants and young children. Pediatr Emerg Care 2006;22(3):145–9.

58. Doan QH, Kissoon N, Dobson S, et al. A randomized, controlled trial of the impact of early and rapid diagnosis of viral infections in children brought to an emergency department with febrile respiratory tract illnesses. J Pediatr 2009;154(1):91–5.

59. Bonner AB, Monroe KW, Talley LI, et al. Impact of the rapid diagnosis of influenza on physician decision-making and patient management in the pediatric emergency department: results of a randomized, prospective, controlled trial. Pediatrics 2003;112(2):363–7.

60. Iyer SB, Gerber MA, Pomerantz WJ, et al. Effect of point-of-care influenza testing on management of febrile children. Acad Emerg Med 2006;13(12): 1259–68.

61. Esposito S, Marchisio P, Morelli P, et al. Effect of a rapid influenza diagnosis. Arch Dis Child 2003;88(6):525–6.
62. Doan Q, Enarson P, Kissoon N, et al. Rapid viral diagnosis for acute febrile respiratory illness in children in the Emergency Department. Cochrane Database Syst Rev 2012;(5):CD006452.
63. Benito-Fernández J, Vázquez-Ronco MA, Morteruel-Aizkuren E, et al. Impact of rapid viral testing for influenza A and B viruses on management of febrile infants without signs of focal infection. Pediatr Infect Dis J 2006;25(12):1153–7.
64. Falsey AR, Murata Y, Walsh EE. Impact of rapid diagnosis on management of adults hospitalized with influenza. Arch Intern Med 2007;167(4):354–60.
65. Byington CL, Castillo H, Gerber K, et al. The effect of rapid respiratory viral diagnostic testing on antibiotic use in a children's hospital. Arch Pediatr Adolesc Med 2002;156(12):1230–4.
66. Mintegi S, Garcia-Garcia JJ, Benito J, et al. Rapid influenza test in young febrile infants for the identification of low-risk patients. Pediatr Infect Dis J 2009;28(11): 1026–8.
67. Barenfanger J, Drake C, Leon N, et al. Clinical and financial benefits of rapid detection of respiratory viruses: an outcomes study. J Clin Microbiol 2000; 38(8):2824–8.
68. Oosterheert JJ, van Loon AM, Schuurman R, et al. Impact of rapid detection of viral and atypical bacterial pathogens by real-time polymerase chain reaction for patients with lower respiratory tract infection. Clin Infect Dis 2005;41(10): 1438–44.
69. Xu M, Qin X, Astion ML, et al. Implementation of FilmArray respiratory viral panel in a core laboratory improves testing turnaround time and patient care. Am J Clin Pathol 2013;139(1):118–23.
70. Rocholl C, Gerber K, Daly J, et al. Adenoviral infections in children: the impact of rapid diagnosis. Pediatrics 2004;113(1 Pt 1):e51–6.

Antiviral Resistance in Influenza Viruses

Laboratory Testing

Jennifer Laplante, BS, Kirsten St. George, MAppSc, PhD*

KEYWORDS

- Pyrosequencing • Matrix gene • Neuraminidase • Inhibition assays

KEY POINTS

- Influenza continues to be a significant health care issue. Although vaccination is the major line of defense, antiviral drugs play an important role in prophylaxis and disease management. Approved drug treatments for influenza are currently limited to those that target the viral matrix protein or neuraminidase enzyme.
- Resistance-associated sequence changes in the genes encoding these proteins have been extensively studied. Available methods for genotypic and phenotypic antiviral susceptibility testing have been expanded and are being further developed and improved.
- Rapid molecular techniques including real-time polymerase chain reaction and pyrosequencing assays can be used to screen large numbers of samples but extensive sequencing and phenotypic assays are required for a more comprehensive assessment of antiviral susceptibility.
- The sporadic emergence of drug-resistant variants and the global spread of resistant strains several times in recent years have demonstrated the ongoing need for vigilant patient testing and surveillance programs.

INTRODUCTION

Influenza continues to be a health care challenge, causing annual epidemics that typically affect 10% to 20% of the population from winter to early spring in temperate climates. In addition, the viruses are rapidly evolving, with the continual emergence of new strains and constant threat of another pandemic. In the last century these have occurred in 1918 with the H1N1 "Spanish influenza," in 1957 with the H2N2 "Asian

Authors were not in receipt of any funding to support the preparation of this article. Laboratory directed by K. St. George is under contract to CDC and APHL to provide antiviral resistance testing support to public health laboratories throughout the United States.
The authors have nothing to disclose.
Laboratory of Viral Diseases, Wadsworth Center, New York State Department of Health, PO Box 22002, Albany, NY 12201-2002, USA
* Corresponding author.
E-mail address: kxs16@health.state.ny.us

Clin Lab Med 34 (2014) 387–408
http://dx.doi.org/10.1016/j.cll.2014.02.010
0272-2712/14/$ – see front matter © 2014 Elsevier Inc. All rights reserved.

influenza," in 1968 with H3N2 "Hong Kong influenza," and most recently in 2009 with the new H1N1 strain that emerged from swine in Mexico. Vaccination is typically the first line of defense against influenza. However, evolutionary changes in the virus during a season can result in suboptimal correlations between vaccine strain antigens and those of the circulating strains, and manufacturing problems may cause delays in vaccine availability, either of which results in poor community protection. Furthermore, even in ideal circumstances, as with all vaccines, efficacy is less than 100%; there are always members of the community who are unable to be vaccinated for medical reasons. Therefore, antiviral drugs play an important role in the prevention of influenza infection and in disease management.

Currently there are only 4 antiviral drugs approved by the Food and Drug Administration (FDA) in the United States for the treatment or prophylaxis of influenza. These drugs include 2 adamantanes, amantadine and rimantadine, which block the M2 protein channel in the virus envelope, and 2 neuraminidase (NA) inhibitors, oseltamivir and zanamivir. Additional drugs that target the NA enzyme as well as those directed at other viral and cell targets are in various stages of development and approval. Although influenza viruses do not readily generate resistance to antiviral drugs, resistant strains can spread rapidly, replacing the susceptible virus population globally within 1 to 2 seasons. Therefore, testing for the presence of resistance is an important component of influenza surveillance as well as an important diagnostic service for patients who are not responding to treatment.

MICROBIOLOGY

Members of the family *Orthomyxoviridae*, influenza viruses, types A, B, and C, infect humans, although type C viruses usually cause insignificant and asymptomatic infections and are not included in this review. Influenza A viruses are further subtyped based on the 2 major glycoproteins in the viral envelope, the hemagglutinin (HA) and the NA. A total of 18 different HA and 9 different NA have been described, and although other influenza A subtypes occasionally infect humans and cause disease, only subtypes H1N1, H1N2, H2N2, and H3N2 circulate in humans, together with influenza B viruses.

Both influenza A and B viruses contain a segmented genome comprising 8 negative-sense RNA fragments. Three of the largest segments encode the proteins of the replication machinery PB1, PB2, and PA and a fourth contains the information for the nucleoprotein, NP. Two other segments encode the HA and NA genes. Finally, 2 smaller segments encode the matrix (M) gene proteins M1 and M2 (or BM2 in influenza B viruses) on one segment and an interferon antagonist and nuclear export protein, NS1 and NEP, on the other segment. A few additional genes have been identified in some segments, not all of which have had their function elucidated. At both ends of all segments are conserved sequences that function as replication and transcription promoters.

Receptor-mediated binding is facilitated by the HA envelope proteins of the virus, which bind to sialic acid residues on glycoprotein or glycolipids on the external cell membrane surface. Following endocytosis, a decrease in pH inside the endosome causes a conformational change in the HA protein. This decrease initiates fusion of the viral and endosomal membranes and results in the release of genomic segments and internal structural proteins into the cell cytoplasm. These viral components are imported into the cell nucleus where replication and transcription occur. As is seen in most RNA viruses, the polymerase has a relatively high error rate, resulting in the frequent generation of sequence changes. In addition, because of the segmented

ruses can undergo reassortment if more than one strain or type of
nd replicates at the same time. Progeny viral ribonucleoprotein
sing viral RNAs, polymerase, and nucleoprotein proteins, are
plasm and assembled with structural viral proteins, and mature
rom the host cell membrane with the assistance of the NA. During
cleaves sialic acid receptors on the cell surface that would other-
n the cell surface.

TRANSMISSION

ruses cause seasonal epidemics in temperate climates, season-
ed in tropical regions where infections are seen year-round. Mul-
late simultaneously, generally at least one each of influenza A
H3N2, as well as one or both of the 2 major lineages of influenza
ead rapidly as a result of the short incubation period and high
latter is due to the large number of viral particles present in res-
cted individuals that are spread during the early days of infection
ezing. Host range is primarily determined by the receptor binding
protein, which recognizes terminal N-acetylsialic acid residues
n oligosaccharides by an $\alpha2,6$-linkage or $\alpha2,3$-linkage. Human
e a higher affinity for $\alpha2,6$-linked residues expressed on human
as avian viruses bind more strongly to $\alpha2,3$-linked residues found
s lining the intestines of many water fowl. Importantly, epithelial
y tract of swine express both configurations and can be infected
avian influenza viruses.

teins are the major determinants of pathogenicity in influenza.
s contain multiple basic amino acid residues at the cleavage
rsor protein, HA0, is cleaved into HA1 and HA2. In human and
ian influenza viruses, changes in the amino acid residue at posi-
plication efficiencies in the upper and lower respiratory tracts of
ditional pathogenesis factors include the NS1 protein that inter-
ses induced by interferon and prevents the activation of innate
thways.

ON

uses can cause a wide range of severity of respiratory illness in
ptomatic to fatal infections. Symptoms typically include fever,
eadache, malaise, myalgia, and anorexia but additional symp-
sentations may be seen. Disease severity depends on virulence

OLOGIC AGENTS
nes

antanes block the M2 ion channel protein complex in the virus membrane,[4] a
protein encoded by the M gene of the virus (**Fig. 1**). The M2 protein is an in-
nbrane protein responsible for controlling ion exchange across the viral
, a function essential for viral uncoating and subsequent virus replication.[5]
nes are only effective against influenza A viruses and are inactive against the
of influenza B. Two drugs in this class, amantadine and rimantadine, have
oval in the United States for the clinical treatment of influenza. In addition,
e is approved as an anti-Parkinson drug. Because the M gene is highly
among influenza A viruses and its function is essential for virus replication,
sidered an ideal target for antiviral therapy. However, shortly after the initi-
nical use of these drugs, various phenotypic and molecular studies clearly
ed mutations in the M2 protein that did not affect viral replication or trans-
ut rendered the viruses drug resistant.[4]

ors

zyme of influenza is a homotetrameric protein, structurally composed of a short
ic tail, transmembrane stalk, and large quadrant head exposed on the outside
particle. The enzyme's active site is a pocket, centrally located in the quadrant

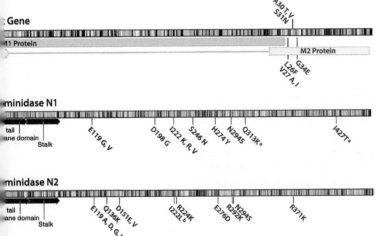

sidues in the pocket are directly involved with cleaving terminal sialic
 influenza HA to aid the release of progeny virus as it buds from the
nown as NA inhibitors (NAIs) fit and bind into the pocket, blocking the
nd preventing enzymatic activity. Consequently, newly formed virus
e cell surface, thereby disrupting subsequent cell infection.[6] This
effective against both influenza A and B viruses. Two NAIs that are
ved for clinical use in the United States are oseltamivir and zanamivir.
istered orally, whereas zanamivir is inhaled.

travenously administered NAI and is in clinical use outside of the
ly in Japan and South Korea.[7] For a short period of time, during
09 pandemic, the FDA granted Emergency Use Authorization for
f peramivir to certain hospitalized influenza patients in the United
ncy Use Authorization expired on June 23, 2010. At the time of this
ical trials have been completed.

NAI, lananimivir, is currently being evaluated in phase 2 clinical
asal dose in humans has been documented to have an elimination
45.7 hours.[8] In comparison, the half-life of oseltamivir is 6 to
tion of the very long half-life of lananimivir has been demonstrated
ncluding one showing protection from H5N1 infection for 7 days
se of the drug.[10]

ets and Drugs

T-705, favipiravir is an RNA polymerase inhibitor that has shown
nst influenza as well as other RNA and DNA viruses. Also of recent
ch targets host cell sites critical to virus replication rather than the
tivating human sialic acid receptors. Current clinical trials will
ential utility of these drugs as well as monitor for resistance mu-
-approved antiviral drugs and those in late-stage clinical trials is

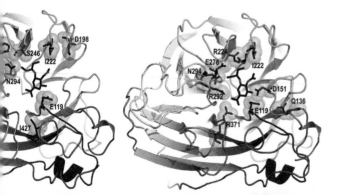

Commercial Name	Target	Administration	Manufacturer	Year of Approval/Current Status
mmetrel	Matrix, M2	Oral	Endo Pharmaceuticals	1966 US FDA approval
umadine	Matrix, M2	Oral	Forest Pharmaceuticals	1993 US FDA approval
elenza	Neuraminidase NA	Inhaled	GlaxoSmithKline	1999 US FDA approval
miflu	Neuraminidase NA	Oral	Roche	1999 US FDA approval
APlACTA[a]	Neuraminidase NA	Intravenous	BioCryst	Post clinical phase 3
eramiFlu[b]				
avir[a]	Neuraminidase NA	Inhaled	Biota	Phase 3 trials
	RNA Polymerase	Intravenous	MediVector	Phase 2 trials
udase	Inhibits virus attachment	Inhaled	NexBio, Inc	Phase 2 trials

in Japan.
in Korea.

RESISTANCE GENETICS

Genetic changes that confer resistance to the M2-inhibitors have been thoroughly studied and well characterized. The M gene in segment 7 of influenza A virus encodes the M1 and M2 proteins. Coding regions for both proteins and key residues involved in antiviral resistance are shown in **Fig. 1**. Resistance is directly linked to amino acid changes at positions 26, 27, 30, 31, and 34 in the M2 gene of influenza A viruses.[11,12] A dramatic increase in the prevalence of adamantane-resistant influenza A strains from 0.4% in the 1994–1995 influenza season to 12.3% in the 2003–2004 season was reported in 2005.[13] Analysis of global isolates from the 2005–2006 season demonstrated that adamantane-resistant strains of influenza A/H3N2 had almost completely replaced circulating susceptible strains in Asia and the United States.[14] Among influenza A/H1N1 strains the prevalence of resistance was estimated to be 15.5% globally in 2005–2006[14] and continued to increase. Both wild-type and resistant strains were subsequently replaced by the emergence of the pandemic H1N1 strain of 2009, which is universally resistant to adamantanes.[15]

The sixth fragment of the influenza genome encodes one protein, the NA enzyme. A linear map of the gene (see **Fig. 1**) shows that a small portion of sequence encodes the cytoplasmic tail inside the membrane at the amino-terminal end of the protein, followed by the transmembrane domain and the stalk, downstream of which most of the gene codes for the large globular head. Amino acid changes associated with NAI resistance are located in and around the enzymatic pocket, formed in the center of the globular head of the tetramer (see **Fig. 2**). Sequence changes that result in altered antiviral susceptibility to NAIs are scattered throughout the NA gene (see **Fig. 1**), although in the folded protein they are located either in the enzyme's active site or in a position where the resultant amino acid change impacts the size or shape of the enzymatic pocket. A comprehensive list of amino acid changes associated with decreased susceptibility or resistance to the NAIs that are in current clinical use for influenza A/H1pdm09, influenza A/H3, and influenza B is shown in **Table 2**. For consistency, amino acid location follows standard N2 numbering throughout the table and this review. The degree of resistance caused by a mutation is assessed in a phenotypic assay. In 2012, the World Health Organization (WHO) Influenza Antiviral Working Group (AVWG) proposed criteria for the classification of resistance-associated amino acid changes, according to their associated phenotypic data, to bring consistency to the reporting of NI susceptibility.[16] The utility of these criteria was reinforced at a subsequent meeting, and they have been used in numerous subsequent publications.[17] In general, they provide the intended benefit of uniformity, and the classification of most mutations listed in **Table 2** of this review follow the WHO AVWG criteria. However, some mutations produce extremely high levels of resistance and these have been referred to as "extremely reduced" or XR in the table. Furthermore, there are a few amino acid changes that are generally considered to be associated with reduced susceptibility, although by strict AVWG criteria they cause changes that should be classified as normal. In **Table 2**, these are indicated as *N with an explanatory footnote.

Most mutations in the table are associated with altered susceptibility to more than one NAI and very few are associated with zanamivir resistance only. Changes at one position that may be associated with high levels of resistance in one type or subtype of influenza may cause no change to antiviral susceptibility in another. An example of this is the widely reported H274Y variant; when present in A/H1N1pdm (or previously in seasonal A/H1N1), it causes a high level of resistance to oseltamivir, but when present in A/H3N2, it has no impact on antiviral susceptibility. In contrast, some variants

Table 2
Amino acid changes in the NA gene associated with reduced antiviral susceptibility

Influenza Subtype	NA Mutation[a]	Antiviral Susceptibility[b]			Source
		Oseltamivir	Zanamivir	Peramivir	
A/H1pdm09	E119G	N	HR	R	96
	E119V	R	HR	R	96
	D198G	R	N	N	96
	I222K	R	N	N	18
	I222R	R	R	Unknown	19,20
	I222V[c]	*N	N	N	96
	S246N[c]	*N	N	N	97
	H274Y	HR	N	HR	19,75,96,98
	N294S	HR	N	R	96
	D198N + H274Y	HR	N	Unknown	37
	I222R + H274Y	XR	R	XR	18
	I222V + H274Y	XR	N	XR	96
	S246N + H274Y	XR	N	HR	97
	Q313K + I427T	R	R	N	99
A/H3N2	E119A	HR	HR	HR	100
	E119D	N	R	N	101
	E119G	N	HR	R	100
	E119I	HR	R	HR	100,102
	E119V	R[d]	N	N	24,102–104
	Q136K	N	R	Unknown	105
	D151E	R	N	Unknown	106
	D151N	N	R	Unknown	107,108
	D151V	N	R	Unknown	107,108
	I222L	*N	N	Unknown	21
	R224K	XR	R	Unknown	106
	E276D	R	HR	Unknown	106
	R292K	XR	R	HR	101,106,109–111
	N294S	HR	*N	N	100,112
	R371K	R	R	Unknown	106
	E119V + I222L	XR	N	Unknown	21
	E119V + I222V	HR	N	N	24,113

(continued on next page)

impact antiviral susceptibility regardless of the type or subtype in which they occur, such as position 222 in the NA. Amino acid changes at this codon are associated with antiviral resistance in A/H1N1pdm09, A/H3N2, and B.[18–22] Reports also indicate that certain combinations of variants have a synergistic effect, resulting in significantly increased resistance to antivirals. Furthermore, although some variants are thought to compromise viral fitness, subsequent "permissive secondary mutations" may compensate[23] and restore growth rates to wild-type levels. Again, genetic variants at position 222 have been shown to have a compensatory role and produce enhanced resistance to NAIs in both A/H1N1pdm09[18] and A/H3N2.[21,24]

INFLUENZA DIAGNOSIS

Several techniques are used for the detection of influenza infection, including direct antigen detection with immunochromatographic or direct immunofluorescence methods, various molecular methods, and virus culture.[25] Of the available detection methods, direct antigen detection with commercially available kits is the most widely

Table 2
(continued)

Influenza Subtype	NA Mutation[a]	Antiviral Susceptibility[b]			Source
		Oseltamivir	Zanamivir	Peramivir	
B	E119A	HR	HR	XR	114
	E119D	HR	HR	XR	114
	E119G	R	HR	XR	64,114
	E119V	HR	N	HR	114
	E152K	HR	N	HR	114,115
	D198E	R	R	R	116–118
	D198N	R	R	*N	108,119
	D198Y	R	R	Unknown	120
	I222T	R	R	Unknown	116,118
	I222V	R	N	R	22
	S250G	N	R	Unknown	118
	R292K	HR	R	HR	114
	N294S	R	N	Unknown	121
	R371K	HR	R	Unknown	108
	G402S	N	R	Unknown	118

[a] Amino acid location follows standard N2 numbering throughout.
[b] Susceptibility assessed in phenotypic assays, by fold increase in IC_{50} above wild type, is generally in accordance with the classification recommended by the WHO AVWG.[16,17] Briefly, for influenza A viruses: fold changes of <10, 10–100, 100–1000, and >1000 are normal susceptibility (N), reduced susceptibility (R), highly reduced (HR), and extremely reduced (XR). For influenza B: <5, 5–50, 50–500, and >500, are N, R, HR, and XR. A classification of *N indicates that reported fold changes generally fall within the WHO AVWG normal range of <10, but the variants detected with this change have been suspected in some reports as having reduced susceptibility to antiviral drug. Classification is based on review of cited references.
[c] Effect on antiviral susceptibility not significant except when mutation present with H274Y, when it exacerbates resistance.
[d] One report of this variant conferring extreme resistance to oseltamivir.[24]

used. Requiring little training or expertise, these tests can be performed in less than 30 minutes and are used in thousands of physician office laboratories and other point-of-care locations.

Direct immunofluorescence offers more sensitive and specific results with a slightly longer testing time; however, a higher level of expertise and scientific knowledge are required to obtain accurate results, in addition to the availability of a fluorescence microscope. Accurate testing using virus culture requires an even higher level of expertise and results can take as long as 2 to 3 weeks. Finally, the diagnosis of influenza with molecular methods may be the most beneficial with regard to antiviral resistance profiling. With the increasing availability of simplified commercial platforms, some molecular techniques can be performed with little scientific background, and the type and subtype of influenza can be ascertained in as little as an hour.

ANTIVIRAL DRUG SUSCEPTIBILITY TESTING
Genotypic Methods

The presence of genomic variants conferring antiviral drug resistance or reduced susceptibility is detected primarily with sequencing assays including pyrosequencing, Sanger dideoxy sequencing, and next-generation sequencing chemistries. Pyrosequencing is a rapid and cost-effective technique[26] that can facilitate the surveillance of small sequence fragments in large numbers of samples. For this method of sequencing on influenza, a one-step reverse-transcriptase (RT) conventional polymerase chain reaction (PCR) is performed, with one primer biotin-labeled. This PCR facilitates isolation of the complementary strand of amplified DNA, by binding to streptavidin-coated beads. During pyrosequencing, the strand complementary to the biotinylated product, is synthesized and pyrophosphate molecules are released as nucleotides are incorporated, enabling luciferase, present in the reaction mixture, to oxidize luciferin, which produces light. The pyrosequencer measures the light produced; a strong light signal indicates the incorporation of that nucleotide. Light intensity is plotted against the nucleotide additions to produce a pyrogram, and signal intensity is proportional to the number of nucleotides incorporated. Two modes of pyrosequencing analysis can be performed: sequence analysis (SQA) involves the addition of nucleotides in a predefined cyclical manner, whereas single nucleotide polymorphism (SNP) analysis uses sequence-specific, directed dispensation of nucleotides. In SNP mode, the software is designed to quantitate the nucleotides at prespecified positions where changes and mixtures might be expected. Analysis of resultant data includes the careful visual inspection of each pyrogram by a trained scientist, because the patterns can be complicated and difficult to interpret. Variations from wild-type sequence, even single-nucleotide changes or mixed bases in the target region, may drastically change the appearance of a pyrogram.

Numerous pyrosequencing assays have been developed that target regions of influenza virus genomes for the detection of sequence variations associated with antiviral drug resistance.[13,27–30] Mixed populations of sensitive and resistant viruses can be accurately quantitated by using the SNP mode of analysis in pyrosequencing instruments, within a documented reliability of 10%.[27,28] However, in homopolymeric regions, inaccuracies can occur in the quantitation.[31]

Sequence changes conferring adamantane resistance are clustered in close proximity in the matrix gene (see **Fig. 1**) and can be tested for quickly and efficiently with pyrosequencing methods.[13] However, circulating human influenza strains are resistant to adamantanes,[32] and the clinical use of these drugs has not been recommended since 2006.[33] Therefore, matrix genotypic testing is generally not useful except in research settings. Several pyrosequencing assays have also been published for the detection of common NAI resistance-associated variants in circulating influenza viruses. These variants include the H274Y change in the NA of influenza A/H1N1pdm09,[29] and multiple changes at codons E119, R292, and S294 in the NA of influenza A/H3N2.[27] In addition, pyrosequencing assays have been published that provide sequence information across several regions of the NA gene, spanning numerous variations associated with NAI resistance in influenza B.[30]

Sanger dideoxy sequencing continues to be considered the gold standard for genotypic resistance analysis, providing more information compared with that obtained with short pyrosequencing fragments. In addition, a wide variety of software is available for dideoxy sequence analysis, some of which is freely accessible on the Internet. For dideoxy sequencing, oligonucleotide primers used for both the amplification and the sequencing portions of the assays are easily modified. Furthermore, the primers are relatively affordable compared with the labeled oligonucleotides required for pyrosequencing. Resulting color-coded chromatograms are more easily interpreted and edited than pyrograms, including the analysis of mixed populations. These assays are useful for detailed genotypic antiviral susceptibility surveillance.[34–36]

Next-generation sequencing technologies for analyzing influenza virus genomes are gaining in popularity and have proven capable of rapidly generating extensive volumes of data. This technology is unmatched in its ability to detect and analyze mixed infections of influenza, as has been clearly demonstrated in the detailed investigation of complex resistance cases.[37] Furthermore, it provides comprehensive genomic information on the virus, with the ultimate potential for genetic phenotyping, although this goal remains a long way off. However, it requires considerably greater computer processing and storage capacity, and a higher level of comprehension and interpretation for analysis, than either pyrosequencing or dideoxy sequencing. At this time, it is considerably more expensive than these alternatives and would require a concerted effort to generate standard methods for testing and analysis practices.

Real-time RT-PCR assays have been developed for the rapid detection of resistance-associated variants and for their quantitation in mixed virus populations, particularly for the H274Y change in A/H1N1pdm09.[38–45] Some assays use a modified RT-PCR with melt curve analysis.[46–50] Other reported methods include single-nucleotide polymorphism extension,[51] rolling circle amplification,[52] cycling probe,[53] RT-PCR restriction fragment length polymorphism,[54] RT-PCR followed by electro-spray ionization,[55] and isolated probe asymmetric amplification.[56] These assays can be used for the rapid screening of large numbers of samples but do not provide the detailed information of sequencing methods. Real-time RT-PCR methods may be suited to laboratories requiring faster turnaround time than can be achieved with current sequencing platforms, or those without sequencing capabilities.

Microarrays using various chemistries have been developed for the detection and subtyping of influenza viruses as well as the detection of adamantane or NAI resistance-associated mutations.[57–61] Although the reported testing has often been on limited sample sizes, sensitivities for some of the arrays have been within acceptable ranges. However, validation of arrays in clinical settings remains problematic. In addition, the need for specialized equipment and technical expertise has rendered them generally impractical for widespread implementation.

Of importance, any molecular assay can be rendered ineffective with as little as a single-nucleotide change that affects oligonucleotide binding. Such changes may not affect resistance profiles or cause amino acid changes, but may drastically alter assay performance. A notable example of this occurred in 2011, when a single-nucleotide substitution in the probe-binding region of the NA gene in A/H1N1pdm09 caused a 100% loss of detection signal in the assay that was being used at the time[62]; this highlights the importance of viral surveillance for the monitoring of sequence changes to inform the appropriate use of molecular methods as well as the utility of antiviral drug susceptibility testing with phenotypic assays that are not reliant on genomic sequence.

Phenotypic Methods

The results generated from genotypic antiviral resistance testing may not give a complete picture of susceptibility. Genotypic testing is targeted to specific gene regions or genes, and other genetic factors in the viral genome can impact overall drug susceptibility. Definitive measurement is tested using phenotypic methods such as NA inhibition assays (NIA). These methods measure the activity of the NA enzyme of the virus and its susceptibility to inhibition by antiviral drugs. Typically, testing is performed on cultured virus incubated with several concentrations of drug. In NIAs, the amount of substrate cleaved by the NA enzyme in the absence of drug is compared with that produced in the presence of drug, a ratio referred to as the 50% inhibitory concentration or IC_{50} value. Higher drug concentrations are needed to inhibit the NA activity to 50% of wild-type levels: therefore, higher IC_{50} levels correspond to more resistant virus. To help overcome biologic variations across assays, results are converted to ratios comparing the IC_{50} of test viruses to that of wild-type virus, to reflect the fold changes in IC_{50} rather than actual IC_{50} values. Although methods using plaque inhibition assays have been published,[63,64] they are tedious and time-consuming and generally unsuitable for clinical testing or routine surveillance work.[65]

Commercially manufactured kits for NIAs are available, which have provided the advantage of reagent consistency for some of the required materials. Drawbacks to the use of NIAs include the inherent delay and required technical expertise for in vitro growth of influenza viruses. Moreover, the cultured viral progeny may not be representative of those in the original sample due to in vitro selection or may vary across isolates from a single sample when different cell lines are used to grow virus from a specimen.[66] In addition, variations in testing methodology continue, with considerable potential for consequent error.[67] Laboratories must obtain their own supply of antiviral drug stocks from the relevant manufacturing company. Initial supplies may vary between lots and are not consistent among users, and methods for reconstitution, dilution, and storage are not standardized. Furthermore, the length of time that virus is incubated with drug, substrate, or other reagents is not standardized, and studies on the binding kinetics of influenza viruses with antiviral drugs have demonstrated that variations in these incubation times dramatically affect IC_{50} values.[68] There have also been significant differences between laboratories on the instruments used for NIA testing and in the methods for analysis of the resultant data. Commercial kits with either chemiluminescent or fluorescent-labeled substrates are available for NIA methods, and each has advantages and disadvantages. For example, the chemiluminescence assay is more expensive but can be used on culture harvests with lower viral titers.[69] In attempts to establish standardized testing methods and provide laboratory guidance, detailed protocols have been published on both types of NIAs.[69,70]

Kits have also been developed for direct NIA testing of primary clinical specimens and have undergone some initial evaluations[71,72] but in general have not been widely implemented as replacements for NIAs on cultured virus. There may be the potential for a point-of-care NIA in the near future: a bioluminescence-based assay has been evaluated against the fluorescence and chemiluminescence NIA[72] and is currently in clinical trials.

The testing of mixed influenza infections for the suspected presence of virus with reduced antiviral susceptibility can be very complicated.[73] Depending on the specific mixture of types or subtypes, more information may be gained by genotypic than phenotypic testing, or it may be necessary to plaque purify viruses to obtain a clear understanding of the situation. The latter is a very time-consuming and lengthy procedure. Overall, such cases should always be referred to an experienced reference laboratory for investigation.

Patient Testing and Surveillance Programs

The testing of influenza-positive specimens collected before the initiation of antiviral treatment, as well as samples collected during or after treatment, is important for the full investigation of suspected cases of drug-resistant influenza. The emergence of resistance has most commonly been observed in immunocompromised individuals[74] and clinicians should be particularly alert to indications of treatment failure in these patients, in whom resistance can develop rapidly.[75–78] Due to the prolonged shedding that can occur in these patients,[79–82] including in unusual sample types such as stool,[83] immunocompromised patients may need to be monitored for very long periods of time. Additional risk factors for the development of drug-resistant virus include chronic pulmonary, cardiovascular, and renal diseases, diabetes, and pregnancy.[74]

The proportion of antiviral-resistant variant in the virus population within an individual may increase or decrease relative to that of the wild-type or drug-susceptible virus over time. In general, the amount of resistant virus will increase under ongoing drug pressure; however, investigators should be aware of potential confounders such as drug absorption, metabolism, tissue distribution, drug interactions, and noncompliance. Resistant variants may emerge during antiviral therapy, whereby increases in the proportion of resistant virus may be observed over time with treatment. Alternatively, the presence of high proportions of a resistant strain in pretreatment samples would strongly suggest that resistance had evolved before infection of that patient.

Surveillance programs for monitoring the emergence of drug-resistant variants in circulating viruses should take into account several factors. Appropriate programs must first be in place for the statistically robust surveillance of influenza infection, ensuring representative sample sizes from relevant cases across age groups and patient types, geographically diverse areas, tested with appropriate methods including those that will detect the presence of novel subtypes. Alternative data sources may be used to assess circulating influenza levels and subtypes, rather than direct testing of samples; however, the reliability of data sources should be carefully evaluated. Randomly selected influenza-positive samples of each subtype should then be investigated for antiviral susceptibility. A balance of techniques should be used, ensuring rapid screening for the most likely variations, and more extensive genotypic and phenotypic testing on a smaller subset of samples.

TREATMENT AND PROGNOSIS

Adamantanes were widely prescribed for influenza A infection until the 2005–2006 influenza season, when a dramatic global increase in adamantane resistance was reported.[13] Following this, the Centers for Disease Control and Prevention recommended that neither amantadine nor rimantadine be used for the prophylaxis or treatment of influenza A for the remainder of the 2005–2006 influenza season[33] and this recommendation has continued. New antiviral agents currently in development that block the M2 channel and may overcome the adamantane-resistance mutations have not demonstrated utility in clinical trials at this time.[84,85] Adamantane-resistant strains of influenza A/H1N1pdm09 and A/H3N2 viruses have continued to dominate in circulating virus populations globally, with NAIs the antiviral drugs of choice for the treatment and prophylaxis of influenza.

Oseltamivir, the most commonly prescribed NAI, is administered orally, whereas zanamivir is inhaled. The most commonly reported adverse effects from oseltamivir are nausea and vomiting and both oseltamivir and zanamivir have been associated with an increased risk of seizures. In addition, there is a risk of bronchospasm from zanamivir treatment if used in patients with asthma or other pulmonary diseases.[86] Oseltamivir resistance emerged in influenza A/seasonal H1N1 and spread rapidly throughout the world during the 2007–2008 influenza season. Secondary mutations in the variant strain resulted in a fitness advantage, even in the absence of drug pressure.[23,87] Occasional clusters of cases of resistant strains of influenza A/H1N1pdm09 and influenza B have been reported,[22,88] also in patients who have not been treated with antiviral drugs.[89] However, the prevalence of NAI resistance has remained low.[90]

Following the diagnosis of influenza, in addition to factors such as recent travel history and relevant animal contact, patients should be evaluated for current disease duration, severity, and the likelihood of progression to more serious outcomes. This evaluation will help determine which, if any, antiviral should be used, based on medication delivery and bioavailability. Dosage and treatment duration will depend on factors including patient age, weight, severity of illness, and immunocompetence.[86] Patients with advanced disease who are intubated or on mechanical ventilators cannot take oral or inhaled medications and therefore must be treated intravenously. Although emergency use authorization was granted for peramivir during the 2009 pandemic, there are no NAIs currently FDA-approved in the United States for intravenous administration. However, intravenous zanamivir is available through enrollment in a phase 3 clinical trial, or compassionate use can be requested from the manufacturer with FDA approval. Extensive clinical recommendations for the treatment of influenza have been published elsewhere.[86]

Several studies have reported on the potential treatment of influenza with combinations of antiviral drugs, compared with single drug regimens. Despite promising results with in vitro systems and predictive mathematical modeling,[91,92] patient trials have not demonstrated a significant advantage to combination therapy over monotherapy.[93,94] In addition, the combination treatment regimens may be challenging for patients to tolerate.[95]

SUMMARY

Antiviral-resistant strains of influenza have emerged and spread globally several times in the last several years. Examples include amantadine-resistant A/H3N2 and oseltamivir-resistant A/seasonal H1N1. Options for the laboratory analysis of antiviral susceptibility have expanded. Screening for genomic changes is possible with techniques such as rapid sequencing assays and real-time PCR. Detailed genomic analysis and phenotypic assays provide a more thorough picture of the susceptibility of the virus.

Although available drugs for influenza treatment remain limited, new NAIs as well as antiviral agents targeting other viral and cellular proteins are in late-stage clinical trials. Meanwhile, there is ongoing concern for the potential emergence and spread of strains that are resistant to the few approved drugs, especially given the possibility of cross-resistant mutations. Therefore, patients not responding to treatment, especially those at high risk for the development of resistant variants, should be investigated promptly, and surveillance for circulating resistant strains continues to be a high priority.

ACKNOWLEDGMENTS

The authors sincerely thank the staff of the Photography and Illustration Unit for their assistance with modifications to **Fig. 1**, and Dr Joachim Jaeger in the Computational and Structural Biology Laboratory at the Wadsworth Center for generating the images in **Fig. 2**.

REFERENCES

1. Dharan NJ, Gubareva LV, Meyer JJ, et al. Infections with oseltamivir-resistant influenza A(H1N1) virus in the United States. JAMA 2009;301(10):1034–41.
2. Ciancio BC, Meerhoff TJ, Kramarz P, et al. Oseltamivir-resistant influenza A(H1N1) viruses detected in Europe during season 2007-8 had epidemiologic and clinical characteristics similar to co-circulating susceptible A(H1N1) viruses. Euro Surveill 2009;14(46). pii:19412.
3. Hauge SH, Dudman S, Borgen K, et al. Oseltamivir-resistant influenza viruses A (H1N1), Norway, 2007-08. Emerg Infect Dis 2009;15(2):155–62.
4. Hayden FG. Antiviral resistance in influenza viruses–implications for management and pandemic response. N Engl J Med 2006;354(8):785–8.

5. Lamb RA, Krug RM. Orthomyxoviridae: the viruses and their replication. In: Fields BN, Knipe DM, Howley PM, et al, editors. Field's virology, vol. 1, 4th edition. Philadelphia: Lippincott Williams & Wilkins; 2001. p. 1487–531.
6. Moscona A. Neuraminidase inhibitors for influenza. N Engl J Med 2005;353(13): 1363–73.
7. Hernandez JE, Adiga R, Armstrong R, et al. Clinical experience in adults and children treated with intravenous peramivir for 2009 influenza A (H1N1) under an Emergency IND program in the United States. Clin Infect Dis 2011;52(6): 695–706.
8. Ishizuka H, Toyama K, Yoshiba S, et al. Intrapulmonary distribution and pharmacokinetics of laninamivir, a neuraminidase inhibitor, after a single inhaled administration of its prodrug, laninamivir octanoate, in healthy volunteers. Antimicrob Agents Chemother 2012;56(7):3873–8.
9. Davies BE. Pharmacokinetics of oseltamivir: an oral antiviral for the treatment and prophylaxis of influenza in diverse populations. J Antimicrob Chemother 2010;65(Suppl 2):ii5–10.
10. Kiso M, Kubo S, Ozawa M, et al. Efficacy of the new neuraminidase inhibitor CS-8958 against H5N1 influenza viruses. PLoS Pathog 2010;6(2):e1000786.
11. Hay AJ, Zambon MC, Wolstenholme AJ, et al. Molecular basis of resistance of influenza A viruses to amantadine. J Antimicrob Chemother 1986;18(Suppl B):19–29.
12. Belshe RB, Smith MH, Hall CB, et al. Genetic basis of resistance to rimantadine emerging during treatment of influenza virus infection. J Virol 1988;62(5):1508–12.
13. Bright RA, Medina MJ, Xu X, et al. Incidence of adamantane resistance among influenza A (H3N2) viruses isolated worldwide from 1994 to 2005: a cause for concern. Lancet 2005;366(9492):1175–81.
14. Deyde VM, Xu X, Bright RA, et al. Surveillance of resistance to adamantanes among influenza A(H3N2) and A(H1N1) viruses isolated worldwide. J Infect Dis 2007;196(2):249–57.
15. Centers for Disease Control and Prevention (CDC). Update: influenza activity—United States, August 30-October 31, 2009. MMWR Morb Mortal Wkly Rep 2009;58(44):1236–41.
16. Meetings of the WHO working group on surveillance of influenza antiviral susceptibility—Geneva, November 2011 and June 2012. Wkly Epidemiol Rec 2012;87(39):369–74.
17. Meeting of the WHO expert working group on surveillance of influenza antiviral susceptibility, Geneva, July 2013. Wkly Epidemiol Rec 2013;88(44–45):477–82.
18. Nguyen HT, Fry AM, Loveless PA, et al. Recovery of a multidrug-resistant strain of pandemic influenza A 2009 (H1N1) virus carrying a dual H275Y/I223R mutation from a child after prolonged treatment with oseltamivir. Clin Infect Dis 2010; 51(8):983–4.
19. van der Vries E, Stelma FF, Boucher CA. Emergence of a multidrug-resistant pandemic influenza A (H1N1) virus. N Engl J Med 2010;363(14):1381–2.
20. Eshaghi A, Patel SN, Sarabia A, et al. Multidrug-resistant pandemic (H1N1) 2009 infection in immunocompetent child. Emerg Infect Dis 2011;17(8):1472–4.
21. Richard M, Ferraris O, Erny A, et al. Combinatorial effect of two framework mutations (E119V and I222L) in the neuraminidase active site of H3N2 influenza virus on resistance to oseltamivir. Antimicrob Agents Chemother 2011;55(6): 2942–52.
22. Sleeman K, Sheu TG, Moore Z, et al. Influenza B viruses with mutation in the neuraminidase active site, North Carolina, USA, 2010-11. Emerg Infect Dis 2011;17(11):2043–6.

23. Bloom JD, Gong LI, Baltimore D. Permissive secondary mutations enable the evolution of influenza oseltamivir resistance. Science 2010;328(5983):1272–5.

24. Simon P, Holder BP, Bouhy X, et al. The I222V neuraminidase mutation has a compensatory role in replication of an oseltamivir-resistant influenza virus A/H3N2 E119V mutant. J Clin Microbiol 2011;49(2):715–7.

25. St. George K. Diagnosis of influenza virus. In: Kawaoka Y, Neumann G, editors. Springer protocols–influenza virus: methods and protocols. New York: Humana; 2012. p. 53–69, iv.

26. Ahmadian A, Ehn M, Hober S. Pyrosequencing: history, biochemistry and future. Clin Chim Acta 2006;363(1–2):83–94.

27. Duwe S, Schweiger B. A new and rapid genotypic assay for the detection of neuraminidase inhibitor resistant influenza A viruses of subtype H1N1, H3N2, and H5N1. J Virol Methods 2008;153(2):134–41.

28. Deyde VM, Okomo-Adhiambo M, Sheu TG, et al. Pyrosequencing as a tool to detect molecular markers of resistance to neuraminidase inhibitors in seasonal influenza A viruses. Antiviral Res 2009;81(1):16–24.

29. Deyde VM, Sheu TG, Trujillo AA, et al. Detection of molecular markers of drug resistance in 2009 pandemic influenza A (H1N1) viruses by pyrosequencing. Antimicrob Agents Chemother 2010;54(3):1102–10.

30. Sheu TG, Deyde VM, Garten RJ, et al. Detection of antiviral resistance and genetic lineage markers in influenza B virus neuraminidase using pyrosequencing. Antiviral Res 2010;85(2):354–60.

31. Deyde VM, Gubareva LV. Influenza genome analysis using pyrosequencing method: current applications for a moving target. Expert Rev Mol Diagn 2009; 9(5):493–509.

32. Nguyen HT, Fry AM, Gubareva LV. Neuraminidase inhibitor resistance in influenza viruses and laboratory testing methods. Antivir Ther 2012;17(1 Pt B): 159–73.

33. Centers for Disease Control and Prevention (CDC). High levels of adamantane resistance among influenza A (H3N2) viruses and interim guidelines for use of antiviral agents–United States, 2005-06 influenza season. MMWR Morb Mortal Wkly Rep 2006;55(2):44–6.

34. Deyde V, Garten R, Sheu T, et al. Genomic events underlying the changes in adamantane resistance among influenza A(H3N2) viruses during 2006-2008. Influenza Other Respir Viruses 2009;3(6):297–314.

35. Laplante JM, Marshall SA, Shudt M, et al. Influenza antiviral resistance testing in New York and Wisconsin, 2006 to 2008: methodology and surveillance data. J Clin Microbiol 2009;47(5):1372–8.

36. Ruiz-Carrascoso G, Casas I, Pozo F, et al. Development and implementation of influenza a virus subtyping and detection of genotypic resistance to neuraminidase inhibitors. J Med Virol 2010;82(5):843–53.

37. Ghedin E, Laplante J, DePasse J, et al. Deep sequencing reveals mixed infection with 2009 pandemic influenza A (H1N1) virus strains and the emergence of oseltamivir resistance. J Infect Dis 2011;203(2):168–74.

38. van der Vries E, Anber J, van der Linden A, et al. Molecular assays for quantitative and qualitative detection of influenza virus and oseltamivir resistance mutations. J Mol Diagn 2013;15(3):347–54.

39. van der Vries E, Jonges M, Herfst S, et al. Evaluation of a rapid molecular algorithm for detection of pandemic influenza A (H1N1) 2009 virus and screening for a key oseltamivir resistance (H275Y) substitution in neuraminidase. J Clin Virol 2010;47(1):34–7.

40. Hindiyeh M, Ram D, Mandelboim M, et al. Rapid detection of influenza A pandemic (H1N1) 2009 virus neuraminidase resistance mutation H275Y by real-time reverse transcriptase PCR. J Clin Microbiol 2010;48(5):1884–7.
41. Renaud C, Kuypers J, Corey L. Diagnostic accuracy of an allele-specific reverse transcriptase-PCR assay targeting the H275Y oseltamivir resistant mutation in 2009 pandemic influenza A/H1N1 virus. J Clin Virol 2010;49(1):21–5.
42. Liu CM, Driebe EM, Schupp J, et al. Rapid quantification of single-nucleotide mutations in mixed influenza A viral populations using allele-specific mixture analysis. J Virol Methods 2010;163(1):109–15.
43. Bennett S, Gunson RN, MacLean A, et al. The validation of a real-time RT-PCR assay which detects influenza A and types simultaneously for influenza A H1N1 (2009) and oseltamivir-resistant (H275Y) influenza A H1N1(2009). J Virol Methods 2011;171(1):86–90.
44. Wong S, Pabbaraju K, Wong A, et al. Development of a real-time RT-PCR assay for detection of resistance to oseltamivir in influenza A pandemic (H1N1) 2009 virus using single nucleotide polymorphism probes. J Virol Methods 2011; 173(2):259–65.
45. Nakauchi M, Ujike M, Obuchi M, et al. Rapid discrimination of oseltamivir-resistant 275Y and -susceptible 275H substitutions in the neuraminidase gene of pandemic influenza A/H1N1 2009 virus by duplex one-step RT-PCR assay. J Med Virol 2011;83(7):1121–7.
46. Operario DJ, Moser MJ, St George K. Highly sensitive and quantitative detection of the H274Y oseltamivir resistance mutation in seasonal A/H1N1 influenza virus. J Clin Microbiol 2010;48(10):3517–24.
47. Tong SY, Dakh F, Hurt AC, et al. Rapid detection of the H275Y oseltamivir resistance mutation in influenza A/H1N1 2009 by single base pair RT-PCR and high-resolution melting. PLoS One 2011;6(6):e21446.
48. Chen N, Pinsky BA, Lee BP, et al. Ultrasensitive detection of drug-resistant pandemic 2009 (H1N1) influenza A virus by rare-variant-sensitive high-resolution melting-curve analysis. J Clin Microbiol 2011;49(7):2602–9.
49. Redlberger-Fritz M, Aberle SW, Strassl R, et al. Rapid identification of neuraminidase inhibitor resistance mutations in seasonal influenza virus A(H1N1), A(H1N1)2009, and A(H3N2) subtypes by melting point analysis. Eur J Clin Microbiol Infect Dis 2012;31(7):1593–601.
50. Takayama I, Nakauchi M, Fujisaki S, et al. Rapid detection of the S247N neuraminidase mutation in influenza A(H1N1)pdm09 virus by one-step duplex RT-PCR assay. J Virol Methods 2013;188(1–2):73–5.
51. Duan S, Boltz DA, Li J, et al. Novel genotyping and quantitative analysis of neuraminidase inhibitor resistance-associated mutations in influenza a viruses by single-nucleotide polymorphism analysis. Antimicrob Agents Chemother 2011; 55(10):4718–27.
52. Steain MC, Dwyer DE, Hurt AC, et al. Detection of influenza A H1N1 and H3N2 mutations conferring resistance to oseltamivir using rolling circle amplification. Antiviral Res 2009;84(3):242–8.
53. Suzuki Y, Saito R, Sato I, et al. Identification of oseltamivir resistance among pandemic and seasonal influenza A (H1N1) viruses by an His275Tyr genotyping assay using the cycling probe method. J Clin Microbiol 2011;49(1): 125–30.
54. Guo L, Garten RJ, Foust AS, et al. Rapid identification of oseltamivir-resistant influenza A(H1N1) viruses with H274Y mutation by RT-PCR/restriction fragment length polymorphism assay. Antiviral Res 2009;82(1):29–33.

55. Deyde VM, Sampath R, Garten RJ, et al. Genomic signature-based identification of influenza A viruses using RT-PCR/electro-spray ionization mass spectrometry (ESI-MS) technology. PLoS One 2010;5(10):e13293.

56. Lee HK, Lee CK, Loh TP, et al. High-resolution melting approach to efficient identification and quantification of H275Y mutant influenza H1N1/2009 virus in mixed-virus-population samples. J Clin Microbiol 2011;49(10):3555–9.

57. Townsend MB, Smagala JA, Dawson ED, et al. Detection of adamantane-resistant influenza on a microarray. J Clin Virol 2008;42(2):117–23.

58. Metzgar D, Myers CA, Russell KL, et al. Single assay for simultaneous detection and differential identification of human and avian influenza virus types, subtypes, and emergent variants. PLoS One 2010;5(2):e8995.

59. Lee CW, Koh CW, Chan YS, et al. Large-scale evolutionary surveillance of the 2009 H1N1 influenza A virus using resequencing arrays. Nucleic Acids Res 2010;38(9):e111.

60. Zhang Y, Liu Q, Wang D, et al. Simultaneous detection of oseltamivir- and amantadine-resistant influenza by oligonucleotide microarray visualization. PLoS One 2013;8(2):e57154.

61. Van Wesenbeeck L, Meeuws H, Van Immerseel A, et al. Comparison of the FilmArray RP, Verigene RV+, and Prodesse ProFLU+/FAST+ multiplex platforms for detection of influenza viruses in clinical samples from the 2011-2012 influenza season in Belgium. J Clin Microbiol 2013;51(9):2977–85.

62. Trevino C, Bihon S, Pinsky BA. A synonymous change in the influenza A virus neuraminidase gene interferes with PCR-based subtyping and oseltamivir resistance mutation detection. J Clin Microbiol 2011;49(8):3101–2.

63. Hayden FG, Cote KM, Douglas RG Jr. Plaque inhibition assay for drug susceptibility testing of influenza viruses. Antimicrob Agents Chemother 1980;17(5):865–70.

64. Blick TJ, Tiong T, Sahasrabudhe A, et al. Generation and characterization of an influenza virus neuraminidase variant with decreased sensitivity to the neuraminidase-specific inhibitor 4-guanidino-Neu5Ac2en. Virology 1995;214(2):475–84.

65. Tisdale M. Monitoring of viral susceptibility: new challenges with the development of influenza NA inhibitors. Rev Med Virol 2000;10(1):45–55.

66. Okomo-Adhiambo M, Nguyen HT, Sleeman K, et al. Host cell selection of influenza neuraminidase variants: implications for drug resistance monitoring in A(H1N1) viruses. Antiviral Res 2010;85(2):381–8.

67. Gubareva LV, Fry AM. Current challenges in the risk assessment of neuraminidase inhibitor-resistant influenza viruses. J Infect Dis 2010;201(5):656–8.

68. Barrett S, Mohr PG, Schmidt PM, et al. Real time enzyme inhibition assays provide insights into differences in binding of neuraminidase inhibitors to wild type and mutant influenza viruses. PLoS One 2011;6(8):e23627.

69. Okomo-Adhiambo M, Sheu TG, Gubareva LV. Assays for monitoring susceptibility of influenza viruses to neuraminidase inhibitors. Influenza Other Respir Viruses 2013;7(Suppl 1):44–9.

70. Hurt AC, Okomo-Adhiambo M, Gubareva LV. The fluorescence neuraminidase inhibition assay: a functional method for detection of influenza virus resistance to the neuraminidase inhibitors. Methods Mol Biol 2012;865:115–25.

71. Murtaugh W, Mahaman L, Healey B, et al. Evaluation of three influenza neuraminidase inhibition assays for use in a public health laboratory setting during the 2011-2012 influenza season. Public Health Rep 2013;128(Suppl 2):75–87.

72. Marjuki H, Mishin VP, Sleeman K, et al. Bioluminescence-based neuraminidase inhibition assay for monitoring influenza virus drug susceptibility in clinical specimens. Antimicrob Agents Chemother 2013;57(11):5209–15.
73. Mohr PG, Geyer H, McKimm-Breschkin JL. Mixed influenza A and B infections complicate the detection of influenza viruses with altered sensitivities to neuraminidase inhibitors. Antiviral Res 2011;91(1):20–2.
74. Graitcer SB, Gubareva L, Kamimoto L, et al. Characteristics of patients with oseltamivir-resistant pandemic (H1N1) 2009, United States. Emerg Infect Dis 2011;17(2):255–7.
75. Memoli MJ, Hrabal RJ, Hassantoufighi A, et al. Rapid selection of oseltamivir- and peramivir-resistant pandemic H1N1 virus during therapy in 2 immunocompromised hosts. Clin Infect Dis 2010;50(9):1252–5.
76. Inoue M, Barkham T, Leo YS, et al. Emergence of oseltamivir-resistant pandemic (H1N1) 2009 virus within 48 hours. Emerg Infect Dis 2010;16(10): 1633–6.
77. Memoli MJ, Hrabal RJ, Hassantoufighi A, et al. Rapid selection of a transmissible multidrug-resistant influenza A/H3N2 virus in an immunocompromised host. J Infect Dis 2010;201(9):1397–403.
78. Valinotto LE, Diez RA, Barrero PR, et al. Emergence of intratreatment resistance to oseltamivir in pandemic influenza A H1N1 2009 virus. Antivir Ther 2010;15(6): 923–7.
79. Piralla A, Gozalo-Marguello M, Fiorina L, et al. Different drug-resistant influenza A(H3N2) variants in two immunocompromised patients treated with oseltamivir during the 2011-2012 influenza season in Italy. J Clin Virol 2013;58(1): 132–7.
80. van der Vries E, Stittelaar KJ, van Amerongen G, et al. Prolonged influenza virus shedding and emergence of antiviral resistance in immunocompromised patients and ferrets. PLoS Pathog 2013;9(5):e1003343.
81. Weinstock DM, Gubareva LV, Zuccotti G. Prolonged shedding of multidrug-resistant influenza A virus in an immunocompromised patient. N Engl J Med 2003;348(9):867–8.
82. Hurt AC, Leang SK, Tiedemann K, et al. Progressive emergence of an oseltamivir-resistant A(H3N2) virus over two courses of oseltamivir treatment in an immunocompromised paediatric patient. Influenza Other Respir Viruses 2013;7(6):904–8.
83. Pinsky BA, Mix S, Rowe J, et al. Long-term shedding of influenza A virus in stool of immunocompromised child. Emerg Infect Dis 2010;16(7):1165–7.
84. Zhao X, Jie Y, Rosenberg MR, et al. Design and synthesis of pinanamine derivatives as anti-influenza A M2 ion channel inhibitors. Antiviral Res 2012;96(2): 91–9.
85. Larson AM, Chen J, Klibanov AM. Conjugation to polymeric chains of influenza drugs targeting M2 ion channels partially restores inhibition of drug-resistant mutants. J Pharm Sci 2013;102(8):2450–9.
86. Fiore AE, Fry A, Shay D, et al. Antiviral agents for the treatment and chemoprophylaxis of influenza – recommendations of the Advisory Committee on Immunization Practices (ACIP). MMWR Recomm Rep 2011;60(1):1–24.
87. Rameix-Welti MA, Munier S, Le Gal S, et al. Neuraminidase of 2007-2008 influenza A(H1N1) viruses shows increased affinity for sialic acids due to the D344N substitution. Antivir Ther 2011;16(4):597–603.
88. Chen LF, Dailey NJ, Rao AK, et al. Cluster of oseltamivir-resistant 2009 pandemic influenza A (H1N1) virus infections on a hospital ward among

immunocompromised patients–North Carolina, 2009. J Infect Dis 2011;203(6): 838–46.

89. Hurt AC, Hardie K, Wilson NJ, et al. Characteristics of a widespread community cluster of H275Y oseltamivir-resistant A(H1N1)pdm09 influenza in Australia. J Infect Dis 2012;206(2):148–57.

90. Centers for Disease Control and Prevention. 2013-2014 Influenza Season Week 2 ending January 11, 2014. Available at: http://www.cdc.gov/flu/weekly/. Accessed January 17, 2014.

91. Nguyen JT, Hoopes JD, Le MH, et al. Triple combination of amantadine, ribavirin, and oseltamivir is highly active and synergistic against drug resistant influenza virus strains in vitro. PLoS One 2010;5(2):e9332.

92. Perelson AS, Rong L, Hayden FG. Combination antiviral therapy for influenza: predictions from modeling of human infections. J Infect Dis 2012;205(11): 1642–5.

93. Kim WY, Young Suh G, Huh JW, et al. Triple-combination antiviral drug for pandemic H1N1 influenza virus infection in critically ill patients on mechanical ventilation. Antimicrob Agents Chemother 2011;55(12):5703–9.

94. Seo S, Englund JA, Nguyen JT, et al. Combination therapy with amantadine, oseltamivir and ribavirin for influenza A infection: safety and pharmacokinetics. Antivir Ther 2013;18(3):377–86.

95. Duval X, van der Werf S, Blanchon T, et al. Efficacy of oseltamivir-zanamivir combination compared to each monotherapy for seasonal influenza: a randomized placebo-controlled trial. PLoS Med 2010;7(11):e1000362.

96. Pizzorno A, Bouhy X, Abed Y, et al. Generation and characterization of recombinant pandemic influenza A(H1N1) viruses resistant to neuraminidase inhibitors. J Infect Dis 2011;203(1):25–31.

97. Hurt AC, Lee RT, Leang SK, et al. Increased detection in Australia and Singapore of a novel influenza A(H1N1)2009 variant with reduced oseltamivir and zanamivir sensitivity due to a S247N neuraminidase mutation. Euro Surveill 2011;16(23). pii:19884.

98. Nguyen HT, Sheu TG, Mishin VP, et al. Assessment of pandemic and seasonal influenza A (H1N1) virus susceptibility to neuraminidase inhibitors in three enzyme activity inhibition assays. Antimicrob Agents Chemother 2010;54(9): 3671–7.

99. Hurt AC, Chotpitayasunondh T, Cox NJ, et al. Antiviral resistance during the 2009 influenza A H1N1 pandemic: public health, laboratory, and clinical perspectives. Lancet Infect Dis 2012;12(3):240–8.

100. McKimm-Breschkin JL. Influenza neuraminidase inhibitors: antiviral action and mechanisms of resistance. Influenza Other Respir Viruses 2012;7(Suppl 1):25–36.

101. Zurcher T, Yates PJ, Daly J, et al. Mutations conferring zanamivir resistance in human influenza virus N2 neuraminidases compromise virus fitness and are not stably maintained in vitro. J Antimicrob Chemother 2006;58(4):723–32.

102. Okomo-Adhiambo M, Demmler-Harrison GJ, Deyde VM, et al. Detection of E119V and E119I mutations in influenza A (H3N2) viruses isolated from an immunocompromised patient: challenges in diagnosis of oseltamivir resistance. Antimicrob Agents Chemother 2010;54(5):1834–41.

103. Tamura D, Sugaya N, Ozawa M, et al. Frequency of drug-resistant viruses and virus shedding in pediatric influenza patients treated with neuraminidase inhibitors. Clin Infect Dis 2011;52(4):432–7.

104. Ison MG, Gubareva LV, Atmar RL, et al. Recovery of drug-resistant influenza virus from immunocompromised patients: a case series. J Infect Dis 2006;193(6):760–4.

105. Dapat C, Suzuki Y, Saito R, et al. Rare influenza A (H3N2) variants with reduced sensitivity to antiviral drugs. Emerg Infect Dis 2010;16(3):493–6.
106. Yen HL, Hoffmann E, Taylor G, et al. Importance of neuraminidase active-site residues to the neuraminidase inhibitor resistance of influenza viruses. J Virol 2006;80(17):8787–95.
107. McKimm-Breschkin J, Trivedi T, Hampson A, et al. Neuraminidase sequence analysis and susceptibilities of influenza virus clinical isolates to zanamivir and oseltamivir. Antimicrob Agents Chemother 2003;47(7):2264–72.
108. Sheu TG, Deyde VM, Okomo-Adhiambo M, et al. Surveillance for neuraminidase inhibitor resistance among human influenza A and B viruses circulating worldwide from 2004 to 2008. Antimicrob Agents Chemother 2008;52(9): 3284–92.
109. Wetherall NT, Trivedi T, Zeller J, et al. Evaluation of neuraminidase enzyme assays using different substrates to measure susceptibility of influenza virus clinical isolates to neuraminidase inhibitors: report of the neuraminidase inhibitor susceptibility network. J Clin Microbiol 2003;41(2):742–50.
110. McKimm-Breschkin JL, Sahasrabudhe A, Blick TJ, et al. Mutations in a conserved residue in the influenza virus neuraminidase active site decreases sensitivity to Neu5Ac2en-derived inhibitors. J Virol 1998;72(3):2456–62.
111. Smith BJ, McKimm-Breshkin JL, McDonald M, et al. Structural studies of the resistance of influenza virus neuramindase to inhibitors. J Med Chem 2002; 45(11):2207–12.
112. Kiso M, Mitamura K, Sakai-Tagawa Y, et al. Resistant influenza A viruses in children treated with oseltamivir: descriptive study. Lancet 2004;364(9436):759–65.
113. Baz M, Abed Y, McDonald J, et al. Characterization of multidrug-resistant influenza A/H3N2 viruses shed during 1 year by an immunocompromised child. Clin Infect Dis 2006;43(12):1555–61.
114. Jackson D, Barclay W, Zurcher T. Characterization of recombinant influenza B viruses with key neuraminidase inhibitor resistance mutations. J Antimicrob Chemother 2005;55(2):162–9.
115. Gubareva LV, Matrosovich MN, Brenner MK, et al. Evidence for zanamivir resistance in an immunocompromised child infected with influenza B virus. J Infect Dis 1998;178(5):1257–62.
116. Monto AS, McKimm-Breschkin JL, Macken C, et al. Detection of influenza viruses resistant to neuraminidase inhibitors in global surveillance during the first 3 years of their use. Antimicrob Agents Chemother 2006;50(7): 2395–402.
117. Hurt AC, Iannello P, Jachno K, et al. Neuraminidase inhibitor-resistant and -sensitive influenza B viruses isolated from an untreated human patient. Antimicrob Agents Chemother 2006;50(5):1872–4.
118. Hatakeyama S, Sugaya N, Ito M, et al. Emergence of influenza B viruses with reduced sensitivity to neuraminidase inhibitors. JAMA 2007;297(13):1435–42.
119. Mishin VP, Hayden FG, Gubareva LV. Susceptibilities of antiviral-resistant influenza viruses to novel neuraminidase inhibitors. Antimicrob Agents Chemother 2005;49(11):4515–20.
120. Escuret V, Frobert E, Bouscambert-Duchamp M, et al. Detection of human influenza A (H1N1) and B strains with reduced sensitivity to neuraminidase inhibitors. J Clin Virol 2008;41(1):25–8.
121. Carr S, Ilyushina NA, Franks J, et al. Oseltamivir-resistant influenza A and B viruses pre- and postantiviral therapy in children and young adults with cancer. Pediatr Infect Dis J 2011;30(4):284–8.

122. Vavricka CJ, Li Q, Wu Y, et al. Structural and functional analysis of laninamivir and its octanoate prodrug reveals group specific mechanisms for influenza NA inhibition. PLoS Pathog 2011;7(10):e1002249.
123. Zhu X, McBride R, Nycholat CM, et al. Influenza virus neuraminidases with reduced enzymatic activity that avidly bind sialic acid receptors. J Virol 2012; 86(24):13371–83.

Emerging Respiratory Viruses Other than Influenza

James J. Dunn, PhD[a],*, Melissa B. Miller, PhD[b]

KEYWORDS

- Respiratory viruses • Middle East respiratory syndrome coronavirus • Adenovirus
- Human rhinovirus • Human bocavirus

KEY POINTS

- Noninfluenza viral respiratory tract infections are a significant cause of morbidity and mortality worldwide.
- Early detection and characterization of novel and emerging viruses is important in limiting further transmission.
- Middle East respiratory syndrome coronavirus infection can cause severe respiratory illness with high mortality rates, and all cases to date have been epidemiologically linked to the Middle East region.
- Adenovirus 14 is associated with outbreaks of acute respiratory disease in military camps and the general population.
- Rhinovirus C and human bocavirus type 1 are commonly detected in infants and young children with respiratory tract illness, and are often associated with severe disease requiring hospitalization.

INTRODUCTION

Viral respiratory tract infections (VRTIs) are some of the most common infections worldwide, and represent a major public health concern. Noninfluenza respiratory viruses cause infections in all age groups and are a major contributing factor to morbidity and mortality. Disease severity can range from mild, common cold-like illness to severe, life-threatening respiratory tract infection. The burden of noninfluenza VRTIs is often more pronounced in individuals with chronic comorbidities or clinical risk factors. Moreover, it is estimated that 500 million noninfluenza VRTIs occur annually in the United States, resulting in combined direct and indirect costs of $40 billion.[1]

[a] Department of Pathology and Laboratory Medicine, Cook Children's Medical Center, 801 Seventh Avenue, Fort Worth, TX 76104, USA; [b] Department of Pathology and Laboratory Medicine, University of North Carolina School of Medicine, Campus Box 7525, Chapel Hill, NC 27599-7525, USA
* Corresponding author.
E-mail address: Jim.Dunn@cookchildrens.org

Clin Lab Med 34 (2014) 409–430
http://dx.doi.org/10.1016/j.cll.2014.02.011
0272-2712/14/$ – see front matter © 2014 Elsevier Inc. All rights reserved.

labmed.theclinics.com

In the past, a significant proportion of respiratory tract disease could not be attributed to a specific pathogen. With the advent of molecular detection and genotyping techniques, there has been a substantial increase in the recognition of several newly identified noninfluenza respiratory viruses involved in disease. These potential pathogens have included severe acute respiratory syndrome coronavirus (SARS-CoV) and Middle East respiratory syndrome coronavirus (MERS-CoV), adenovirus type 14 (Ad14), human rhinovirus species C (RV-C), and human bocaviruses. Diagnostic testing for these and other viruses is important because many of the signs and symptoms of infection overlap those of other viruses such as influenza, and would otherwise be ascribed to cases of influenza-like illness without an etiologic assessment.

Coronaviruses are ubiquitous worldwide and were associated with relatively mild respiratory disease (eg, the common cold) up to the emergence of the SARS-CoV in China in 2002. The SARS epidemic spread to 29 countries and infected more than 8000 people, with a case-fatality rate of approximately 10%. However, additional cases have not been documented since 2004. Nearly 10 years later, another virulent coronavirus, MERS-CoV, emerged. The index case of MERS-CoV occurred in Saudi Arabia in June 2012.[2] As of November 20, 2013, there have been 157 laboratory-confirmed cases and 66 deaths reported from 9 countries (**Fig. 1**).

Adenovirus-associated respiratory disease is most often associated with species B and C, with serotypes 3, 4, 7, and 21 being associated with outbreaks of acute febrile respiratory illness, particularly in military trainees. Vaccines against adenoviruses Ad4 and Ad7 were available for military recruits from 1971 to 1999, which decreased the burden of adenovirus-associated acute respiratory disease (ARD) in that population. Before vaccination efforts, adenovirus reportedly infected 10% to 20% of trainees and caused 90% of pneumonia cases at military training camps.[3,4] Ad14 (species B) has emerged as a new source of ARD in military trainees and the general public. Ad14 ARD was first described in 1955 in Dutch military recruits, but had been rarely reported since until 2 major outbreaks at military training centers in the United States occurred in 2007. Ad14 is now known to cause potentially severe acute respiratory illness in both military and civilian individuals.

RV-C and human bocavirus type 1 (HBoV1), recently identified by molecular methods, have been found to be prevalent, widely distributed geographically, and frequently associated with severe respiratory disease following primary infections, particularly in young children. RV-C is also an exacerbating factor in asthma and other chronic obstructive airway diseases. Serologic and quantitative polymerase chain reaction (PCR) analyses have provided compelling evidence for HBoV1 being the etiologic agent of several forms of respiratory tract disease.

This review details the virologic, epidemiologic, clinical, and diagnostic aspects of these viral species.

MICROBIOLOGY
MERS-CoV

Coronaviruses are enveloped, single-stranded, positive-sense RNA viruses with a relatively large genome (27–32 kb). The spike (S) glycoprotein protrudes from the virion, giving the virus its characteristic crown-like (ie, "corona") appearance under electron microscopy. Only 6 coronaviruses have been described that infect humans, all belonging to the Alphacoronavirus and Betacoronavirus genera. CoV 229E and NL63 are alphacoronaviruses, whereas OC43, HKU1, SARS, and MERS are betacoronaviruses.[5] Both 229E and OC43 were identified by viral culture in the mid-1960s. NL63 and HKU1 were not described until after the SARS epidemic in

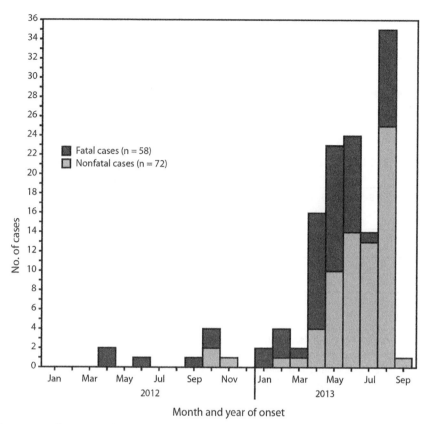

Fig. 1. Cumulative worldwide cases of Middle East respiratory syndrome coronavirus as of September 20, 2013 reported by month of illness onset. (*From* Centers for Disease Control and Prevention. Updated information on the epidemiology of Middle East respiratory syndrome coronavirus (MERS-CoV) infection and guidance for the public, clinicians, and public health authorities, 2012–2013. Morb Mortal Wkly Rep 2013;62:793–6.)

2003, and were detected by nucleic acid methods. However, studies have shown these viruses, unlike SARS-CoV and MERS-CoV, were not recently introduced to the human population. All human CoV have been cultured in vitro with the exception of HKU1.[5]

Ad14

Adenoviruses are large (70–90 nM) double-stranded DNA viruses. As a nonenveloped virus, adenovirus is stable in the environment, and is somewhat resistant to detergents and adverse environmental conditions. The linear DNA genome is associated with 2 core proteins and has a terminal protein covalently attached to each 5′ end. The adenovirus icosahedral capsid is formed by 7 structural proteins, including the hexon, penton base, and fiber.[6] The fiber protein is a spike-like projection with a terminal knob that interacts with host cell receptors along with the penton base. There are 7 species (A–G) of adenovirus that are grouped by oncogenic potential in rodents, hemagglutination properties, and DNA homology. Using serum neutralization and/or hexon gene sequencing, species are further characterized into serotypes. More than 60 serotypes have been described, which cause a variety of clinical syndromes (**Table 1**).

Table 1
Adenovirus species and serotypes, and associated clinical syndromes

Species	Serotypes	Clinical Syndromes
A	12, 18, 31, 61	Unknown; oncogenic in hamsters
B	3, 7, 11, 14, 16, 21, 34, 35, 50, 55	Respiratory infections (7, 14, 21 particularly in military recruits), conjunctivitis, hemorrhagic cystitis (7, 11, 21), myocarditis (7, 21), meningoencephalitis (7), disseminated disease (11, 34, 35)
C	1, 2, 5, 6, 57	Respiratory infections, intussusception, disseminated disease (1, 2, 5)
D	8–10, 13, 15, 17, 19, 20, 22–30, 32, 33, 36–39, 42–49, 51, 53, 54, 56, 58, 59, 60, 62–65	Respiratory infections, conjunctivitis
E	4	Respiratory infections (particularly in military recruits), conjunctivitis
F	40, 41	Gastroenteritis
G	52	Gastroenteritis

RV-C

A series of studies published in 2006 and 2007 described a novel clade of RVs detected in respiratory specimens from patients with acute respiratory illness, asthma, and influenza-like illness that were genetically distinct from existing rhinoviruses,[7–9] subsequently designated RV-C. RVs are now divided into 3 species based on phylogenetic analyses: 2 well-characterized species, A and B, and the novel RV-C species. Although newly described, there are indications that RV-C has been circulating for decades.[10] It seems that RV-C went undetected for years because it does not propagate using traditional virus-isolation methods.[9,11–13] Historically, RVs have been classified according to serotype, which is based on phenotypic characteristics. However, variants of RV-C are not currently assigned to serotypes, as methods for their in vitro culture have not been successful to date and their cross-neutralization properties remain unknown. RV-A currently comprises 77 different serotypes and RV-B 30 types, and, based on genotypic relatedness, RV-C can be separated into at least 60 (geno) types.[14] RVs are small, nonenveloped viruses of approximately 30 nm in diameter with a single-stranded, positive-sense RNA genome of approximately 7.1 kb, which belong to the genus Enterovirus within the family Picornaviridae. The genome organization of all RVs consists of a 5′ untranslated region (UTR), a single open reading frame encoding a single polyprotein, and a 3′ UTR before a polyadenylated tract (**Fig. 2**). RV-Cs are more genetically diverse than the other RV species, and the RV-C genome is the shortest among other reported RVs and human enteroviruses.[9,11] There are also several unique genetic elements that distinguish RV-C from the other species.[9,15]

HBoV1

HBoV1 was first identified in 2005 from respiratory secretions from patients who had pneumonia.[16] Although most commonly detected in the respiratory tract and sometimes in stool, it can also be found in blood, cerebrospinal fluid, and tonsillar tissues. HBoVs are members of the proposed genus Bocaparvovirus in the family Parvoviridae. These small, nonenveloped, icosahedral viruses are approximately 25 nm diameter with a 5.3-kb single-stranded DNA genome containing 3 open reading frames

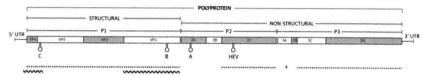

Fig. 2. The approximately 7200-nucleotide, positive-sense, single-stranded RNA genome of rhinovirus C. Regions sequenced for speciating are indicated by the dashed line, and those more commonly used by the wavy line. HEV, human enterovirus; UTR, untranslated region. (*Adapted from* McErlean P, Shackelton LA, Andrews E, et al. Distinguishing molecular features and clinical characteristics of a putative new rhinovirus species, human rhinovirus C (HRV C). PLoS One 2008;3(4):e1847.)

(ORFs). The first 2 sequential ORFs encode nonstructural proteins NS1 and NP1, and the third downstream ORF encodes 2 viral capsid proteins, VP1 and VP2.[16,17] Virus replication depends on the host cell machinery (eg, DNA polymerase). By 2010, 3 additional genotypes, HBoV2, 3, and 4, had been identified in human stool samples from children with gastrointestinal illness[18,19] and have since been rarely detected in respiratory specimens.[20,21] There are some data linking HBoV2 with gastroenteritis,[19] but HBoV3 and HBoV4 have not been conclusively associated with any clinical illness.

EPIDEMIOLOGY
MERS-CoV

To date, all human cases of MERS have had an epidemiologic link to the Middle East (Jordan, Saudi Arabia, United Arab Emirates, or Qatar) (**Fig. 3**). Both health care–associated and familial transmissions have been documented. MERS-CoV is closely related to other betacoronaviruses that have been recovered from bats in Hong Kong, Mexico, Europe, and Africa.[2,22] In addition, serologic studies have determined that dromedary camels in Oman have been exposed to MERS-CoV, possibly linking camels to the transmission cycle.[23]

Ad14

Adenovirus species B can be further subdivided into B1 and B2. Species B1 (3, 7, 16, 21, 50) are generally associated with respiratory disease, whereas members of species B2 (11, 14, 34, 35) tend to infect the genitourinary and/or respiratory tracts. Adenoviruses are transmitted by respiratory droplets and the fecal-oral route as well as by fomites. Military recruits are highly susceptible to adenovirus infections, including pneumonia and ARD likely attributable to crowding and numerous stressors.[3] Ad14 was first described in 1955 during an outbreak of ARD at a military training facility in the Netherlands. Rare outbreaks were described in the 1950s and 1960s in Great Britain, Uzbekistan, and Czechoslovakia, but there were no further described cases or outbreaks caused by Ad14 until sporadic cases were described in United States military recruits in 2006.[24] Outbreaks of Ad14 occurred in the United States at 3 military training facilities in 2007. In the landmark outbreak in San Antonio, approximately 550 trainees were infected with Ad14, although not all individuals had severe disease.[25] Subsequently, Ad14 was detected in 5 additional military bases and in civilians in Washington, Oregon, Alaska, Wisconsin, Pennsylvania, New York, and California.[26–28] From March to June 2007, 140 Ad14 cases were confirmed in 4 states, including 38% hospitalizations (17% intensive care) and 5% mortality.[26] The sequences of the Ad14 viruses from these outbreaks were identical but different from the 1955 virus from the Netherlands, suggesting the emergence of a new

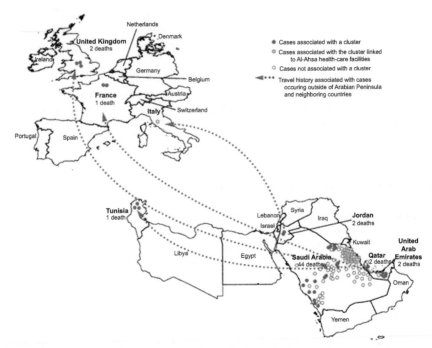

Fig. 3. The first 55 confirmed cases of Middle East respiratory syndrome coronavirus and associated travel history within 14 days of illness onset. (*From* Centers for Disease Control and Prevention. Updated information on the epidemiology of Middle East respiratory syndrome coronavirus (MERS-CoV) infection and guidance for the public, clinicians, and public health authorities, 2012–2013. Morb Mortal Wkly Rep 2013;62:793–6.)

variant.[26] It is likely that the cessation of adenovirus vaccination efforts in the US Military in 1999 likely contributed to the reemergence of adenovirus-associated ARD on military bases, including Ad14-associated disease.

RV-C

Similarly to other RVs, it is thought that RV-C can be transmitted person to person by both direct and indirect contact with aerosolized virus, and infection is efficiently initiated by intranasal and conjunctival inoculation.[29] RV-Cs have been detected on all continents throughout the world and often show seasonal patterns of infection similar to that identified for RVs in general, with high incidence peaks in early fall and late spring in most temperate or subtropical countries, and during the rainy season in the tropics.[9–11,30–34] In some areas, they may peak in winter or be evenly distributed year-round. RV-A and RV-C often cocirculate in near-equivalent proportions or may alternate as the most common RV species at different times of the year.[35,36] RV-B infections typically occur less frequently. The overall prevalence of RV-C in published studies of adults and children with respiratory symptoms ranges from 1.4% to 30.9%, with RV-C accounting for 14% to 81% of all RVs tested.[8,10,13,32,37–42] Differences among patient groups, specimen types, and detection methods may account for the broad range in reported prevalence.

The VP4/VP2 region has been most commonly used for genetic characterization of RVs in clinical samples,[43,44] and more recent phylogenetic analyses suggest that nearly full VP1 region sequencing can reliably separate the clades.[14] Use of the

5′ UTR sequences alone in species determination is sometimes problematic because of recombination events that affect the region.[43,45,46] Using molecular dating analysis of sequences of the VP4/VP2 coding regions, it is projected that RV-Cs have been circulating for at least 250 years, with an estimated evolutionary rate of 6.6×10^{-4} substitutions per site per year.[10]

HBoV1

The modes of transmission for HBoV1 are largely unknown, but may be similar to those of other parvoviruses that can be transmitted by various routes, including respiratory, urine, and fecal-oral.[47] Seroepidemiology studies indicate that HBoV1 is distributed worldwide and that more than 90% of individuals have been exposed, often early in life.[48,49] HBoV genotypes 2 to 4 may also be distributed globally, but their seroepidemiology has been complicated by cross-reactivity.[50] HBoV1 seropositivity is common in infants younger than 2 months owing to transfer of maternal antibody, after which it declines and then increases again because of primary infections, until 6 years of age when most children are seropositive.[48,51–55] The prevalence of HBoV1 in respiratory infections ranges from 1.6% to 21.5%, mainly in children younger than 3 years during the winter and spring months.[16,55–59] HBoV1 is detected infrequently in older age groups including adults,[58,60] although most have antibodies to HBoV1.[48,54,61] HBoV1 is estimated to be among the 4 most prevalent viruses along with respiratory syncytial virus (RSV), rhinoviruses, and adenoviruses in children hospitalized for respiratory disease.[54,62–64] However, serologic studies have shown that the mere presence of HBoV1 DNA in the respiratory tract is not proof of an acute primary infection.[48,50,65] Prolonged viral shedding could explain why some studies found HBoV1 DNA more frequently in asymptomatic than symptomatic cases,[58,66,67] and the high percentage of coinfections.[55,60] HBoV1 DNA has been detected in stool samples in 0% to 13% of patients with or without gastroenteritis[55] and in 0% to 44% of respiratory specimens from asymptomatic individuals.[55,58,68]

CLINICAL PRESENTATION
MERS-CoV

Individuals infected with MERS-CoV typically present with rapidly progressive pneumonia, with abnormal chest radiographs ranging from mild to extensive unilateral and bilateral opacities.[69] In addition, a significant number of cases also present with or develop acute renal failure. A case series of 47 patients indicated that 98% had fever, 83% cough, 72% dyspnea, and 32% myalgia. Gastrointestinal symptoms were also noted, with 26% having diarrhea, 21% vomiting, and 17% abdominal pain. Interestingly 96% of patients had comorbidities, including diabetes (68%), hypertension (34%), chronic heart disease (28%), and chronic renal disease (49%).[69] The mortality rate of MERS is approximately 50%, which is much higher than the 10% mortality reported for SARS, and the case-fatality rate appears to increase with age. Mild and asymptomatic cases have also been identified, bringing the full spectrum of disease caused by MERS-CoV into question.[70]

Ad14

Similar to Ad4, Ad7, and Ad21, Ad14 primarily causes febrile respiratory illness (FRI) in the outbreak setting. FRI is defined as fever (≥38°C/100.5°F) plus one other sign of respiratory illness or diagnosis of pneumonia. The most common presentation reported is pneumonia.[24] Cases of pharyngoconjunctival fever caused by Ad14 have also been reported. One of the military-associated outbreaks found the most common symptoms of Ad14 infection to be cough (89%), sputum production (78%), chills (56%), dyspnea (56%), and sore throat and nausea (44%).[3] Chest radiographs typically show patchy or interstitial infiltrates, with occasional cases of lobar consolidation.[3,27] The patient's white blood cell count is typically normal (89%), although a neutrophilic and monocytic predominance has been noted. The primary risk factor is military training, although one outbreak also demonstrated smoking, advanced age (≥65 years), and Alaskan Native heritage as risk factors.[27]

RV-C

Like other respiratory viruses, the clinical syndromes associated with RV-C range from mild or even asymptomatic infections to acute lower respiratory tract illnesses including pneumonia, recurrent wheezing, and bronchitis. RV-C has been detected in patients with acute illness of upper respiratory tract and lower respiratory tract,[9,11,12,71,72] wheezing,[9,37,39,45,73] bronchiolitis,[11,74,75] asthma exacerbations,[9,13,45,72,76,77] exacerbations of chronic obstructive pulmonary disease, pneumonia,[9,30,32,74,78–80] common cold and flu-like illness,[38] pharyngitis[74] and croup-like cough,[15] rhinitis, nasal congestion, bronchitis, and dyspnea.[74] Nonrespiratory symptoms in RV-C–positive patients include fever, febrile convulsion,[15] otitis media,[81] pericarditis,[80] poor appetite, and apparent life-threatening events.[75] Data suggest that RV-Cs are more frequently detected in older children than are RV-As.[13,72,82] RV-C has been detected in blood samples of children with severe respiratory infection, and viremia was associated with a significantly higher concentration of virus in the nasopharynx.[83,84] In fact, higher RV-C viral loads in respiratory specimens have been associated with severe upper and lower respiratory tract disease, and the median peak viral load in patients with RV-C infection has been shown to be higher than in those patients with RV-A or RV-B infection.[40,85] Stool specimens have also revealed the presence of RV-C and other RV species with viral loads comparable with those of enteroviruses, sometimes along with other gastrointestinal pathogens.[86–88] The clinical significance of RVs in fecal samples remains unclear. In patients hospitalized with disseminated disease, RV-C was detected in respiratory, stool, pericardial effusion, urine, and plasma specimens.[78,80] Health care–associated outbreaks of respiratory infections have been attributed to RV-C in a neonatal intensive care unit[89] and a long-term care facility.[90]

Several studies have demonstrated clinically significant differences among patients infected with RV-C in comparison with those infected with other RV species. Such differences prevail in acute upper and lower respiratory tract infections,[11,12,30,41,44,71,74,79,91–95] wheezing,[9,37,39,45] asthma,[9,13,32,45,72,76,77] and cystic fibrosis exacerbations.[96] On the other hand, some investigators report no significant differences between RV-C and RV-A with respect to disease manifestations.[33,35,42,92,97–99] Confounding this issue is the fact that RV-C may be found in coinfections with other respiratory viruses in up to 42% of cases.[32,35,79,92,94] Nevertheless, as evidenced by cases of RV-C monoinfection, this species contributes substantially to respiratory tract infections, many of which require hospitalization.[32,79,94]

HBoV1

The clinical manifestations of HBoV1 respiratory tract infection have ranged from mild upper respiratory disease to severe, life-threatening pneumonia. However, the direct impact of HBoV1 infection of the respiratory tract is often difficult to assess because of its frequent detection in asymptomatic children[58,66,67] and coinfection with other respiratory viruses in symptomatic children; a rate of up to 83% in respiratory samples.[55] Many studies have demonstrated a positive correlation between respiratory illness and high copy numbers of HBoV1 DNA or the presence of HBoV1 monoinfection,[53,54,56,59,62,100,101] with monoinfection being associated with higher viral load than coinfection. Likewise, detection of HBoV1 viremia is distinctly associated with respiratory symptoms, but not in asymptomatic individuals.[48,62] Infections in patients with HBoV1 viremia, serologic evidence of acute infection, high (>10^4 copies/mL) viral load or mRNA in respiratory secretions, and/or monoinfection include pneumonia,[52,54,56,59,64,101–106] acute wheezing,[48,62,104,107,108] bronchitis/bronchiolitis,[48,52,54,56,64,109,110] asthma,[54,56,64] and acute otitis media (**Table 2**).[49,52,104,111,112] Reports of severe respiratory disease found a significant association between HBoV1 and otherwise unexplained lower respiratory tract infections.[101,113–115] In children, HBoV1 may cause encephalitis and life-threatening complications.[113,114,116,117] HBoV1 can be detected in tonsillar lymphocytes and adenoids of pediatric patients, suggesting a role in the pathogenesis of chronic tonsillar diseases.[118,119] Compared with other viruses known to cause respiratory illness in young children, patients with HBoV1 monoinfection may be older than those with RSV[48,56,64,103,109] or human metapneumovirus[56] infection. In some studies, HBoV1 monoinfection was associated with shorter duration of hospitalization,[56,110] higher C-reactive protein levels[64,109] and white blood cell counts,[64] lower clinical severity score,[110] and less frequent hypoxia compared with RSV-monoinfected patients (**Table 3**).[107]

PATHOGENESIS
MERS-CoV

Cell culture–based experiments have shown that the MERS-CoV receptor is different from the one used by SARS-CoV, and has been identified as DDP4 (dipeptidyl peptidase 4), which interacts with the viral S protein.[120] MERS-CoV also appears to have a broader host range than that of SARS-CoV, infecting human, primate, porcine, and bat cell lines.[120] Because there is not yet a small animal model for MERS-CoV infection, the pathogenesis has not been fully elucidated. However, viral antigen has been localized to the ciliated bronchial epithelium and unciliated cells of terminal bronchi. MERS-CoV replication has also been demonstrated in both type I and type II pneumocytes. Thus, it appears that MERS-CoV affects the alveoli and gas exchange as well as surfactant production and tissue repair.[121]

Ad14

The tissue tropism of adenovirus varies by species and serotype, and is thought to be mediated by specific fiber-receptor interactions. Species C and E, and some species B viruses infect the respiratory tract while other species B viruses infect the urinary tract; species A and F replicate in the gastrointestinal tract, and species D in the eyes.[122] Ad14 belongs to species B2 along with Ad11, Ad34, and Ad35, which have a predilection for the respiratory epithelium. Replication in the respiratory epithelium leads to cell death in the host; however, it is not clear whether the cytopathic effect of adenovirus is due to viral pathogenesis or the host immune response.[123] Adenoviruses also evade the host immune response by inhibiting interferon activity, apoptosis, and expression of major histocompatibility complex class I.[123] These immunomodulatory functions may also play a role in the development of latency or persistence for some of the adenovirus species (namely, species C).

RV-C

Early experiments have shown that RVs have a relatively low optimal temperature for growth (33°C), which may reflect their adaptation to the human nasopharynx and

Table 2
Number (%) of patients with indicated clinical and laboratory findings and human bocavirus type 1 (HBoV1) infection diagnosed serologically, as monoinfection, DNAemia, or mRNA in respiratory samples

N	CXR	Fever	Cough	Wheeze	Tachypnea	Dyspnea	AOM	Hosp.	Mean Age (y)	Serology	DNAemia	mRNA	>10⁴ cop/mL	Monoinfection	Ref.
15	15 (100)	14 (93.3)	13 (86.7)	8 (53.3)	—	—	—	11 (73.3)	1.8	—	—	—	—	15	103
12	—	5 (41.7)	12 (100)	12 (100)	9 (75)	9 (75)	—	12 (100)	—	—	—	—	—	12	108
10	—	5 (50)	9 (90)	4 (40)	9 (75)	4 (40)	2 (20)	7 (70)	0.8	—	—	10	9	6	104
28	8 (28.6)	18 (64.3)	—	28 (100)	—	—	—	28 (100)	1.6	—	—	—	—	28	107
12	—	10 (83.3)	11 (91.7)	—	5 (41.7)	—	—	7 (58.3)	2.3	12	—	—	—	7	102
14	5 (35.7)	9 (64.3)	—	14 (100)	—	—	—	14 (100)	0.8	—	—	—	—	14	109
12	9 (75)	—	—	11 (91.7)	—	—	5 (41.7)	—	1.3	—	12	—	10	12	48,62
Occ.ᵃ	56.1%	67.0%	91.8%	84.6%	58.3%	59.1%	31.8%	86.8%	—	—	—	—	—	—	—

Serology: detection of antibodies to HBoV1 consistent with primary infection.

DNAemia, detection of HBoV1 DNA in blood.

>10⁴ cop/mL, greater than 10⁴ copies/mL of HBoV1 DNA in respiratory samples.

Abbreviations: AOM, acute otitis media; CXR, abnormal chest radiograph; Hosp., hospitalized patients; N, number evaluated in each study.

ᵃ Percent occurrence of finding among all studies.

Table 3
Clinical and laboratory findings in patients with monoinfection with HBoV1, RSV, hMPV, and RV

Finding	HBoV1	RSV	hMPV	RV
Male	62.2%	55.9%	58.7%	63.1%
Fever	71.7%	77.9%	85.7%	60.9%
Abnormal chest radiograph	54.9%	50.9%	48.1%	40.5%
O_2 saturation <95%	55.5%	65.9%	56.2%	48.8%
Antibiotics administered	33.7%	34.0%	66.7%	42.3%
Range of mean age (mo)	4.9–21.6	2–18	5.9–33.6	3.1–46.8
Range of mean hospitalization (d)	1.3–5.6	1.6–7.2	3.5–6.2	0.8–6.9
Range of mean WBC ($\times 10^3$ cells/mm^3)	8.5–14.8	9.4–12.3	9.5–15.4	11.8–17.3
Range of mean CRP (mg/L)	7.5–50.1	8–35.8	15.3–56	18–77.6

Abbreviations: CRP, C-reactive protein level; HBoV1, human bocavirus type 1; hMPV, human metapneumovirus; RSV, respiratory syncytial virus; RV, rhinovirus; WBC, peripheral white blood cell count.
Data from Refs.[48,56,62,64,103,107,109,110]

association with upper respiratory tract infections. However, later experiments determined that there were minimal differences in replication capacities at 33°C and 37°C for several RVs.[124] RVs have been shown to replicate in the nasal epithelium and nasopharynx and, unlike influenza virus and RSV, do not cause destructive cytopathology of the upper respiratory tract. In the lower respiratory tract, RVs have been shown to cause changes in both interstitial and alveolar processes with inflammatory findings. RV-B and most RV-A variants use the intracellular adhesion molecule 1 receptor for cell entry, whereas a subset of RV-A types use the low-density lipoprotein receptor. The receptor used by RV-C types is currently unknown. The predicted capsid structure of RV-C differs significantly from those of RV-A and RV-B, particularly in regions relating to receptor and antiviral binding footprints.[11,15] RV-Cs do not grow in typical cell-culture lines but have recently been grown in vitro using sinus mucosal tissue or fully differentiated human airway epithelial cells, and the virus appears to use a cellular receptor distinct from that of RV-A and RV-B.[125,126] In general, shedding of RV-C does not extend beyond 3 weeks after resolution of symptoms,[45,82] but immunocompromised patients may shed virus for extended periods.[40]

HBoV1

HBoV1, like RV-C, is difficult to cultivate in vitro, and no definitive animal model of HBoV1 infection has been established. Thus, the mechanisms of virus replication and related host immune response remain largely unknown. Studies on children with pneumonia, acute wheezing, asthma, or bronchiolitis suggest that HBoV1 is able to infect the lower airways down to the bronchioles.[51,62,64,107] In some patients, HBoV1 infection may be systemic because viral DNA can be detected in blood and cerebrospinal fluid.[48,52,54,59,62,116] HBoV1 has recently been cultured in differentiated human airway epithelial cells, with documented productive infection causing cytopathogenesis.[127–129] Apical and basolateral infection of cultured epithelial cells results in disruption of the tight junction barrier, loss of cilia, and cell hypertrophy.[130] Recent studies have implied that HBoV DNA can exist episomally in infected human tissues and can likely establish persistent infection in the host.[131] It is not currently known whether this represents a latent state that can be reactivated, but HBoV1 has been detected frequently in tonsillar and adenoid tissues,[118,119,132] suggesting that lymphatic tissue might represent a site of persistent infection, as well as in sinus mucosal tissues.[133] HBoV1 DNA has been detected for up to 6 months in serial nasopharyngeal specimens from otherwise healthy infants and young children,[68,134,135] and in respiratory samples for up to 5 months in immunocompromised pediatric patients.[136,137] Prolonged replication or passive persistence may account for the frequent presence of HBoV1 in both symptomatic and asymptomatic children.

DIAGNOSIS

For most VRTIs, diagnosis of the specific cause cannot be made based solely on clinical signs and symptoms. Establishing the viral etiology of infection is highly dependent on appropriate and accurate diagnostic methods. For many newly identified or emerging viruses, the prevalence of infections may have historically been underestimated owing to the lack of sensitive detection methods.

MERS-CoV can be cultured in LLC-MK2 and Vero E6 cell cultures,[2] although commercially available reagents are not available to identify the MERS-CoV virus in positive cultures. Furthermore, commercially available molecular tests (even those that detect other human CoVs) will not detect the MERS-CoV. However, the Centers for Disease Control and Prevention (CDC) have developed and validated laboratory-developed molecular tests for the detection of MERS-CoV.[138] The Food and Drug Administration (FDA) has issued an Emergency Use Authorization for the CDC real-time reverse transcriptase (RT)-PCR assay, and this test has been distributed to the Laboratory Response Network to aid in the identification of potential cases in the United States. The definition of a confirmed MERS case requires a positive RT-PCR test for at least 2 specific MERS-CoV targets, or a positive single target test with sequencing of a second target.

Respiratory infections caused by adenovirus are generally diagnosed using direct fluorescent antigen detection (DFA), viral culture, or nucleic acid amplification tests (NAATs). Several FDA-cleared NAAT-based tests that include adenovirus detection are currently available. DFA, culture, and NAATs all have a wide range of reported sensitivities because of the large number of serotypes and the genetic heterogeneity seen among adenoviruses. Ad14-specific NAATs have been described, but are generally used only for epidemiologic studies.[139]

RVs are best identified by RT-PCR targeting the 5' UTR performed on respiratory secretions from infected individuals. Although relatively highly conserved in comparison with RV coding regions, sequence variation in the 5' UTR between different RV types creates difficulties in designing primer pairs that can satisfactorily detect all RV types and species.[140] Specific identification of RVs using RT-PCR targeting the 5' UTR is also complicated by the fact that enterovirus detection assays often cross-react with RVs because of sequence similarity in this region.[87] The high sensitivity of PCR can also be a limitation because the presence of viral nucleic acid in respiratory secretions of a patient with respiratory symptoms does not necessarily connote causality. RV-C, and other RVs, have been identified by RT-PCR in respiratory specimens from a high proportion of asymptomatic individuals,[55] possibly leading to an overestimation of the disease burden. However, one study that included asymptomatic controls identified RV-C more often in sick than in well patients, with RVs detected in only 3 of 93 asymptomatic individuals.[38] There is also some evidence that RV-C may interfere with infection by other viruses.[71,82] Co-detections of multiple viruses in respiratory infections have been seen more frequently as a result of the increased availability of multiplex and microarray detection assays.[141] The high co-detection rate also adds to the difficulty of differentiating RV-C as a true pathogen.

Some reports have indicated a correlation between higher viral loads and symptomatic disease.[85,142] However, quantitative RT-PCR testing is not readily available, and there is no standard for the quantification of all RV types. In general, accurate viral load testing of respiratory specimens can be challenging because of the various types of samples, collection techniques, and patient populations assessed.[143] Identification of the infecting species or serotype is of importance diagnostically for the detection of mixed infections or a reinfection with different RV serotypes, as well as in broader clinical investigations of the relationship between a serotype or species with disease severity and in epidemiologic investigations of the circulation and turnover of RVs.

HBoV1 can readily be detected by PCR assays targeting the NS, NP, or VP genes. However, as HBoV1 can be shed in respiratory secretions for weeks to months following primary infection or detected in asymptomatic individuals, detection of anti-HBoV1 antibodies in serum in addition to HBoV1 DNA detection can differentiate primary infection from long-term postinfectious shedding.[68] Serologic methods have been developed to detect HBoV1-specific immunoglobulin (Ig)M and IgG antibodies using recombinant capsid antigens or virus-like particles.[48,51–53,144] It is known that antibodies to HBoV2-4 can cross-react with HBoV1 antigens, so reliable detection of an HBoV1-specific response may best be achieved by depletion of reactive antibodies to the other genotypes.[50] An IgG-avidity enzyme immunoassay has been used to distinguish between acute and past infections, or between primary and secondary infections,[53] although the same antigenic cross-reactions may occur. Detection of HBoV1 DNA in blood is more closely associated with symptoms than are positive respiratory samples alone,[62,106] and higher viral loads in respiratory specimens correlate with acute infections, fewer coinfections, and increased disease severity.[48,51,52,54,56,59,101,108] Therefore, acute HBoV1 infection can more accurately be made by detection of DNA in serum or high viral load ($>10^4$ HBoV1 copies/mL) in respiratory samples along with detection of IgM antibodies or an increase in IgG response in paired serum samples.[48] To overcome the ambiguity and limitations of qualitative HBoV1 DNA detection in respiratory specimens, it has also been shown that the presence of HBoV1 mRNA (ie, actively transcribing virus) is more likely to indicate a causative role of the virus in acute respiratory tract disease.[104,105]

TREATMENT AND PROGNOSIS

As for many respiratory viruses, there is no definitive treatment for CoV-associated illness, which is generally not needed owing to the mild nature of most CoV infections (eg, 229E, OC43, NL63, and HKU1). However, the severe disease and increased mortality caused by both SARS-CoV and MERS-CoV demonstrates the need for antiviral options. Interferon-α2b in combination with ribavirin has been shown to reduce viral replication, moderate host immunologic response, and improve outcomes in rhesus macaques infected with MERS-CoV.[145] In addition, in vitro data have demonstrated that ribavirin, interferon-α, interferon-β, and mycophenolic acid have activity against MERS-CoV.[22] However, many of these drugs are nephrotoxic and may not be an appropriate choice for patients infected with MERS-CoV, which can also cause acute renal failure.

Although no specific treatment exists for adenovirus, both cidofovir and ribavirin show in vitro activity as well as limited clinical efficacy.[122] Cidofovir is an acyclic nucleoside phosphate with activity against several DNA viruses. Ribavirin, a nucleoside analogue, has broad antiviral properties, but clinical data on its efficacy are conflicting. Owing to the paucity of clinical efficacy data and side effects of treatment, off-label use of either drug for adenovirus treatment is generally reserved for disseminated infections in immunocompromised patients. Treatment of ARD in immunocompetent patients is generally only supportive in nature. A live, attenuated vaccine for Ad4 and Ad7 was approved in 2011 for use in military recruits aged 17 to 50 years entering basic training, which may provide some cross-protection against other adenovirus serotypes.

There are no specific antiviral treatments for RV-C or HBoV1 infections. Therapy is supportive, just as for most respiratory virus infections. Vaccines have not been successfully developed for these viruses. For RVs, this is primarily due to the numerous serotypes and limited cross-protections between serotypes. For RV-C and HBoV1, standard precautions should be taken to limit transmission by respiratory secretions.

SUMMARY

Novel viruses are continuously discovered with surveillance programs and the application of new molecular techniques. Moreover, new introductions of viruses in areas where they had never been previously detected represent a challenge for diagnostic virology laboratories. To date the MERS epidemic is localized to the Middle East. However, MERS-CoV is the second CoV to emerge as a major human respiratory pathogen in the last 10 years. Further studies are needed to ascertain the full scope of disease and epidemiologic risk factors. Research aimed at refining the pathogenesis of MERS-CoV will be important in informing potential chemotherapy and interventional strategies. Although much was learned through the SARS epidemic, MERS-CoV belongs to a different lineage and appears to be more pathogenic. Surveillance efforts will need to continue to identify novel coronaviruses in bats and other potential hosts. Early detection of novel viruses, including coronaviruses, is an important strategy in limiting the spread of newly emerging viruses.

The combination of an immunologically naïve population and the emergence of an adenovirus with greater virulence and transmissibility has led to both military and civilian outbreaks involving Ad14. It is clear that Ad14 can cause outbreaks of respiratory disease that are largely recognizable by the severity of disease and increase in pneumonia and mortality. Mild respiratory infections attributable to Ad14 may go undiagnosed, because of either lack of testing altogether or lack of type-specific testing for Ad14. Therefore, it will be important to continue surveillance efforts, including adenovirus serotyping, to assess the full spectrum of Ad14-associated disease.

Until recently most VRTIs in infants and young children were attributed to established pathogens such as RSV, parainfluenza virus, and adenovirus. There is now evidence that newly identified species such as RV-C and viruses such as HBoV1 can be significant respiratory pathogens in young children. RV-C has been detected sometimes as a passenger and sometimes as a pathogen in acute respiratory tract disease; with monoinfection associated with high rates of morbidity. The pathogenic role of HBoV1 has been challenged, but diagnosis of acute infection using a combination of methods, including PCR of blood, quantitative PCR or detection of mRNA in respiratory secretions, and serology, has demonstrated that HBoV1 is responsible for a significant amount of respiratory tract disease in young children. The ability of newer diagnostic assays to simultaneously detect multiple respiratory viruses, including the newly identified ones, will help to clarify virus-host interactions that are still partially unknown, elucidate appropriate infection control measures, and monitor for respiratory outbreaks.

Accurate and timely diagnosis of viral infections is key to optimizing patient management, appropriate use of antivirals, reducing unnecessary tests and superfluous antibiotics, and implementing infection control precautions. Identification and genotyping of novel viral pathogens also affects public health initiatives aimed at curtailing widespread outbreaks.

REFERENCES

1. Fendrick AM, Monto AS, Nightengale B, et al. The economic burden of non-influenza-related viral respiratory tract infection in the United States. Arch Intern Med 2003;163:487–94.
2. Zaki AM, van Boheemen S, Bestebroer TM, et al. Isolation of a novel coronavirus from a man with pneumonia in Saudi Arabia. N Engl J Med 2012;367:1814–20.
3. Brosch L, Tchandja J, Marconi V, et al. Adenovirus serotype 14 pneumonia at a basic military training site in the United States, spring 2007: a case series. Mil Med 2009;174:1295–9.
4. Metzgar D, Osuna M, Kajon AE, et al. Abrupt emergence of diverse species B adenoviruses at US military recruit training centers. J Infect Dis 2007;196:1465–73.
5. Pabbaraju K, Fox JD. Coronaviruses. In: Versalovic J, Carroll KC, Funke G, et al, editors. Manual of clinical microbiology, vol. 2, 10th edition. Washington, DC: ASM Press; 2011. p. 1410–22.
6. Robinson C, Echavarria M. Adenoviruses. In: Versalovic J, Carroll KC, Funke G, et al, editors. Manual of clinical microbiology, vol. 2, 10th edition. Washington, DC: ASM Press; 2011. p. 1600–11.
7. Arden KE, McErlean P, Nissen MD, et al. Frequent detection of human rhinoviruses, paramyxoviruses, coronaviruses, and bocavirus during acute respiratory tract infections. J Med Virol 2006;78:1232–40.
8. Lamson D, Renwick N, Kapoor V, et al. MassTag polymerase-chain-reaction detection of respiratory pathogens, including a new rhinovirus genotype, that caused influenza-like illness in New York State during 2004-2005. J Infect Dis 2006;194:1398–402.
9. Lau SK, Yip CC, Tsoi H, et al. Clinical features and complete genome characterization of a distinct human rhinovirus (HRV) genetic cluster, probably representing a previously undetected HRV species, HRV-C, associated with acute respiratory illness in children. J Clin Microbiol 2007;45:3655–64.
10. Briese T, Renwick N, Venter M, et al. Global distribution of novel rhinovirus genotype. Emerg Infect Dis 2008;14:944–7.
11. McErlean P, Shackelton LA, Lambert SB, et al. Characterisation of a newly identified human rhinovirus, HRV-QPM, discovered in infants with bronchiolitis. J Clin Virol 2007;39:67–75.
12. Lee WM, Lemanske RF, Evans MD, et al. Human rhinovirus species and season of infection determine illness severity. Am J Respir Crit Care Med 2012;186:886–91.
13. Miller EK, Edwards KM, Weinberg GA, et al. A novel group of rhinoviruses is associated with asthma hospitalizations. J Allergy Clin Immunol 2009;123:98–104.
14. McIntyre CL, Knowles NJ, Simmonds P. Proposals for the classification of human rhinovirus species A, B and C into genotypically assigned types. J Gen Virol 2013;94:1791–806.
15. McErlean P, Shackelton L, Andrews E, et al. Distinguishing molecular features and clinical characteristics of a putative new rhinovirus species, human rhinovirus C (HRV C). PLoS One 2008;3:e1847.
16. Allander T, Tammi MT, Eriksson M, et al. Cloning of a human parvovirus by molecular screening of respiratory tract samples. Proc Natl Acad Sci U S A 2005;102:12891–6.

17. Chen AY, Cheng F, Lou S, et al. Characterization of the gene expression profile of human bocavirus. Virology 2010;403:145–54.
18. Arthur JL, Higgins GD, Davidson GP, et al. A novel bocavirus associated with acute gastroenteritis in Australian children. PLoS Pathog 2009;5:e1000391.
19. Kapoor A, Simmonds P, Slikas E, et al. Human bocaviruses are highly diverse, dispersed, recombination prone, and prevalent in enteric infections. J Infect Dis 2010;201:1633–43.
20. Han TH, Chunk JY, Hwang ES. Human bocavirus 2 in children, South Korea. Emerg Infect Dis 2009;15:1698–700.
21. Koseki N, Teramoto S, Kaiho M, et al. Detection of human bocavirus 1 to 4 from nasopharyngeal swab samples collected from patients with respiratory tract infections. J Clin Microbiol 2012;50:2118–21.
22. Chan JF, Chan KH, Kao RY, et al. Broad-spectrum antivirals for the emerging Middle East respiratory syndrome coronavirus. J Infect 2013;67:606–16.
23. Reusken CB, Haagmans BL, Muller MA, et al. Middle East respiratory syndrome coronavirus neutralising serum antibodies in dromedary camels: a comparative serological study. Lancet Infect Dis 2013;13:859–66.
24. Kajon AE, Lu X, Erdman DD, et al. Molecular epidemiology and brief history of emerging adenovirus 14-associated respiratory disease in the United States. J Infect Dis 2010;202:93–103.
25. Tate JE, Bunning ML, Lott L, et al. Outbreak of severe respiratory disease associated with emergent human adenovirus serotype 14 at a US air force training facility in 2007. J Infect Dis 2009;199:1419–26.
26. Centers for Disease Control and Prevention. Acute respiratory disease associated with adenovirus serotype 14–four states, 2006-2007. Morb Mortal Wkly Rep 2007;56:1181–4.
27. Centers for Disease Control and Prevention. Outbreak of adenovirus 14 respiratory illness—Prince of Wales Island, Alaska, 2008. Morb Mortal Wkly Rep 2010; 59:6–10.
28. Louie JK, Kajon AE, Holodniy M, et al. Severe pneumonia due to adenovirus serotype 14: a new respiratory threat? Clin Infect Dis 2008;46:421–5.
29. Jacobs SE, Lamson DM, St. George K, et al. Human rhinoviruses. Clin Microbiol Rev 2013;26:135–61.
30. Lau SK, Yip CC, Lin AW, et al. Clinical and molecular epidemiology of human rhinovirus C in children and adults in Hong Kong reveals a possible distinct human rhinovirus C subgroup. J Infect Dis 2009;200:1096–103.
31. Xiang Z, Gonzalez R, Xie Z, et al. Human rhinovirus group C infection in children with lower respiratory tract infection. Emerg Infect Dis 2008;14:1665–7.
32. Linsuwanon P, Payungporn S, Samransamruajkit R, et al. High prevalence of human rhinovirus C infection in Thai children with acute lower respiratory tract disease. J Infect 2009;59:115–21.
33. Watanabe A, Carraro E, Kamikawa J, et al. Rhinovirus species and their clinical presentation among different risk groups of non-hospitalized patients. J Med Virol 2010;82:2110–5.
34. Piralla A, Baldanti F, Gerna G. Phylogenetic patterns of human respiratory picornavirus species, including the newly identified group C rhinoviruses, during a 1-year surveillance of a hospitalized patient population in Italy. J Clin Microbiol 2011;49:373–6.
35. Xiang Z, Gonzalez R, Xie Z, et al. Human rhinovirus C infections mirror those of human rhinovirus A in children with community-acquired pneumonia. J Clin Virol 2010;49:94–9.

36. Arakawa M, Okamoto-Nakagawa R, Toda S, et al. Molecular epidemiological study of human rhinovirus species A, B, and C from patients with acute respiratory illnesses in Japan. J Med Microbiol 2012;61:410–9.
37. Miller EK, Khuri-Bulos N, Williams JV, et al. Human rhinovirus C associated with wheezing in hospitalized children in the Middle East. J Clin Virol 2009;46:85–9.
38. Piotrowska Z, Vazquez M, Shapiro E, et al. Rhinoviruses are a major cause of wheezing and hospitalization in children less than 2 years of age. Pediatr Infect Dis J 2009;28:25–9.
39. Linsuwanon P, Payungporn S, Samransamruajkit R, et al. Recurrent human rhinovirus infections in infants with refractory wheezing. Emerg Infect Dis 2009;15:978–80.
40. Piralla A, Rovida F, Campanini G, et al. Clinical severity and molecular typing of human rhinovirus C strains during a fall outbreak affecting hospitalized patients. J Clin Virol 2009;45:311–7.
41. Dominquez SR, Briese T, Palacios G, et al. Multiplex MassTag-PCR for respiratory pathogens in pediatric nasopharyngeal washes negative by conventional diagnostic testing shows a high prevalence of viruses belonging to a newly recognized rhinovirus clade. J Clin Virol 2008;43:219–22.
42. Khetsuriani N, Lu X, Teague W, et al. Novel human rhinoviruses and exacerbation of asthma in children. Emerg Infect Dis 2008;14:1793–6.
43. Savolainen-Kopra C, Blomqvist S, Smura T, et al. 5′ noncoding region alone does not unequivocally determine genetic type of human rhinovirus strains. J Clin Microbiol 2009;47:1278–80.
44. Wisdom A, Leitch E, Gaunt E, et al. Screening respiratory samples for detection of human rhinoviruses (HRVs) and enteroviruses: comprehensive VP4-VP2 typing reveals high incidence and genetic diversity of HRV species C. J Clin Microbiol 2009;47:3958–67.
45. Arden KE, Faux CE, O'Neill NT, et al. Molecular characterization and distinguishing features of a novel human rhinovirus (HRV) C, HRVC-QCE, detected in children with fever, cough and wheeze during 2003. J Clin Virol 2010;47:219–23.
46. McIntyre CL, Leitch EC, Savolainen-Kopra C, et al. Analysis of genetic diversity and sites of recombination in human rhinovirus species C. J Virol 2010;84:10297–310.
47. Berns K, Parrish C. Parvoviridae. In: Knipe DM, Howley PM, editors. Fields' virology. 6th edition. Philadelphia: Wolters Kluwer health/Lippincott Williams & Wilkins; 2013. p. 1768–91.
48. Soderlund-Venermo M, Lahtinen A, Jartti T, et al. Clinical assessment and improved diagnosis of bocavirus-induced wheezing in children, Finland. Emerg Infect Dis 2009;15:1423–30.
49. Meriluoto M, Hedman L, Tanner L, et al. Association of human bocavirus 1 infection with respiratory disease in childhood follow-up study, Finland. Emerg Infect Dis 2012;18:264–71.
50. Kantola K, Hedman L, Arthur J, et al. Seroepidemiology of human bocaviruses 1-4. J Infect Dis 2011;204:403–12.
51. Kantola K, Hedman L, Allander T, et al. Serodiagnosis of human bocavirus infection. Clin Infect Dis 2008;46:540–6.
52. Karalar L, Lindner J, Schimanski S, et al. Prevalence and clinical aspects of human bocavirus infections in children. Clin Microbiol Infect 2010;16:633–9.
53. Hedman L, Soderlund-Venermo M, Jartti T, et al. Dating of human bocavirus infection with protein-denaturing IgG-avidity assays—secondary immune activations are ubiquitous in immunocompetent adults. J Clin Virol 2010;48:44–8.

54. Wang K, Wang W, Yan H, et al. Correlation between bocavirus infection and humoral response, and co-infection with other respiratory viruses in children with acute respiratory infection. J Clin Virol 2010;47:148–55.

55. Jartti T, Hedman K, Jartti L, et al. Human bocavirus—the first 5 years. Rev Med Virol 2012;22:46–64.

56. Brieu N, Guyon G, Rodiere M, et al. Human bocavirus infection in children with respiratory tract disease. Pediatr Infect Dis J 2008;27:969–73.

57. Garcia-Garcia M, Calvo C, Pozo F, et al. Human bocavirus detection in nasopharyngeal aspirates of children without clinical symptoms of respiratory infection. Pediatr Infect Dis J 2008;27:358–60.

58. Longtin J, Bastien M, Gilca R, et al. Human bocavirus infections in hospitalized children and adults. Emerg Infect Dis 2008;14:217–21.

59. Christensen A, Nordbo SA, Krokstad S, et al. Human bocavirus in children: mono-detection, high viral load and viraemia are associated with respiratory tract infection. J Clin Virol 2010;49:158–62.

60. Chow B, Esper F. The human bocaviruses: a review and discussion of their role in infection. Clin Lab Med 2009;29:695–713.

61. Cecchini S, Negrete A, Virag T, et al. Evidence of prior exposure to human bocavirus as determined by a retrospective serological study of 404 serum samples from adults in the United States. Clin Vaccine Immunol 2009;16:597–604.

62. Allander T, Jartti T, Gupta S, et al. Human bocavirus and acute wheezing in children. Clin Infect Dis 2007;44:904–10.

63. Pozo F, Garcia-Garcia M, Calvo C, et al. High incidence of human bocavirus infection in children in Spain. J Clin Virol 2007;40:224–8.

64. Calvo C, Garcia-Garcia M, Pozo F, et al. Clinical characteristics of human bocavirus infections compared with other respiratory viruses in Spanish children. Pediatr Infect Dis J 2008;27:677–80.

65. Don M, Soderlund-Venermo M, Hedman K, et al. Don't forget serum in the diagnosis of human bocavirus infection. J Infect Dis 2011;203:1031–2.

66. Schildgen O, Muller A, Allander T, et al. Human bocavirus: passenger or pathogen in acute respiratory tract infections? Clin Microbiol Rev 2008;21:291–304.

67. von Linstow ML, Hogh M, Hogh B. Clinical and epidemiologic characteristics of human bocavirus in Danish infants: results from a prospective birth cohort study. Pediatr Infect Dis J 2008;27:897–902.

68. Martin ET, Fairchok MP, Kuypers J, et al. Frequent and prolonged shedding of bocavirus in young children attending daycare. J Infect Dis 2010;201:1625–32.

69. Assiri A, Al-Tawfiq JA, Al-Rabeeah AA, et al. Epidemiological, demographic, and clinical characteristics of 47 cases of Middle East respiratory syndrome coronavirus disease from Saudi Arabia: a descriptive study. Lancet Infect Dis 2013;13:752–61.

70. Assiri A, McGeer A, Perl TM, et al. Hospital outbreak of Middle East respiratory syndrome coronavirus. N Engl J Med 2013;369:407–16.

71. Wisdom A, Kutkowska A, Leitch E, et al. Genetics, recombination and clinical features of human rhinovirus species C (HRV-C) infections; interactions of HRV-C with other respiratory viruses. PLoS One 2009;4:e8518.

72. Linder JE, Kraft DC, Mohamed Y, et al. Human rhinovirus C: age, season, and lower respiratory illness over the past 3 decades. J Allergy Clin Immunol 2013;131:69–77.

73. Moreira LP, Kamikawa J, Watanabe A, et al. Frequency of human rhinovirus species in outpatient children with acute respiratory infections at primary care level in Brazil. Pediatr Infect Dis J 2011;30:612–4.

74. Renwick N, Schweiger B, Kapoor V, et al. A recently identified rhinovirus genotype is associated with severe respiratory-tract infection in children in Germany. J Infect Dis 2007;196:1754–60.
75. Calvo C, Garcia ML, Pozo F, et al. Role of rhinovirus C in apparently life-threatening events in infants, Spain. Emerg Infect Dis 2009;15:1506–8.
76. Mak R, Tse L, Lam W, et al. Clinical spectrum of human rhinovirus infections in hospitalized Hong Kong children. Pediatr Infect Dis J 2011;30:749–53.
77. Bizzintino J, Lee W, Laing IA, et al. Association between human rhinovirus C and severity of acute asthma in children. Eur Respir J 2011;37:1037–42.
78. Broberg E, Niemela J, Lahti E, et al. Human rhinovirus C-associated severe pneumonia in a neonate. J Clin Virol 2011;51:79–82.
79. Jin Y, Yuan X, Xie Z, et al. Prevalence and clinical characterization of a newly identified human rhinovirus C species in children with acute respiratory tract infections. J Clin Microbiol 2009;47:2895–900.
80. Tapparel C, L'Huillier A, Rougemont A, et al. Pneumonia and pericarditis in a child with HRV-C infection: a case report. J Clin Virol 2009;45:157–60.
81. Savolainen-Kopra C, Blomqvist S, Kilpi T, et al. Novel species of human rhinoviruses in acute otitis media. Pediatr Infect Dis J 2009;28:59–61.
82. Mackay IM, Lambert SB, Faux CE, et al. Community-wide, contemporaneous circulation of a broad spectrum of human rhinoviruses in healthy Australian preschool-aged children during a 12-month period. J Infect Dis 2012;207:1433–41.
83. Fuji N, Suzuki A, Lupisan S, et al. Detection of human rhinovirus C viral genome in blood among children with severe respiratory infections in the Philippines. PLoS One 2011;6:e27247.
84. Esposito S, Daleno C, Scala A, et al. Impact of rhinovirus nasopharyngeal viral load and viremia on severity of respiratory infections in children. Eur J Clin Microbiol Infect Dis 2014;33(1):41–8.
85. Gerna G, Piralla A, Rovida F, et al. Correlation of rhinovirus load in the respiratory tract and clinical symptoms in hospitalized immunocompetent and immunocompromised patients. J Med Virol 2009;81:1498–507.
86. Lau SK, Yip CC, Lung DC, et al. Detection of human rhinovirus C in fecal samples of children with gastroenteritis. J Clin Virol 2012;53:290–6.
87. Harvala H, McIntyre CL, McLeish NJ, et al. High detection frequency and viral loads of human rhinovirus species A to C in fecal samples; diagnostic and clinical implications. J Med Virol 2012;84:536–42.
88. Honkanen H, Oikarinen S, Peltonen P, et al. Human rhinoviruses including group C are common in stool samples of young Finnish children. J Clin Virol 2013;56:250–4.
89. Reid AB, Anderson TL, Cooley L, et al. An outbreak of human rhinovirus species C infections in a neonatal intensive care unit. Pediatr Infect Dis J 2011;30:1096–8.
90. Longtin J, Marchand-Austin A, Winter AL, et al. Rhinovirus outbreaks in long-term care facilities, Ontario, Canada. Emerg Infect Dis 2010;16:1463–5.
91. da Silva ER, Watanabe A, Carraro E, et al. Rhinovirus genetic diversity among immunosuppressed and immunocompetent patients presenting with a severe respiratory infection. J Clin Virol 2013;56:82–3.
92. Fry AM, Lu X, Olsen SJ, et al. Human rhinovirus infections in rural Thailand: epidemiologic evidence for rhinovirus as both pathogen and bystander. PLoS One 2011;6:e17780.
93. Ferguson PE, Gilroy NM, Faux CE, et al. Human rhinovirus C in adult haematopoietic stem cell transplant recipients with respiratory illness. J Clin Virol 2013;56:255–9.

94. Lauinger IL, Bible JM, Halligan EP, et al. Patient characteristics and severity of human rhinovirus infections in children. J Clin Virol 2013;58:216–20.

95. Annamalay AA, Khoo SK, Jacoby P, et al. Prevalence of and risk factors for human rhinovirus infection in healthy aboriginal and non-aboriginal Western Australian children. Pediatr Infect Dis J 2012;31:673–9.

96. de Almeida MB, Zerbinati RM, Tateno AF, et al. Rhinovirus C and respiratory exacerbations in children with cystic fibrosis. Emerg Infect Dis 2010;16: 996–9.

97. Calvo C, Casas I, Garcia-Garcia ML, et al. Role of rhinovirus C respiratory infections in sick and healthy children in Spain. Pediatr Infect Dis J 2010;29: 717–20.

98. Iwane MK, Prill MM, Lu X, et al. Human rhinovirus species associated with hospitalization for acute respiratory illness in young US children. J Infect Dis 2011; 204:1702–10.

99. Arden KE, Chang AB, Lambert SB, et al. Newly identified respiratory viruses in children with asthma exacerbation not requiring admission to hospital. J Med Virol 2010;82:1458–61.

100. Gerna G, Piralla A, Campanini G, et al. The human bocavirus role in acute respiratory tract infections of pediatric patients as defined by viral load quantification. New Microbiol 2007;30:383–92.

101. Zhao B, Yu X, Wang C, et al. High human bocavirus viral load is associated with disease severity in children under five years of age. PLoS One 2013;8:e62318.

102. Don M, Soderlund-Venermo M, Valent F, et al. Serologically verified human bocavirus pneumonia in children. Pediatr Pulmonol 2010;45:120–6.

103. Esposito S, Daleno C, Prunotto G, et al. Impact of viral infections in children with community-acquired pneumonia: results of a study of 17 respiratory viruses. Influenza Other Respir Viruses 2013;7:18–26.

104. Proenca-Modena JL, Gagliardi TB, de Paula FE, et al. Detection of human bocavirus mRNA in respiratory secretions correlates with high viral load and concurrent diarrhea. PLoS One 2011;6:e21083.

105. Christensen A, Dollner H, Skanke L, et al. Detection of spliced mRNA from human bocavirus 1 in clinical samples from children with respiratory tract infections. Emerg Infect Dis 2013;19:574–80.

106. Jula A, Waris M, Kantola K, et al. Primary and secondary human bocavirus 1 infections in a family, Finland. Emerg Infect Dis 2013;19:1328–31.

107. Garcia-Garcia ML, Calvo C, Falcon A, et al. Role of emerging respiratory viruses in children with severe acute wheezing. Pediatr Pulmonol 2010;45:585–91.

108. Deng Y, Gu X, Zhao X, et al. High viral load of human bocavirus correlates with duration of wheezing in children with severe lower respiratory tract infection. PLoS One 2012;7:e34353.

109. Calvo C, Pozo F, Garcia-Garcia ML, et al. Detection of new respiratory viruses in hospitalized infants with bronchiolitis: a three-year prospective study. Acta Paediatr 2010;99:883–7.

110. Midulla F, Scagnolari C, Bonci E, et al. Respiratory syncytial virus, human bocavirus, and rhinovirus bronchiolitis in infants. Arch Dis Child 2010;95:35–41.

111. Beder LB, Hotomi M, Ogami M, et al. Clinical and microbiological impact of human bocavirus on children with acute otitis media. Eur J Pediatr 2009;168: 1365–72.

112. Rezes S, Soderlund-Venermo M, Roivainen M, et al. Human bocavirus and rhino-enteroviruses in childhood otitis media with effusion. J Clin Virol 2009; 46:234–7.

113. Edner N, Catillo-Rodas P, Falk L, et al. Life-threatening respiratory tract disease with human bocavirus-1 infection in a 4-year-old child. J Clin Microbiol 2012;50:531–2.

114. Korner R, Soderlund-Venermo M, van Koningsbruggen-Rietschel S, et al. Severe human bocavirus infection, Germany. Emerg Infect Dis 2011;17:2303–5.

115. Sadeghi M, Kantola K, Finnegan D, et al. Possible involvement of human bocavirus 1 in the death of a middle-aged immunosuppressed patient. J Clin Microbiol 2013;51:3461–3.

116. Mitui MT, Tabib SM, Matsumoto T, et al. Detection of human bocavirus in the cerebrospinal fluid of children with encephalitis. Clin Infect Dis 2012;54:964–7.

117. Ursic T, Steyer A, Kopriva S, et al. Human bocavirus as the cause of a life-threatening infection. J Clin Microbiol 2011;49:1179–81.

118. Lu X, Gooding LR, Erdman DD. Human bocavirus in tonsillar lymphocytes. Emerg Infect Dis 2008;14:1332–4.

119. Proenca-Modena JL, Valera FC, Jacob MG, et al. High rates of detection of respiratory viruses in tonsillar tissues from children with chronic adenotonsillar disease. PLoS One 2012;7:e42136.

120. Coleman CM, Frieman MB. Emergence of the Middle East respiratory syndrome coronavirus. PLoS Pathog 2013;9:e1003595.

121. Hocke AC, Becher A, Knepper J, et al. Emerging human Middle East respiratory syndrome coronavirus causes widespread infection and alveolar damage in human lungs. Am J Respir Crit Care Med 2013;188:882–6.

122. Lenaerts L, De Clercq E, Naesens L. Clinical features and treatment of adenovirus infections. Rev Med Virol 2008;18:357–74.

123. Echavarria M. Adenoviruses in immunocompromised hosts. Clin Microbiol Rev 2008;21:704–15.

124. Papadopoulos NG, Sanderson G, Hunter J, et al. Rhinoviruses replicate effectively at lower airway temperatures. J Med Virol 1999;58:100–4.

125. Bochkov YA, Palmenberg AC, Lee WM, et al. Molecular modeling, organ culture and reverse genetics for a newly identified human rhinovirus C. Nat Med 2011; 17:627–32.

126. Hao W, Bernard K, Patel N, et al. Infection and propagation of human rhinovirus C in human airway epithelial cells. J Virol 2012;86:13524–32.

127. Dijkman R, Koekkoek S, Molenkamp R, et al. Human bocavirus can be cultured in differentiated human airway epithelial cells. J Virol 2009;83:7739–48.

128. Huang Q, Deng X, Yan Z, et al. Establishment of a reverse genetics system for studying human bocavirus in human airway epithelia. PLoS Pathog 2012;8: e1002899.

129. Deng X, Li Y, Qiu J. Human bocavirus 1 infects commercially available primary human airway epithelium cultures productively. J Virol Methods 2014;195:112–9.

130. Deng X, Yan Z, Luo Y, et al. In vitro modeling of human bocavirus 1 infection of polarized primary human airway epithelia. J Virol 2013;87:4097–102.

131. Kapoor A, Hornig M, Asokan A, et al. Bocavirus episome in infected human tissue contains non-identical termini. PLoS One 2011;6:e21362.

132. Herberhold S, Eis-Hubinger A, Panning M. Frequent detection of respiratory viruses by real-time PCR in adenoid samples from asymptomatic children. J Clin Microbiol 2009;47:2682–3.

133. Falcone V, Ridder GJ, Panning M, et al. Human bocavirus DNA in paranasal sinus mucosa. Emerg Infect Dis 2011;17:1564–5.

134. Blessing K, Neske F, Herre U, et al. Prolonged detection of human bocavirus DNA in nasopharyngeal aspirates of children with respiratory tract disease. Pediatr Infect Dis J 2009;28:1018–9.

135. Lehtoranta L, Soderlund-Venermo M, Nokso-Koivisto J, et al. Human bocavirus in the nasopharynx of otitis-prone children. Int J Pediatr Otorhinolaryngol 2012; 76:206–11.

136. Koskenvuo M, Mottonen M, Waris M, et al. Human bocavirus in children with acute lymphoblastic leukemia. Eur J Pediatr 2008;167:1011–5.

137. Schenk T, Maier B, Hufnagel M, et al. Persistence of human bocavirus DNA in immunocompromised children. Pediatr Infect Dis J 2011;30:82–4.

138. Lu X, Whitaker B, Sakthivel S, et al. Real-time reverse transcription polymerase chain reaction assay panel for Middle East respiratory syndrome coronavirus. J Clin Microbiol 2013;52(1):67–75. http://dx.doi.org/10.1128/JCM.02533-13.

139. Metzgar D, Skochko G, Gibbins C, et al. Evaluation and validation of a real-time PCR assay for detection and quantitation of human adenovirus 14 from clinical samples. PLoS One 2009;4:e7081.

140. Faux CE, Arden KE, Lambert SB, et al. Usefulness of published PCR primers in detecting human rhinovirus infection. Emerg Infect Dis 2011;17:296–8.

141. Mahony JB, Petrich A, Smieja M. Molecular diagnosis of respiratory virus infections. Crit Rev Clin Lab Sci 2011;48:217–49.

142. Utokaparch S, Marchant D, Gosselink J, et al. The relationship between respiratory viral loads and diagnosis in children presenting to a pediatric hospital emergency department. Pediatr Infect Dis J 2011;30:e18–23.

143. Schibler M, Yerly S, Vieille G, et al. Critical analysis of rhinovirus RNA load quantification by real-time reverse transcription-PCR. J Clin Microbiol 2012;50: 2868–72.

144. Kahn JS, Kesebir D, Cotmore SF, et al. Seroepidemiology of human bocavirus defined using recombinant virus-like particles. J Infect Dis 2008;198:41–50.

145. Falzarano D, de Wit E, Rasmussen AL, et al. Treatment with interferon-alpha2b and ribavirin improves outcome in MERS-CoV-infected rhesus macaques. Nat Med 2013;19:1313–7.

Index

Note: Page numbers of article titles are in **boldface** type.

A

Clin Lab Med 34 (2014) 431–442
http://dx.doi.org/10.1016/S0272-2712(14)00035-3
0272-2712/14/$ – see front matter © 2014 Elsevier Inc. All rights reserved.

labmed.theclinics.com

Moving?

Make sure your subscription moves with you!

To notify us of your new address, find your **Clinics Account Number** (located on your mailing label above your name), and contact customer service at:

Email: journalscustomerservice-usa@elsevier.com

800-654-2452 (subscribers in the U.S. & Canada)
314-447-8871 (subscribers outside of the U.S. & Canada)

Fax number: 314-447-8029

Elsevier Health Sciences Division
Subscription Customer Service
3251 Riverport Lane
Maryland Heights, MO 63043

*To ensure uninterrupted delivery of your subscription, please notify us at least 4 weeks in advance of move.

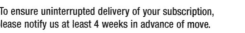
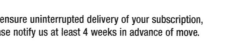

Printed and bound by CPI Group (UK) Ltd, Croydon, CR0 4YY

03/10/2024

01040496-0006